The Cranial Arteries of Mammals

The Cranial Arteries of Mammals

by G H du Boulay
MB BS FRCP FFR

and P M Verity MSR

The Nuffield Institute of Comparative Medicine
Zoological Society of London
Regent's Park

William Heinemann Medical Books Limited

First Published 1973

© G H du Boulay and P M Verity 1973

ISBN 0 433 07850 2

Printed by The Whitefriars Press Ltd.
London and Tonbridge

Contents

Preface

In 1965 very shortly after the opening of the Nuffield Institute of Comparative Medicine at the Zoological Society of London, we received a grant from the Wellcome Foundation to found an animal X-Ray Museum. It was this generous support which gave us both the idea and the opportunity of making a comparative anatomical study of the cranial arteries of mammals. In order, however, to understand the limitations of our study, it is necessary to explain something about the material made available by our grant and by our many friends at the Zoo. In the natural course of events in any zoo, a great variety of mammals come suddenly to the ends of their lives, their deaths are unheralded and their skeletons and soft tissues are valuable to many different workers. Consequently our studies had to be performed without prior notice, but usually after a routine autopsy. It was rarely permissible to open the skull or carry out any helpful dissection of the head. Many of the animals, particularly the smaller ones, had been dead for more than 24 hours before they could be injected, some had been dead for very much longer than this.

With all its limitations the material could still, we felt, provide useful guide lines for an overall understanding of the comparative anatomy for ourselves, and for other researchers who wished to choose a suitable species for their work. It seemed wasteful not to make what we could of the available animals. We regret the poor representation of some orders, notably the bats, and the complete absence of monotremes, flying lemurs, elephants and sirenians.

As Tandler (1899) was at such pains to point out and as Davis and Story (1943) and Daniel et al. (1953) have also confirmed, there is a common basic pattern both of the major trunks of the cranial arteries and of the peripheral networks, though from species to species there are variations in the chief connections between the proximal and the distal sets of vessels. There is also a general pattern which in its main characteristics tends to recur throughout a family or order.

Where anatomists have previously described the courses of the vessels and named them in a particular species, our task of identification has been comparatively easy. Sometimes we have had to allow for individual variations, occasionally we have disagreed fundamentally with previous descriptions. When, however, as in the majority, no previous description could be found, we have named the vessels to the best of our ability by comparison. In order to help us we had not only the lateral and ventro-dorsal views published here, but also stereoscopic pictures and radiographs showing the progress and direction of the advancing bolus of injected material.

Nomenclature has presented us with many problems. In the first place there are a number of animals whose previous descriptions date from the last century and were often written in German, principally by Tandler (1899) and by Hofmann (1900). Tandler's nomenclature differs from the standard B.N.A. in several respects. Hofmann's major contribution, apart from the actual descriptions of the intracranial arteries

of several animals, was a systemisation of the posterior cerebral artery variations (see "Nomenclature of Intracranial Arteries page 1) which we have adopted whenever possible because it makes good sense of the anomalies seen sometimes in man. Hofmann also performed the same service for the cerebellar arteries and this too we have attempted to follow. Some of our illustrations and text combine Hofmann's classification with the names in current medical usage.

We ourselves are guilty of some inconsistencies and have tended to move away from archaic nomenclature as we progressed from the marsupials and through the insectivores. For this we apologise but take some comfort in the fact that anatomists will be able to see the arteries in question for themselves since the atlas consists of photographic reproductions of the actual injection radiographs rather than drawings and interpretations of dissections. For this reason it also contains a great deal of accurate, detailed, but unsignposted information for those who wish to study the subject in depth.

The nomenclatural difficulties of which we are aware chiefly concern the smaller arteries of the face, the orbit and the ethmoidal region. For instance, we have sometimes used "ophthalmic artery" to mean "internal ophthalmic artery" and "orbital branch of internal maxillary" where in some cases "external ophthalmic artery" might have been better.

We are aware of a problem in the naming of the buccal, buccinator or bucco-labial artery. In some animals it does not reach the lips.

Where both anterior and posterior deep temporal vessels are recognisable we have named them so; but if only one deep temporal is visible we have not specified which it may be.

The main trunks of the occipital, posterior auricular and superficial temporal arteries are usually clearly recognisable but their peripheral complement of branches often including a transverse facial artery, permutate their central connections and peripheral anastomoses. Because we have sometimes had doubts about the sense of using the term "posterior auricular artery" when it is evidently the major trunk from which both posterior and anterior branches arise we have consistently written simply "auricular artery" throughout. We have changed from using the term "inferior alveolar" to "inferior dental" artery early in the book, even for the homologous artery in the Edentates. Our difficulty with the facial (external maxillary) artery in Carnivora will be obvious from the text.

So many of the animals had had their necks opened at autopsy that we have made no attempt to name cervical branches. The autopsy incisions, the occasional prior removal of the eyes, the occasional skinning and the onset of decomposition in some specimens are responsible for extravasation of contrast material where it occurs.

During the collection of these post-mortem radiographs we have also had the opportunity of performing diagnostic angiography by percutaneous needle and catheter techniques upon a variety of living mammals including Leopard, Caracal Lynx, Cheetah, Dog, Goat, Rabbit and several species of Monkey. One or two of these are also illustrated but because of the necessity for less opaque contrast material and for rapid serial radiography the smaller vessels do not show up so well. The success of these diagnostic procedures emphasises the potential value of knowing what the anatomy should look like.

Previous literature about the anatomy of the cranial arteries is exceedingly hard to trace but The Zoological record published by The Zoological Society of London has been extremely helpful. We are sure nevertheless that we have overlooked many helpful references and we apologise, hoping that this shortcoming too will be excused by the fact of our publishing our actual material.

The radiographs themselves are filed in the Wellcome Animal X-Ray Museum for future reference and for inspection (by appointment). The opportunity will be taken to fill in gaps in the collection whenever it occurs and if this volume proves useful it may eventually be possible to produce another.

We have not been able to publish all our work. Some animals defeated the combined efforts of ourselves and our friends. From the elephant's head, inverted and positioned with car-jacks we could obtain a montage of seven 17×14 inch plates (without the trunk). Alas, the brain which is 8 inches long is surrounded by a skull twice as thick again, consisting largely of air-sinuses so that the arteries, filled by jugfulls through a funnel are scarcely visible even on the original radiographs.

Injection and radiography are not the only technical processes required. The photographic skill necessary to render the enormous range of contrast acceptable for printing is difficult and very time-consuming. Mr. Derrick Taylor and his assistant are as much responsible for the existence of the atlas as we are ourselves. Had we been able to make subtraction radiographs, the photographic work might have been a little easier, but the many manipulations necessary during injection ruled out that technique.

We know also that to set up a single specimen as the anatomical norm for any species would be ridiculous. In a few cases we have injected two or three individuals of one kind, but it was our intention to make a unique collection generally available and not to make judgments about the range of anatomical variants in a single species.

Acknowledgements

We have spoken of our indebtedness to the Trustees of The Wellcome Foundation in the Preface and there, also, have mentioned Mr. Derrick Taylor and his assistants. Without financial support and without especial photographic skill this book would never have been published.

Equally, we are grateful to Dr. Ian Keymer for permitting us to inject most of the specimens and to his staff and the staff of The Nuffield Institute of Comparative Medicine for transporting them. Many other people have provided us with specimens, too, Mr. Richard Fiennes, Dr. Christine Hawkey, Dr. Barbara Weir, Miss Christine Scott at the Zoo and its Institutes; Dr. Ross Russell and Dr. Harrison at The National Hospital, Queen Square, and Bill Kirby of Christ's Hospital, who first interested one of us in comparative anatomy during the 1930's, has encouraged him ever since and provided the beautiful specimen of a badger which unwisely went courting over the electric railway line by Sharpenhurst.

Some of the most rewarding and interesting angiograms were carried out for diagnostic purposes with Mr. Malcolm Hime.

Dr. L. G. Goodwin's tireless enthusiasm for our project has kept us going. Pat Wright has saved us from administrative worries and Peter Wallace has solved innumerable technical problems.

Miss Evelyn Monson and, later, Miss Marianne Darling both carried out a share of the injecting and X-raying of the specimens. Miss Monson, in particular helped with the organisation of the material into a manageable form and Miss Darling assisted in searching the literature.

Many of the more important works have been in German. Miss Rosemary Pyle relieved us of a considerable part of the task of reading these papers by translating much of Tandler's famous monograph.

We are very grateful indeed to Miss Marcia Edwards for checking the nomenclature of the animals and to Miss Ileen C. M. Parker and Miss Johns for typing the text and arranging the bibliography.

The publishers, themselves, also deserve our thanks for the way in which they have shouldered the responsibility for a highly specialised monograph. Lastly, we would like to record the skill, which would otherwise be anonymous, of the artist who converted all the names and identifying pointers for the arteries on all the pictures into clear lettering and lines. They were originally scribbled in pen in a shaking and illegible hand on glossy photographs during hundreds of train journeys, not infrequently at 90 miles an hour. His name is Mr. Graham Maisey of Reproduction Drawing Ltd.

Nomenclature of intracranial arteries

In mammals it is usual to describe the cerebral carotid as dividing into a cranial and a caudal ramus or anterior and posterior branch. This may confuse those familiar only with human anatomy; but the step is easy if one substitutes in one's mind the term "posterior communicating artery" for "caudal ramus of carotid".

The anatomy of the cerebral arteries of mammals cannot be described wholly in human terminology for several reasons. In the first place most of the best anatomical studies were completed before the crystallisation of modern nomenclature. In the second place there are radical variations for which no human anatomical names are available. In this short account it was considered reasonable to adopt the following general plan.

The terms "Artery of Sylvian Fissure" (or "Fossa") and "Middle Cerebral Artery" are sometimes used synonymously, as are "Artery of Corpus Callosum" and "Anterior Cerebral Artery".

The posterior cerebral arteries and the cerebellar vessels differ in their arrangements and numbers. Happily Hofmann (1900) gives a detailed classification for posterior cerebral arteries into α, β, γ and δ types and for cerebellar arteries into α, β, γ, δ and ε. The nearest human analogy is sometimes used where Hofmann himself has no note. Hofmann's general principles are as follows:

Posterior cerebral α. This usually arises from the cranial ramus of the carotid, more rarely from the caudal ramus near its point of origin, runs along the lateral side of the optic tract and ends in man and some other animals as the anterior choroidal artery. Hofmann gives it as supplying the choroid plexus of the 3rd ventricle. One suspects that this is a manuscript error. It supplies the choroid plexus of the temporal horn, but may, in man at least, also send a major branch to continue around the pulvinar to the 3rd ventricle plexus. In frogs, some reptiles and birds and in occasional mammals such as individual species of deer, it may be much larger and correspond more obviously to a posterior cerebral artery, supplying part of the cerebral hemisphere.

Posterior cerebral β. This springs from the beginning of the caudal ramus of the cerebral carotid, runs laterally in front of the medial geniculate body and behind the pulvinar, both of which it supplies and there it may end. In some mammals, for example guinea pigs, some deer and horses, it becomes, however, a major posterior cerebral artery.

Posterior cerebral γ. This arises close to the oculomotor nerve commonly with the artery for the anterior corpus quadrigeminum and also runs in front of the medial geniculate body where it regularly anastomoses with the posterior cerebral artery β. It may be very small and then a branch of the posterior cerebral artery δ may supply the medial geniculate body. On the other hand, the anastomoses between β, γ and δ may be so wide that the δ artery derives some of its blood supply even from the β as is described in the dog and occurs in other carnivora and many horses. Sometimes, as in horses, two posterior cerebral arteries may thus be found close together. The simultaneous presence of two such arteries dictates that β and γ arteries require separate names.

Posterior cerebral δ. This commonly arises with both the posterior cerebral γ and the artery for the anterior corpus quadrigeminum from the caudal ramus of the carotid. It runs in front of the oculomotor nerve but behind the medial geniculate body against the pineal and ends as the medial posterior choroidal artery of the 3rd ventricle. It may be hypertrophied as in the hedgehog and supply the posterior part of the cerebral hemisphere in preference to α, β and γ arteries. The variability and multiplicity of so-called posterior cerebral arteries in the mammalia goes some way to explain the conflicting accounts of the numbers and origins of the posterior choroidal artery in man.

Cerebellar artery α. This springs from the cranial end of the basilar or the caudal ramus of the internal carotid and runs around the pons to the cerebellum. It supplies a small branch to the posterior corpus quadrigeminum and continues on to the superior vermis and a portion of the cerebellar hemisphere. It anastomoses with one of the more posterior arteries.

This artery is absent in birds but nearly always large in mammals. In guinea pigs and squirrels it supplies the whole of the cerebellum.

The cerebellar artery β. This runs between the pons and the corpus trapezoidium in front of the sixth nerve.

In those mammals in whom the basilar gets most of its blood from the carotids, this artery tends to be large and it anastomosis with the cerebellar artery α.

Where, however, the basilar fills from below the β artery rarely reaches the cerebellum but in its place there is a cerebellar artery γ.

The cerebellar artery γ. This runs to the cerebellum between the corpus trapezoideum and the medulla. It usually supplies an internal auditory artery. With the α artery it supplies the cerebellum in rabbit, hedgehog, weasel, otter, pig and horse. Hofmann illustrates a stag's brain in which on one side the β artery supplies the cerebellum and on the other the γ performs this function.

The cerebellar artery δ. This arises from the basilar as that artery runs over the medulla oblongata. In dogs it shares the supply of the cerebellum with the cerebellar artery α. In them the β and γ arteries are very small.

Cerebellar artery ε. This artery, the posterior inferior cerebellar, according to Hofmann is only found in man. It arises from the vertebral artery and represents the dorsal ramus of the first spinal nerve artery. Its existence in man is probably related to the fact that the cerebellum completely covers the medulla oblongata, while in most animals the medulla protrudes well below the cerebellum. We have shown it in several other mammals.

Monotremata

References in the literature to the arrangement of the cranial arteries of Monotremes are extremely scanty and we have not been able to inject a specimen, but for completeness this book ought to begin with some account of their anatomy.

Shellshear (1929) published a detailed description of the major cerebral vessels of *Echidna aculeata*, now *Tachyglossus aculeatus*, with clear illustrations; but was unable to examine any of the arteries outside the arachnoid. Hyrtl (1853) gave quite detailed accounts of the other arteries of the head and neck of *Ornithorhynchus anatinus* and *Echidna setosa*, now *Tachyglossus setosa*, but the nomenclature is so strange that it is almost certain his understanding of the homologies was at fault. If one ignores his interpretation of what he drew and described, however, and puts names to the vessels which seem reasonable by the standards of present knowledge, one is left not knowing exactly where the internal carotid artery becomes a separate vessel. Hyrtl believed that the "internal carotid" formed one of the two terminal branches of the common carotid, that it then gave rise in turn to the occipital artery and the internal maxillary before proceeding as the "true internal carotid" in close relationship with the dorsal wall of the pharynx, which it supplied. It entered the skull "through a canal in the joint between the anterior and posterior sphenoid, the carotid foramen". One is led to conclude that he mistook the stapedial artery for the internal maxillary; he clearly described the connections of this vessel with the orbital and middle meningeal branches. He probably confused the ascending pharyngeal with the internal carotid. The internal carotid itself is likely to begin as a separate vessel after giving off the stapedial within the temporal bone in a similar way to that found in Insectivores.

Tandler (1899), as on many other occasions, straightened out Hyrtl's confusion and gave clear and reasonable description of *Ornithorhynchus* and *Echidna setosa*.

If one accepts his findings and re-interpretation, the arrangement is as follows. The common carotid divides into two main stems. One of these, the external carotid, gives rise to an extremely tortuous, large lingual artery (it was only large on one side, the right, the left sided artery was little more than a twig). The external carotid then supplies an external maxillary, masseteric, pterygoid arteries, a leash of temporal vessels and an auricular artery, a large branch to the sub-mandibular gland, a sublingual branch and an internal maxillary artery (but not necessarily in that order). This latter gives origin to the middle meningeal and to an external ophthalmic which anastomoses with the orbital and ethmoidal arteries of the inferior division of the stapedial. Two ethmoid arteries are described, the infra-oribital facial is the main continuity of the stapedial/internal maxillary and gives rise to nasal arteries.

The other terminal branch of the common carotid supplies the occipital, a large ascending pharyngeal and a common trunk for the internal carotid and the stapedial artery.

The internal carotid within the head has the following branches: posterior communicating, anterior choroidal, perforating arteries, anterior cerebral and, slightly larger than the anterior cerebral, the middle cerebral artery.

The anterior cerebrals of the two sides fuse to form a common trunk, but are often of unequal size. Heubner's artery was identified by Shellshear in his specimen.

The vertebral arteries are connected with both the anterior and posterior spinal arterial networks. They each give off a posterior inferior cerbellar branch and join to form the basilar.

The branches of the basilar are medullary, anterior inferior cerebellar vessels (internal auditory arteries being separate from the cerebellar arteries β of Hoffman's classification) and superior cerebellar. The posterior cerebral arteries are connected both with the basilar and the posterior communicating vessels; but their exact classification by Hoffman's terminology is unknown.

Marsupialia

Tandler (1899) provided a very complete description of the cranial arteries derived from dissections of five specimens of *Halmaturus giganteus* and one specimen of *Halmaturus ruficollis* (*Macropus rufus*). He appears to have been misled in his estimate of the connections of and flow through the vertebral arteries at the cranio-vertebral junction.

He says of the cervical vertebral artery, "In the region of the atlas, by far the greater portion of the vessel is drawn off as the cervical vertebral branch to the muscles of the neck and the occiput, replacing the almost rudimentary occipital artery. Only a very small branch (of the vertebral) runs as the cerebral vertebral through the occipital foramen into the skull and anastomoses with the similarly named vessel of the other side to become the basilar artery. It is to be noted that the basilar artery diminishes in calibre from front to rear; it therefore derives its blood not from the vertebral but from the carotid".

(Author's translation).

The injection studies show that in *Macropus rufus* this is an overstatement. It is realised that post-mortem injection can give little information about the relative sizes of branches during life. (Witness the greater calibre of the carotid on the injected side due to the pressure of the injection.) Nevertheless the route from the cervical vertebral to the basilar artery is established as a main and effective pathway in *Macropus rufus*, *Wallabia rufogrisea frutica* and in *Marmosa*. The basilar artery does not appear to taper from front to rear in quite the way which Tandler described.

The nomenclature of the posterior cerebral artery, the posterior communicating artery and the caudal ramus of the internal carotid artery is fraught with difficulty.

By analogy with man, the caudal ramus of the internal carotid may be regarded as the posterior communicating artery. The posterior cerebral artery may derive much of its blood supply from the basilar as in *Megaleia rufa* and *Marmosa*, or almost all from the carotid arteries as in *Wallabia rufogrisea frutica* and *Phascolomis ursinus*. In functional terms the former arrangement is more like man than the latter. *Bettongia penicillata* is somewhere intermediate between the two extremes. The pictures strongly suggest that in many cases the attachment of the posterior cerebral artery to the basilar provides the pathway through which blood from the carotid artery usually supplies the superior cerebellar artery. Because of reservations about the suitability of the name "posterior communicating artery" it has not been used. In preference to this there is "posterior or caudal branch of internal carotid artery" (following Tandler's example) and, where appropriate, "posterior stem of posterior cerebral artery" for the portion attached to the basilar, even though the attachment to the basilar may be an indirect one through what appears to be the stem of the superior cerebellar artery.

In every case where the cerebellar arteries have been outlined these have been of Hofmann's (1900) "α" type, with additional supply from "β" or "γ" cerebellar arteries.

These have sometimes been called the "superior" and "inferior" cerebellar arteries in the illustrations, by analogy with man's "superior and anterior-inferior" cerebellar vessels.

Marmosa sp.
Mouse Opossum

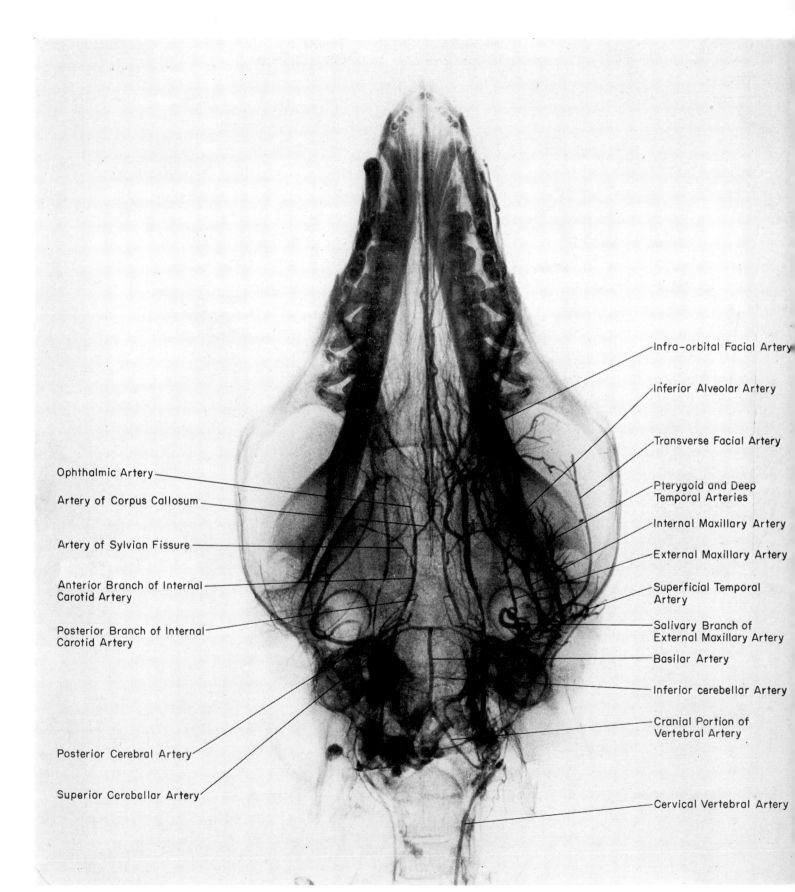

Infra-orbital Facial Artery

Inferior Alveolar Artery

Transverse Facial Artery

Pterygoid and Deep Temporal Arteries

Internal Maxillary Artery

External Maxillary Artery

Superficial Temporal Artery

Salivary Branch of External Maxillary Artery

Basilar Artery

Inferior cerebellar Artery

Cranial Portion of Vertebral Artery

Cervical Vertebral Artery

Ophthalmic Artery

Artery of Corpus Callosum

Artery of Sylvian Fissure

Anterior Branch of Internal Carotid Artery

Posterior Branch of Internal Carotid Artery

Posterior Cerebral Artery

Superior Cerebellar Artery

× 5·0

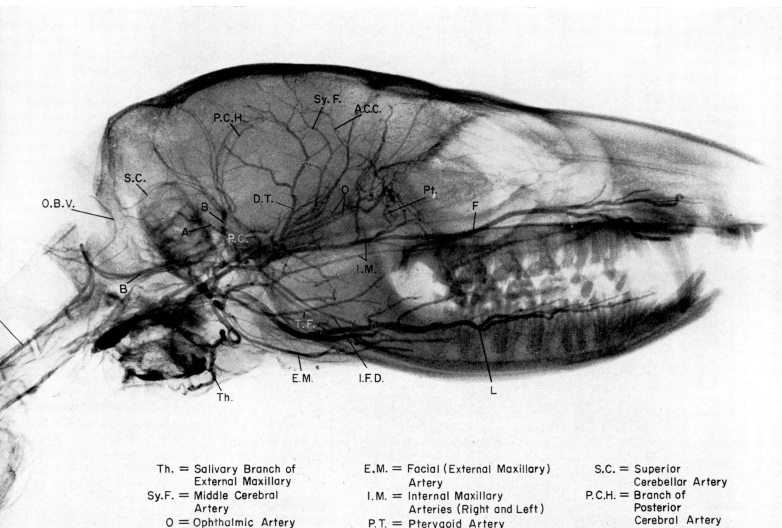

Th. = Salivary Branch of
      External Maxillary
Sy.F. = Middle Cerebral
      Artery
O = Ophthalmic Artery
      (Right and Left)
A = (Probably) Auricular
      Artery
T.F. = Transverse Facial
      Artery
L = Lingual Arteries

E.M. = Facial (External Maxillary)
      Artery
I.M. = Internal Maxillary
      Arteries (Right and Left)
P.T. = Pterygoid Artery
D.T. = Deep Temporal Artery
A.C.C. = Anterior Cerebral
      Artery
V. = Cervical Vertebral
O.B.V. = Occipital Branch of
      Vertebral Artery

S.C. = Superior
      Cerebellar Artery
P.C.H. = Branch of
      Posterior
      Cerebral Artery
S.T. = Superficial
      Temporal Artery
F. = Infra-Orbital
      Facial Artery
I.F.D. = Inferior Alveolar
      Artery
B. = Basilar Artery

× 5·0

The lingual artery is very large, so is the salivary branch of the external maxillary. There is a well-developed transverse facial artery but the bucco-labial has not been identified. There are two branches of the infra-orbital facial or internal maxillary which ramify around the orbital margins but have not been identified as named arteries.

The vertebro-basilar system is well-developed. The posterior branch of the internal carotid is small and the posterior cerebrals receive an equal supply from the basilar artery.

In Hofmann's terminology the posterior cerebral artery is probably of "δ" type.

Lutreolina crassicaudata
Thick-tailed Opossum

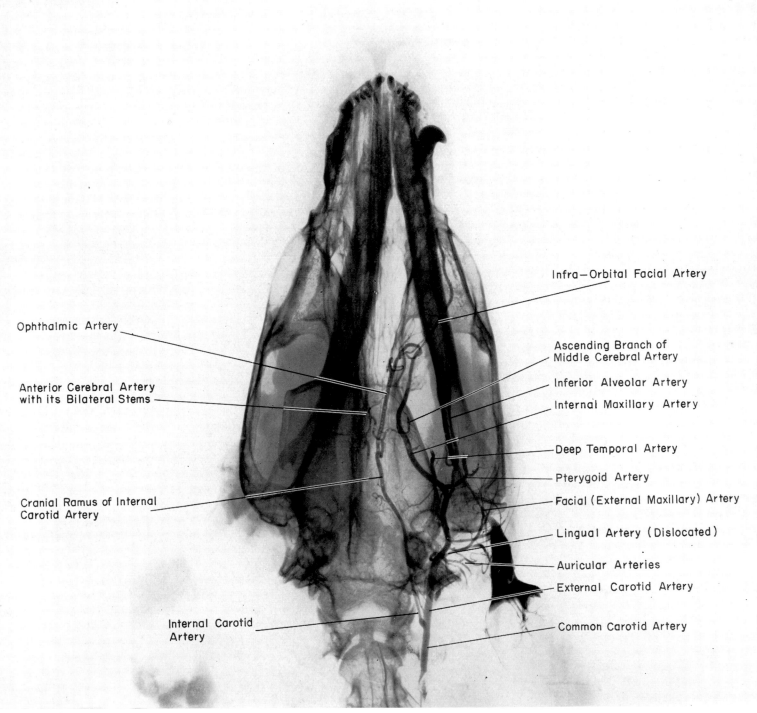

Infra—Orbital Facial Artery

Ophthalmic Artery

Ascending Branch of
Middle Cerebral Artery

Inferior Alveolar Artery

Anterior Cerebral Artery
with its Bilateral Stems

Internal Maxillary Artery

Deep Temporal Artery

Pterygoid Artery

Cranial Ramus of Internal
Carotid Artery

Facial (External Maxillary) Artery

Lingual Artery (Dislocated)

Auricular Arteries

External Carotid Artery

Internal Carotid
Artery

Common Carotid Artery

× 1·7

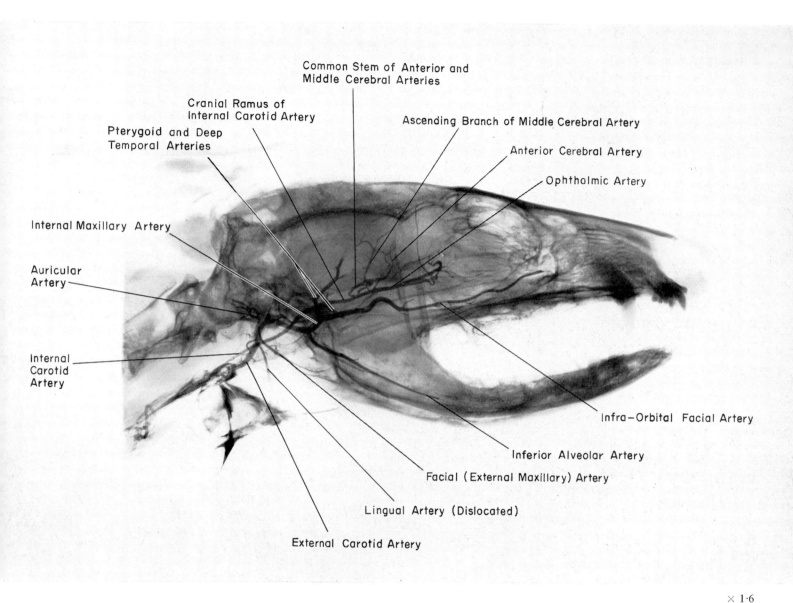

Common Stem of Anterior and
Middle Cerebral Arteries

Cranial Ramus of
Internal Carotid Artery

Ascending Branch of Middle Cerebral Artery

Pterygoid and Deep
Temporal Arteries

Anterior Cerebral Artery

Ophthalmic Artery

Internal Maxillary Artery

Auricular
Artery

Internal
Carotid
Artery

Infra—Orbital Facial Artery

Inferior Alveolar Artery

Facial (External Maxillary) Artery

Lingual Artery (Dislocated)

External Carotid Artery

× 1·6

In this very damaged specimen the relative positions of the
lingual artery and other vessels in the upper part of the neck
have been disturbed.

Only parts of the intracranial arteries have been filled.
There is no filling of the vertebro-basilar circulation.

Note the enormous size of the ophthalmic artery.

Petaurus norfolcensis
Squirrel-like Flying Phalanger

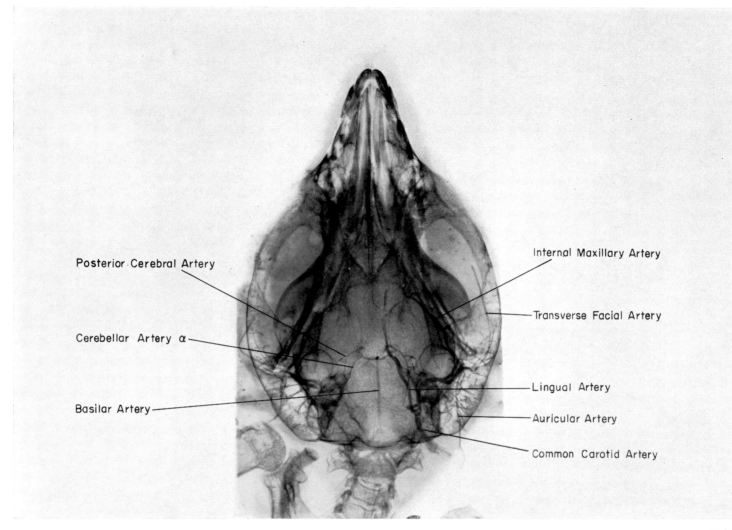

Posterior Cerebral Artery

Cerebellar Artery α

Basilar Artery

Internal Maxillary Artery

Transverse Facial Artery

Lingual Artery

Auricular Artery

Common Carotid Artery

× 2·0

Only a few of the vessels have been shown and it is not clear by which route barium has reached the Circle of Willis.

There is probably a cerebellar artery β as well as a cerebellar artery α.

Phascolomis ursinus
Common Wombat

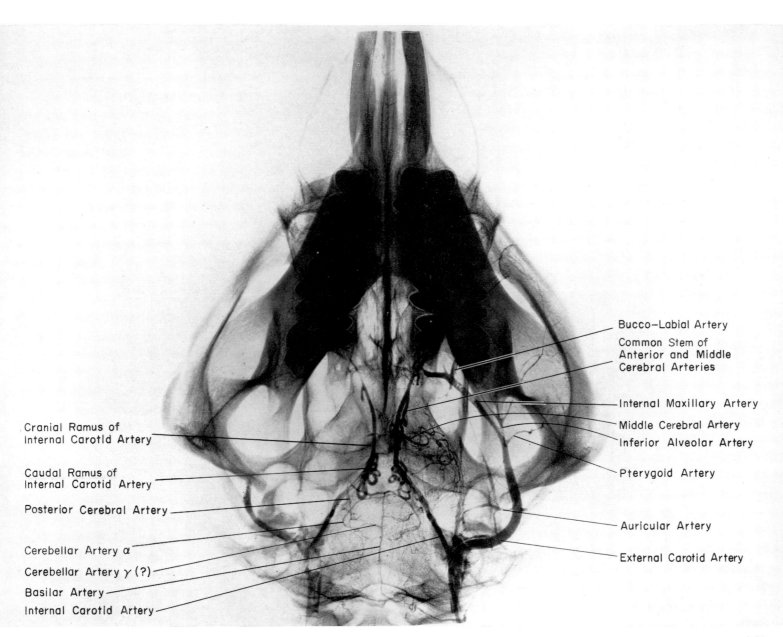

Bucco–Labial Artery

Common Stem of
Anterior and Middle
Cerebral Arteries

Internal Maxillary Artery

Middle Cerebral Artery

Inferior Alveolar Artery

Pterygoid Artery

Cranial Ramus of
Internal Carotid Artery

Caudal Ramus of
Internal Carotid Artery

Posterior Cerebral Artery

Auricular Artery

Cerebellar Artery α

External Carotid Artery

Cerebellar Artery γ (?)

Basilar Artery

Internal Carotid Artery

× 0·82

Branches of the external carotid and internal maxillary arteries are difficult to identify, the enormous development of the jaws making the relationships very different from those to be seen in *Megaleia rufa*.

For reasons not understood the posterior branch of the internal carotid and the common stem of the arteries of the Sylvian fissure and of the corpus callosum are extremely tortuous.

The artery of the corpus callosum in this study is so thin that no label has been attached in the ventro-dorsal view.

The arrangement of the vertebral arteries corresponds rather more closely to the description given by Tandler for *Halmaturus giganteus* than it does to *Megaleia rufa* in our injection, but even through the multiple small channels at the cranio-vertebral junction there is a free flow of barium from cranial to cervical vertebral arteries.

The branches of the artery of the Sylvian fissure are extremely well filled.

The posterior cerebral artery may be of Hofmann's type "γ" or "δ".

In the lateral view there is superimposition of the main arteries of the two sides.

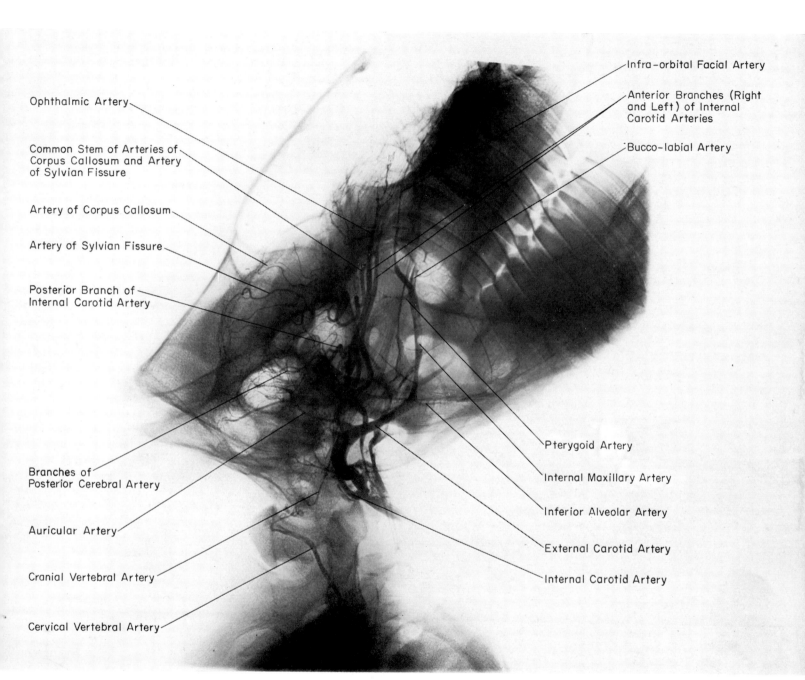

Ophthalmic Artery

Common Stem of Arteries of
Corpus Callosum and Artery
of Sylvian Fissure

Artery of Corpus Callosum

Artery of Sylvian Fissure

Posterior Branch of
Internal Carotid Artery

Branches of
Posterior Cerebral Artery

Auricular Artery

Cranial Vertebral Artery

Cervical Vertebral Artery

Infra-orbital Facial Artery

Anterior Branches (Right
and Left) of Internal
Carotid Arteries

Bucco-labial Artery

Pterygoid Artery

Internal Maxillary Artery

Inferior Alveolar Artery

External Carotid Artery

Internal Carotid Artery

× 0·82

Wallabia rufogrisea frutica
Bennett's Wallaby

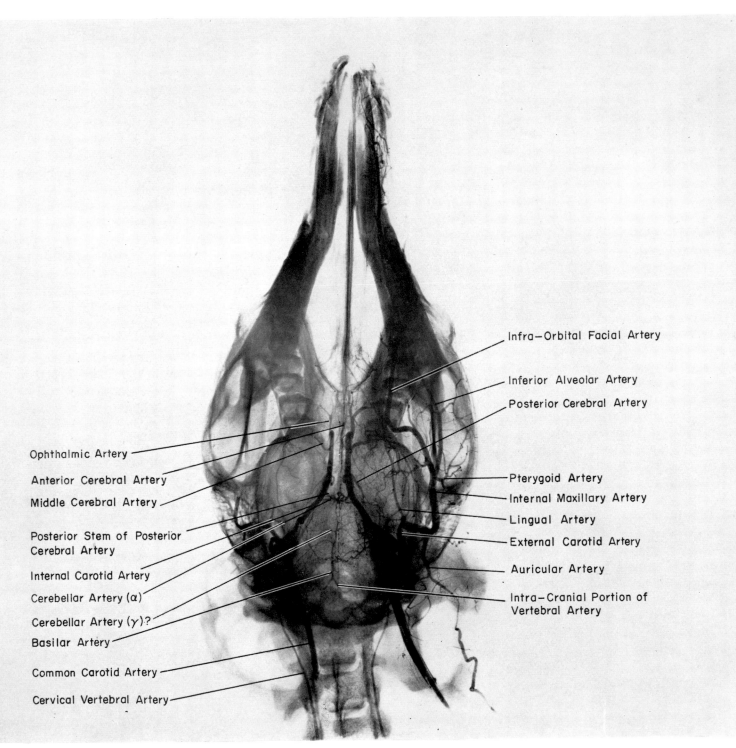

Infra—Orbital Facial Artery

Inferior Alveolar Artery

Posterior Cerebral Artery

Ophthalmic Artery

Anterior Cerebral Artery

Middle Cerebral Artery

Pterygoid Artery

Internal Maxillary Artery

Lingual Artery

Posterior Stem of Posterior
Cerebral Artery

External Carotid Artery

Internal Carotid Artery

Cerebellar Artery (α)

Auricular Artery

Cerebellar Artery (γ)?

Intra—Cranial Portion of
Vertebral Artery

Basilar Artery

Common Carotid Artery

Cervical Vertebral Artery

× 1·15

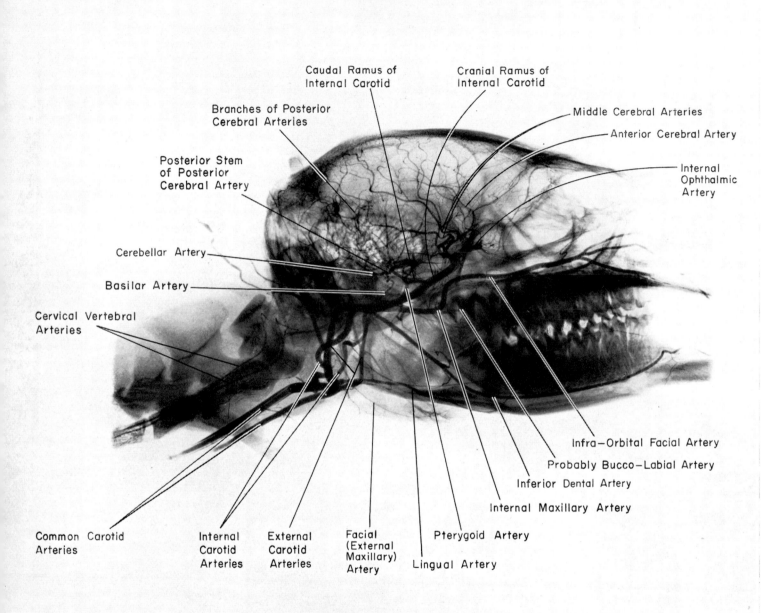

Caudal Ramus of Internal Carotid

Cranial Ramus of Internal Carotid

Branches of Posterior Cerebral Arteries

Middle Cerebral Arteries

Anterior Cerebral Artery

Posterior Stem of Posterior Cerebral Artery

Internal Ophthalmic Artery

Cerebellar Artery

Basilar Artery

Cervical Vertebral Arteries

Infra—Orbital Facial Artery

Probably Bucco—Labial Artery

Inferior Dental Artery

Internal Maxillary Artery

Common Carotid Arteries

Internal Carotid Arteries

External Carotid Arteries

Facial (External Maxillary) Artery

Pterygoid Artery

Lingual Artery

× 1·00

The external maxillary has not been identified in the ventro-dorsal view.

The superficial temporal artery appears to be very small.

The deep temporal artery probably arises separately from the internal maxillary and is visible in the ventro-dorsal view. There is also a moderately large unlabelled artery seen in the ventro-dorsal view running medially from the internal maxillary close to the origin of the inferior alveolar artery. It is probably the middle meningeal artery.

The bucco-labial artery is only very tentatively identified.

The division of the internal carotid into its anterior and posterior branches is superimposed in the ventro-dorsal view upon the main trunk of the carotid and cannot, therefore, be labelled.

The posterior cerebral artery may well be of Hofmann's "γ" type and there is probably an "α" posterior cerebral artery as well.

In lateral view both right and left carotid arterial trees are superimposed on each other.

Macropus rufus
Red Kangaroo

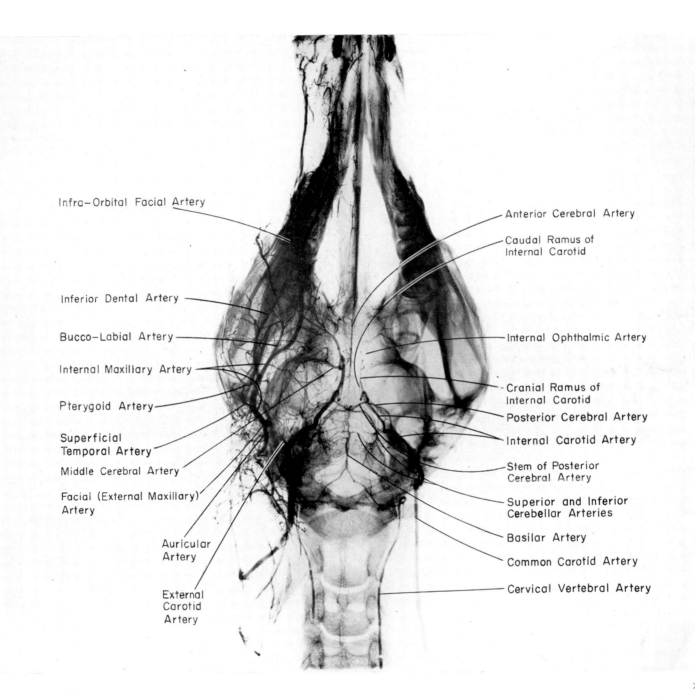

Infra–Orbital Facial Artery

Inferior Dental Artery

Bucco–Labial Artery

Internal Maxillary Artery

Pterygoid Artery

Superficial Temporal Artery

Middle Cerebral Artery

Facial (External Maxillary) Artery

Auricular Artery

External Carotid Artery

Anterior Cerebral Artery

Caudal Ramus of Internal Carotid

Internal Ophthalmic Artery

Cranial Ramus of Internal Carotid

Posterior Cerebral Artery

Internal Carotid Artery

Stem of Posterior Cerebral Artery

Superior and Inferior Cerebellar Arteries

Basilar Artery

Common Carotid Artery

Cervical Vertebral Artery

× 0·9

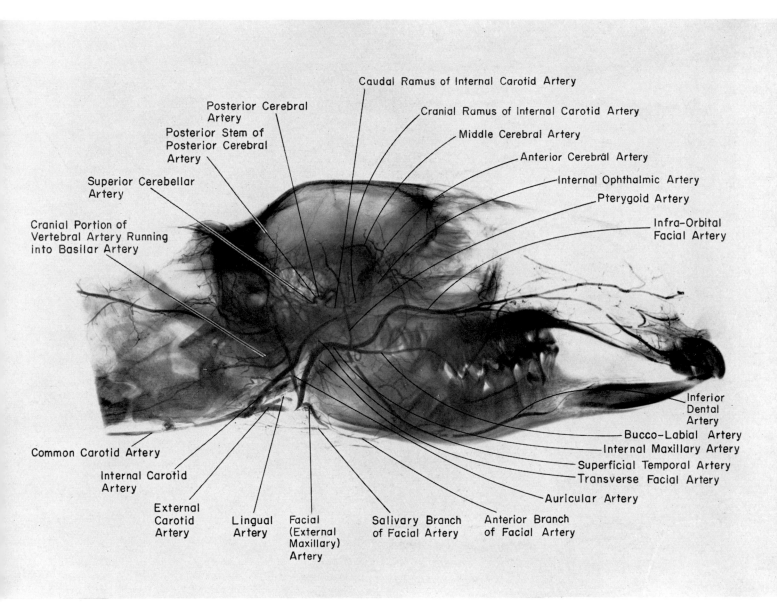

Caudal Ramus of Internal Carotid Artery

Posterior Cerebral Artery

Cranial Ramus of Internal Carotid Artery

Posterior Stem of Posterior Cerebral Artery

Middle Cerebral Artery

Anterior Cerebral Artery

Superior Cerebellar Artery

Internal Ophthalmic Artery

Pterygoid Artery

Cranial Portion of Vertebral Artery Running into Basilar Artery

Infra-Orbital Facial Artery

Inferior Dental Artery

Common Carotid Artery

Bucco-Labial Artery

Internal Maxillary Artery

Internal Carotid Artery

Superficial Temporal Artery

Transverse Facial Artery

Auricular Artery

External Carotid Artery

Lingual Artery

Facial (External Maxillary) Artery

Salivary Branch of Facial Artery

Anterior Branch of Facial Artery

× 0·9

Labels on the right-hand side in the ventro-dorsal view, point to the very faintly outlined branches of the internal carotid. The better filled branches on the left are free of superimposed arrows to allow them to be seen more clearly.

In the ventro-dorsal view the lingual artery is invisible because it is so poorly filled.

The deep temporal artery and the pterygoid arise from a common stem.

Bettongia penicillata
Brush-tailed Rat Kangaroo

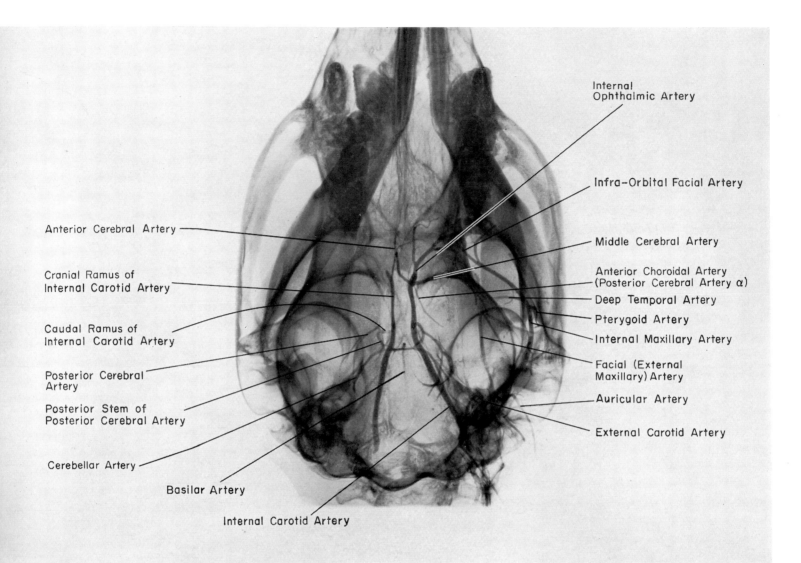

Internal
Ophthalmic Artery

Infra-Orbital Facial Artery

Anterior Cerebral Artery

Middle Cerebral Artery

Cranial Ramus of
Internal Carotid Artery

Anterior Choroidal Artery
(Posterior Cerebral Artery α)

Deep Temporal Artery

Pterygoid Artery

Caudal Ramus of
Internal Carotid Artery

Internal Maxillary Artery

Posterior Cerebral
Artery

Facial (External
Maxillary) Artery

Posterior Stem of
Posterior Cerebral Artery

Auricular Artery

External Carotid Artery

Cerebellar Artery

Basilar Artery

Internal Carotid Artery

× 2·5

The supratentorial intracranial arteries are here filled better than any others.

Note the usual division of the internal carotid into an anterior and posterior branch, the anterior giving rise to the large ophthalmic artery and the common stem for the arteries of the corpus callosum and of the Sylvian fissure.

Note also a vessel which appears to be the anterior choroidal artery. (Hofmann's posterior cerebral "α").

The main continuation of the posterior cerebral artery is clearly seen running around the posterior surface of the thalamus. This artery is perhaps a posterior cerebral "γ".

A major part of the blood supply to the superior cerebellar arteries apparently comes from the carotid via the posterior cerebral. The branching of the basilar into what look like superior cerebellar arteries and their communications with the posterior stem of the posterior cerebral are asymmetrical on the two sides.

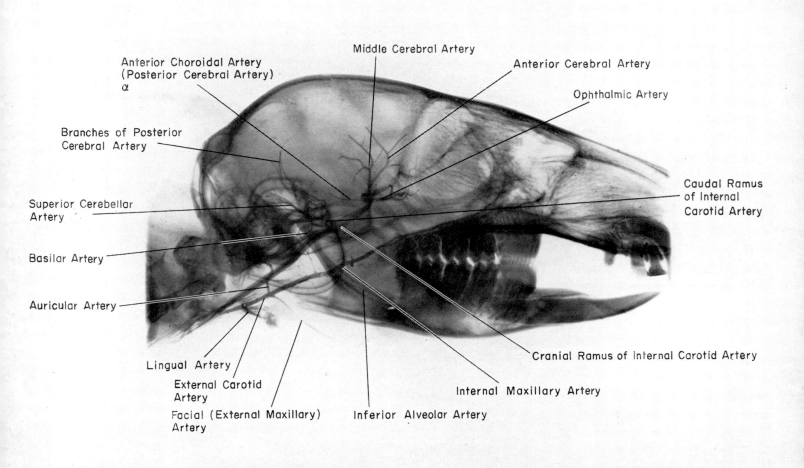

Anterior Choroidal Artery
(Posterior Cerebral Artery)
α

Middle Cerebral Artery

Anterior Cerebral Artery

Ophthalmic Artery

Branches of Posterior
Cerebral Artery

Caudal Ramus
of Internal
Carotid Artery

Superior Cerebellar
Artery

Basilar Artery

Auricular Artery

Cranial Ramus of Internal Carotid Artery

Lingual Artery

External Carotid
Artery

Internal Maxillary Artery

Facial (External Maxillary)
Artery

Inferior Alveolar Artery

× 1·7

Insectivora

The stapedial artery is very large. From it arise many of those arteries of the face and orbit which in other mammals have gained a secondary origin from the external carotid.

Hofmann has described the anatomy of the intracranial vessels of *Erinaceus europaeus*.

"Each cerebral carotid divides after giving off the large ophthalmic artery, into a cranial branch which appears to be the continuation of the main stem and a thin caudal branch.

"The cranial branch runs over the side of the infundibulum and the optic tract proximal to the optic nerve. It converges with that from the other side and turns anteriorly in the longitudinal cerebral fissure, where the two unite. This single anterior cerebral artery gives off a large medial artery of the olfactory bulb which runs for the most part on the medial surface of the hemisphere. The anterior cerebral then divides into two arteries which follow the surface of the corpus callosum giving branches to the medial surfaces of the cerebral hemispheres, finally anastomosing with branches of the posterior cerebral on the splenium. In addition to small branches to the infundibulum, the chiasm and the optic tract, the cranial branch of the cerebral carotid gives rise to the middle cerebral, which supplies the outer surface of the cerebrum with three or four branches, from one of which a small branch runs to the uncus.

"Soon after the origin of the middle cerebral, the anterior cerebral artery gives off an ethmoidal branch which runs cranially over the lamina cribrosa and anastomoses with the rete ethmoidalis, which lies partly subdurally and partly intradurally. This rete is connected through an ethmoidal foramen with the orbital arteries and also sends small branches with the olfactory fibres into the nasal cavity.

"The caudal branch of the cerebral carotid, analogous to the posterior communicating artery of man, is much diminished up to the point of origin of the posterior cerebral (δ) arteries, so that these derive their blood from the basilar. The caudal part of the caudal branch, from where the posterior cerebral artery is given off, is greatly enlarged so that the posterior cerebral gets its blood from the basilar which derives it from the large first spinal nerve arteries. The posterior communicating artery forms a narrow side branch which runs in the groove between the medial geniculate body and the optic thalamus and here breaks up into twigs.

"The posterior cerebral artery (δ) runs laterally giving a small branch in front of the medial geniculate body to anastomose with the posterior cerebral artery (β), so that a bigger vessel is formed. This comes to lie in the groove between the medial geniculate body and the anterior corpus quadrigeminum on the dorsal side of the brain near the midline. Here it gives off a medial posterior choroidal artery to the plexus of the IIIrd ventricle, while the posterior part of the cerebrum both on the outer and medial surfaces is supplied by a series of small vessels from which one anastomoses with the artery of the corpus callosum. The root of the posterior cerebral artery (δ) is closely related to the caudal ramus of the cerebral carotid which gives numerous small branches to the posterior perforated substance and to the infundibulum.

"Just behind the origin of the oculo-motor nerves, the cerebellar arteries (α) arise from the basilar, run laterally on the basal surface of the cerebral peduncles, then return nearly into the midline where each gives a small branch to the posterior corpus quadrigeminum. The main stem, however, breaks up into a series of large branches running caudally in the parasagittal plane to the hind brain and the superior vermis. These anastomose with the end branches of the cerebellar artery (δ).

"The basilar artery often has a very tortuous course or lies entirely on one side or other. In addition, in three injections the basilar was reduplicated over the pons.

"The caudal end of the basilar artery formed by conjunction of the greatly dilated vertebrals is variable in position.

"The basilar artery gives rise (1) to a series of branches to the pons and corpus trapesoideum. Posterior to these lies a small artery to the root of the trigeminal nerve. The basilar also supplies (2) a cerebellar artery (α) and this usually runs in the groove between the corpus trapesoideum and the medulla, occasionally giving off an internal auditory artery and several small branches to the underside of the root of the trigeminal nerve. The main stem, however, branches on the cerebellar hemisphere and anastomoses with the cerebellar artery (α). Usually one can see three end branches on either side of the hind brain. The most lateral runs in the groove between bedullar and cerebellum, the middle between the flocculus and the cerebellar hemisphere and the medial between the hemisphere and the superior vermis. (3) There is a series of branches to the medulla oblongata, from which a few finally end on the restiform body. (4) The basilar gives rise to a central artery in the substance of the spinal cord.

"Each of the two large first spinal nerve arteries (veterbral arteries) divides into a dorsal and ventral branch. The ventral, which has the same direction as the stem, joins with the similar branch from the other side to form the basilar artery.

"The smaller dorsal branch, however, runs over the dorsal surface of the cord and divides into a small cranial and a large caudal twig, which helps to form the dorsal spinal tract by joining its upper end.

"The ventral spinal tract springs by two or more roots from the vertebral arteries as they approach each other, runs tortuously backwards and sometimes makes a series of networks in the ventral fissure of the cord, where it supplies the spinal cord with small branches. It is reinforced by two or three large ventral spinal nerve arteries. By means of dorsal rami it unites with the dorsal spinal tract."

(Author's free translation.)

N.B. Hofmann's "ethmoidal rete" does not correspond with the retia of *felidae* and Artiodactyla.

Echinosorex gymnurus
Moon Rat

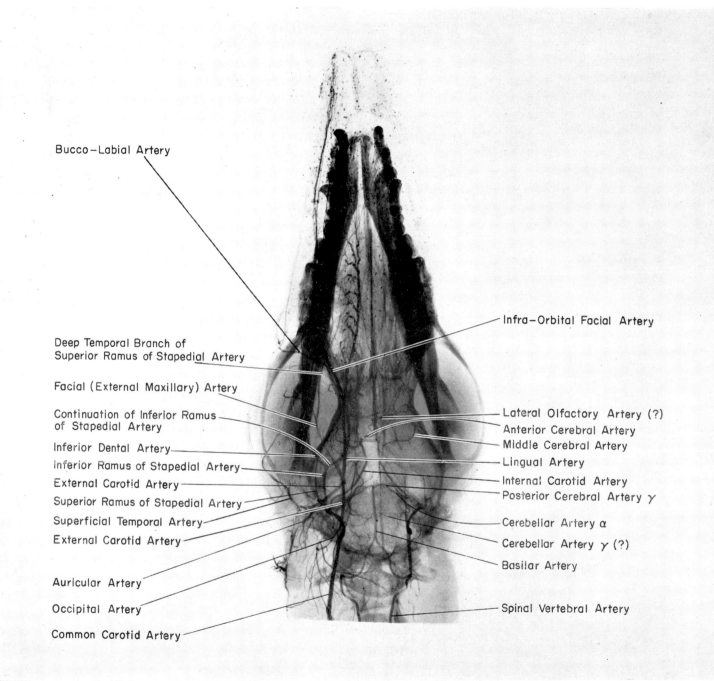

Bucco–Labial Artery

Deep Temporal Branch of
Superior Ramus of Stapedial Artery

Facial (External Maxillary) Artery

Continuation of Inferior Ramus
of Stapedial Artery

Inferior Dental Artery

Inferior Ramus of Stapedial Artery

External Carotid Artery

Superior Ramus of Stapedial Artery

Superficial Temporal Artery

External Carotid Artery

Auricular Artery

Occipital Artery

Common Carotid Artery

Infra–Orbital Facial Artery

Lateral Olfactory Artery (?)

Anterior Cerebral Artery

Middle Cerebral Artery

Lingual Artery

Internal Carotid Artery

Posterior Cerebral Artery γ

Cerebellar Artery α

Cerebellar Artery γ (?)

Basilar Artery

Spinal Vertebral Artery

× 1·5

The general arrangement resembles the mole, but there are some differences in detail.

The lingual artery appears to be the direct continuation of the external carotid. After leaving the lingual the much diminished parent vessel turns backwards and laterally and divides into a large auricular artery and a small superficial temporal.

The stapedial artery presents a superior ramus from which arises another superficial temporal artery. As far as the superficial temporal arteries are concerned, therefore, the moon rat combines the characteristics of the mole and hedgehog.

The inferior ramus divides solely into the inferior dental and the infra-orbital facial arteries. As in the mole the terminal branches of the superior ramus of the stapedial artery are frontal and external ethmoidal, the terminal branches of the inferior ramus are orbital and nasal.

From the anterior cerebral arteries large branches run

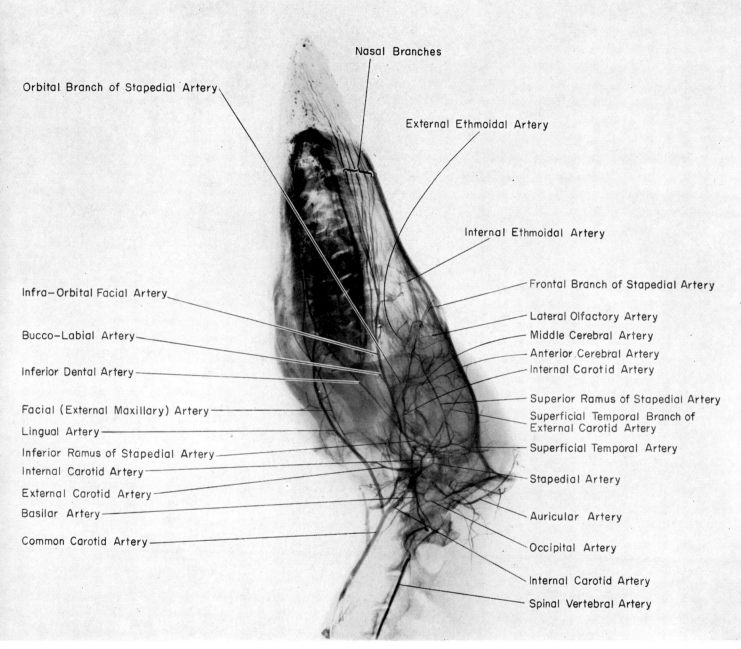

Nasal Branches

Orbital Branch of Stapedial Artery

External Ethmoidal Artery

Internal Ethmoidal Artery

Frontal Branch of Stapedial Artery

Infra-Orbital Facial Artery

Lateral Olfactory Artery

Middle Cerebral Artery

Bucco-Labial Artery

Anterior Cerebral Artery

Inferior Dental Artery

Internal Carotid Artery

Superior Ramus of Stapedial Artery

Facial (External Maxillary) Artery

Superficial Temporal Branch of External Carotid Artery

Lingual Artery

Inferior Ramus of Stapedial Artery

Superficial Temporal Artery

Internal Carotid Artery

External Carotid Artery

Stapedial Artery

Basilar Artery

Auricular Artery

Common Carotid Artery

Occipital Artery

Internal Carotid Artery

Spinal Vertebral Artery

× 1·5

laterally under and then around the lateral aspect of the olfactory lobes.

The posterior cerebral arteries (probably γ) are visible in the lateral view, but have not been arrowed because of the numerous other overlying shadows.

Erinaceus europaeus
Hedgehog

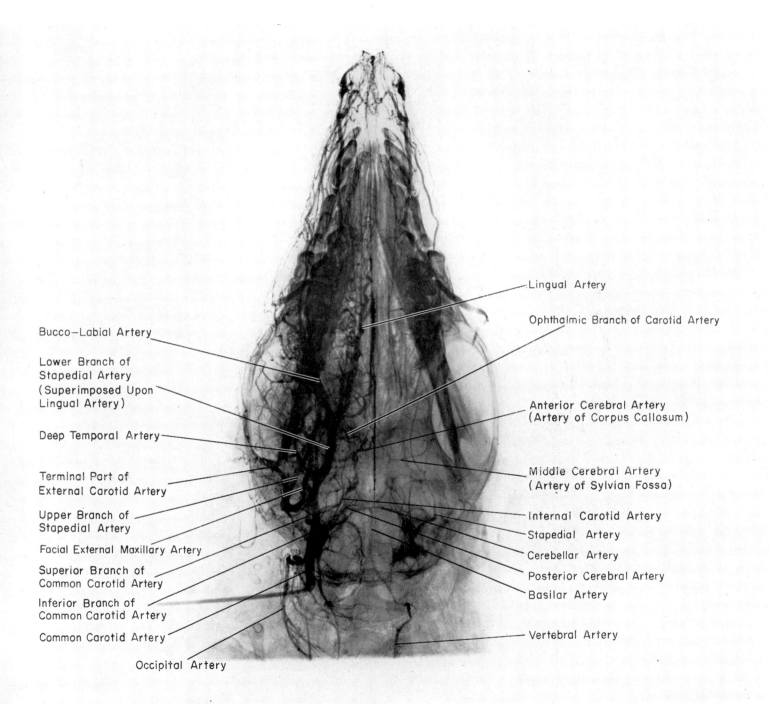

Lingual Artery

Ophthalmic Branch of Carotid Artery

Bucco—Labial Artery

Lower Branch of
Stapedial Artery
(Superimposed Upon
Lingual Artery)

Anterior Cerebral Artery
(Artery of Corpus Callosum)

Deep Temporal Artery

Middle Cerebral Artery
(Artery of Sylvian Fossa)

Terminal Part of
External Carotid Artery

Internal Carotid Artery

Upper Branch of
Stapedial Artery

Stapedial Artery

Cerebellar Artery

Facial External Maxillary Artery

Posterior Cerebral Artery

Superior Branch of
Common Carotid Artery

Basilar Artery

Inferior Branch of
Common Carotid Artery

Common Carotid Artery

Vertebral Artery

Occipital Artery

× 2·0

In *Erinaceus europaeus* the radiographic problem is to avoid confusion due to the shadows of the spines. In this particular hedgehog the injected micropaque had penetrated through to the veins of the nose.

The complexity of shadows in the orbit hides the anastomosis between the upper branch of the stapedial artery and the orbital ramus of the lower branch. The lachrymal and ethmoidal branches of the upper part of the stapedial artery are also filled, but not labelled.

In the lateral view the terminal part of the external carotid artery is superimposed upon the lower branch of the stapedial artery where that vessel gives origin to the inferior dental and deep temporal arteries. The auricular branches of the external carotid emerge from behind the superior branch of the stapedial artery looking as though they were derived from it.

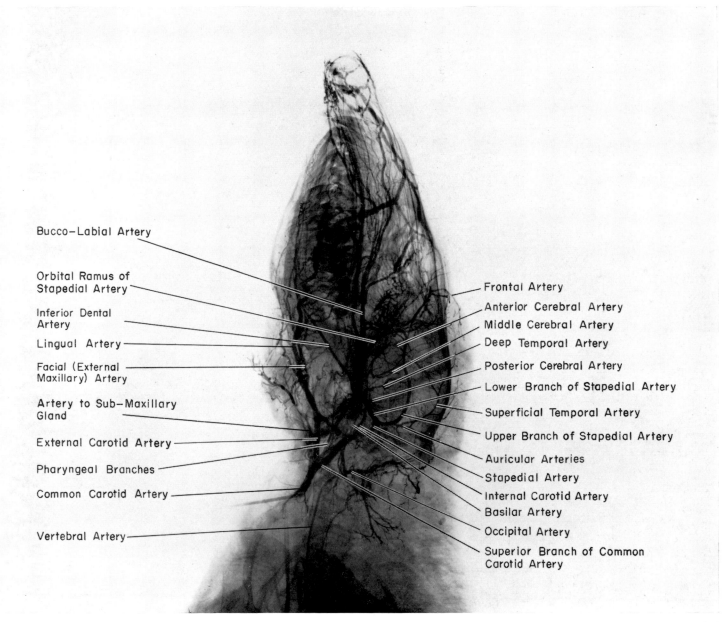

Bucco-Labial Artery

Orbital Ramus of
Stapedial Artery

Inferior Dental
Artery

Lingual Artery

Facial (External
Maxillary) Artery

Artery to Sub-Maxillary
Gland

External Carotid Artery

Pharyngeal Branches

Common Carotid Artery

Vertebral Artery

Frontal Artery

Anterior Cerebral Artery

Middle Cerebral Artery

Deep Temporal Artery

Posterior Cerebral Artery

Lower Branch of Stapedial Artery

Superficial Temporal Artery

Upper Branch of Stapedial Artery

Auricular Arteries

Stapedial Artery

Internal Carotid Artery

Basilar Artery

Occipital Artery

Superior Branch of Common
Carotid Artery

× 1·5

Petrodromus tetradactylus
Elephant Shrew

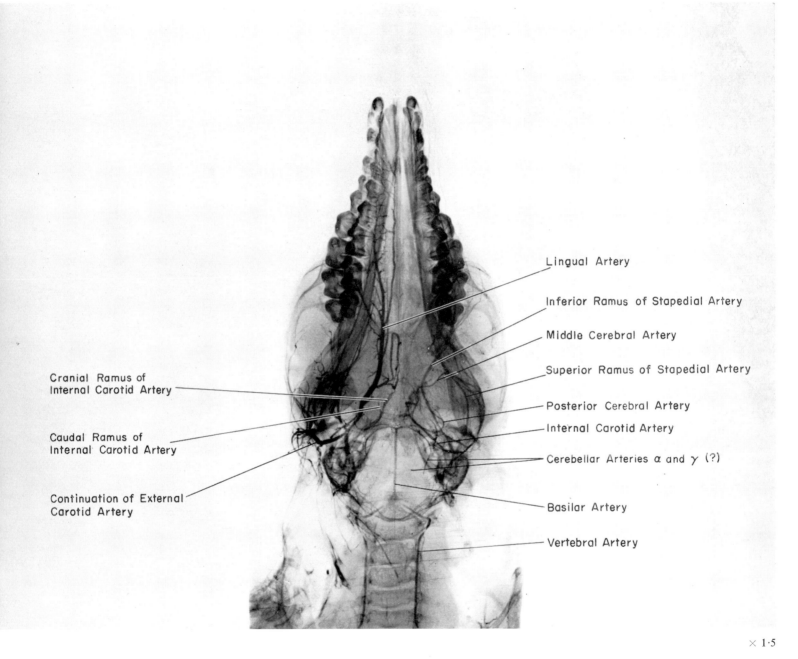

Lingual Artery

Inferior Ramus of Stapedial Artery

Middle Cerebral Artery

Superior Ramus of Stapedial Artery

Posterior Cerebral Artery

Internal Carotid Artery

Cerebellar Arteries α and γ (?)

Basilar Artery

Vertebral Artery

Cranial Ramus of
Internal Carotid Artery

Caudal Ramus of
Internal Carotid Artery

Continuation of External
Carotid Artery

× 1·5

Injection is incomplete. On one side in the ventrodorsal view the superior and inferior rami of the stapedial artery (but not their branches) are filled, as well as the cerebral part of the internal carotid. On the other side some branches only of the inferior ramus are shown. There, the inferior dental artery and the bucco-labial artery are superimposed upon the external maxillary and the deep temporal, and have not been labelled.

In the lateral view the superior ramus of the stapedial artery is not filled.

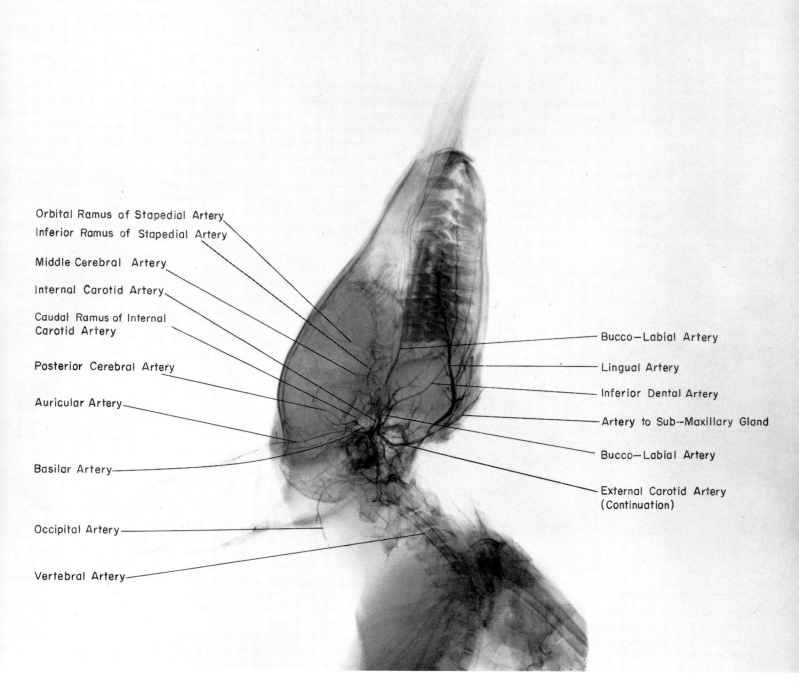

Orbital Ramus of Stapedial Artery

Inferior Ramus of Stapedial Artery

Middle Cerebral Artery

Internal Carotid Artery

Caudal Ramus of Internal Carotid Artery

Posterior Cerebral Artery

Auricular Artery

Basilar Artery

Occipital Artery

Vertebral Artery

Bucco—Labial Artery

Lingual Artery

Inferior Dental Artery

Artery to Sub--Maxillary Gland

Bucco—Labial Artery

External Carotid Artery (Continuation)

× 1·5

Dermoptera

We have been unable to find any account in the literature of the cranial arteries of flying lemurs. A study of the vessels would be of great interest because of the affinities of these animals to the insectivores.

Cabrera (1925) states that the brain is more like that of bats than insectivores or primates. He also gives our only reference to the carotid artery "Las arterias carotidas y subclavias están dispuestas como en el hombre".

Chiroptera

The bats are somewhat like Insectivora in the arrangement of their cranial arteries; but the stapedial artery has partially retrogressed. According to Tandler, who took most of his description of the three species with which he dealt from the work of his colleague Dr. Grosser (1901), this retrogression is variable from one species to another.

Tandler (1899) as he frequently does about other animals, takes issue with previous authors on the anatomy of the cranial arteries of bats. He cites Otto: De animalium quorundam per hymem dormentium vasis cephalicis and Hyrtl: (Vergleichend-anatomische Untersuchungen über das innere Gehörorgan des Menschen und der Säugethiere") only to disagree with them.

In *Pteropus edulis*, he says, the main trunk of the stapedial artery has become obliterated and the inferior ramus has acquired a new origin from the internal maxillary just posterior to the pterygoid "canal". (In this case a groove without a bony roof.) The inferior ramus gives origin to the infra-orbital facial and the external ophthalmic arteries. The latter unites with the internal ophthalmic to supply the eye.

The middle meningeal artery consists of a horizontal portion which begins at the junction of the internal maxillary artery and the erstwhile inferior ramus of the stapedial, and a more vertical continuation. Developmentally speaking, the horizontal portion must be the beginning of the inferior ramus of the stapedial artery, along which flow is now reversed. The vertical portion is probably the beginning of the superior ramus. The rest of the superior ramus has disappeared and the arteries in the upper part of the orbit now come from the inferior ramus.

It is worth noting that the common anomaly in man whereby the anterior division of the middle meningeal derives its blood supply from the lachrymal artery is probably due to persistance of a portion of the superior ramus of the stapedial artery. In many ways the arrangement of remnants of the stapedial artery in *Pteropus edulis* resembles that of a great variety of mammals including man.

The external carotid and its branches are also of the "standard" pattern except that the occipital artery is derived from the point where external and internal carotids both arise.

The internal carotid, however, is only a small vessel and most of the supply to the Circle of Willis comes from the large vertebral arteries.

In *Vespertilio murinus*, Tandler says, the main trunk of the stapedial artery is large, larger than the cerebral internal carotid, is prolonged as the superior ramus and after supplying the middle meningeal artery, continues as the external ethmoidal. The inferior ramus of the stapedial, however, has lost its connection with the main trunk and derives its blood supply, very much as in *Pteropus edulis*, from the internal maxillary artery. The external carotid is not altogether standard in its arrangement of branches since according to Tandler the external maxillary (facial) artery is given off after the posterior auricular. It may be, however, that the so-called external maxillary is really the transverse facial. The internal carotid gives off the occipital artery. After losing the stapedial artery it becomes very small and the main supply to the Circle of Willis is again from the vertebrals.

According to Tandler *Rhinolophus hipposideros* is similar to *Vespertilio murinus* except that the external maxillary (facial) artery has its origin in the usual place just after the lingual.

The cerebral internal carotid is only a minute thread.

Buchanan and Arata (1969) have described the cranial arterial system of *Artibeus lituratus*, a neo-tropical fruit-eating bat. After an account of the intraosseous canal, which passes from the post-glenoid foramen towards the supra-occipital-parietal junction in microchiropterans of the families *Phyllostomatidae*, *Noctilionidae*, *Desmodontidae*, *Emballonuridae*, *Molossidae* and *Vespertilionoidea*, they point out that a similar canal is present in the megachiropteran genera *Pteropus*, *Eidolon* and *Epomops* though it may resemble more closely in them the neonatal form of *Artibeus lituratus* (Buchanan and Arata, 1967). This canal in Artibeus contains the middle temporal artery (one of the two major branches of the stapedial artery, the other being the middle meningeal).

Neither the internal carotid nor its branches supply blood to the cerebral vessels, which are fed purely by the vertebral arteries.

The internal carotid arches dorso-cranially from its origin to beneath the tympanum, then continues via an anastomotic connection of essentially undiminished calibre to join the vertebral above the foramen transversarium of the atlas. This anastomosis may represent a first cervical intersegmental or pro-atlantal artery.

The proximal internal carotid provides an ascending pharyngeal and a muscular artery before supplying the stapedial. Apart from the major branches of the stapedial already described, there may also be a small anastomotic connection between it, the alleged pro-atlantal and the auricular branch of the external carotid.

The external carotid, as big as the common, supplies a lingual artery, an auricular/occipital branch and then, medial to the mandible, gives off two branches which Buchanan and Arata speak of as mandibular and pterygoid portions. The mandibular portion supplies the sublingual region. The pterygoid portion gives off the inferior alveolar, the deep temporal and a third branch which turns medially and enters the alisphenoid canal. This last anastomoses within the orbit with the internal ophthalmic artery and supplies ciliary vessels to the eye. The main continuation of the pterygoid portion of the internal maxillary artery gives rise to a pterygoid and buccinator branch and divides into the infra-orbital facial and a superior orbital artery which anastomoses by frontal and supra-orbital branches with the middle meningeal.

Buchanan and Arata describe the terminal portion of the external carotid as supplying the superficial temporal and two arteries to the cheek and face.

An interpretation of their findings, more consistent with the usual mammalian arrangement, would be that the pterygoid portion is the internal maxillary, the mandibular portion is a sublingual artery and what they call the terminal portion of the external carotid is the common stem of superficial temporal and transverse facial arteries.

Desmodus rotundus
Vampire Bat

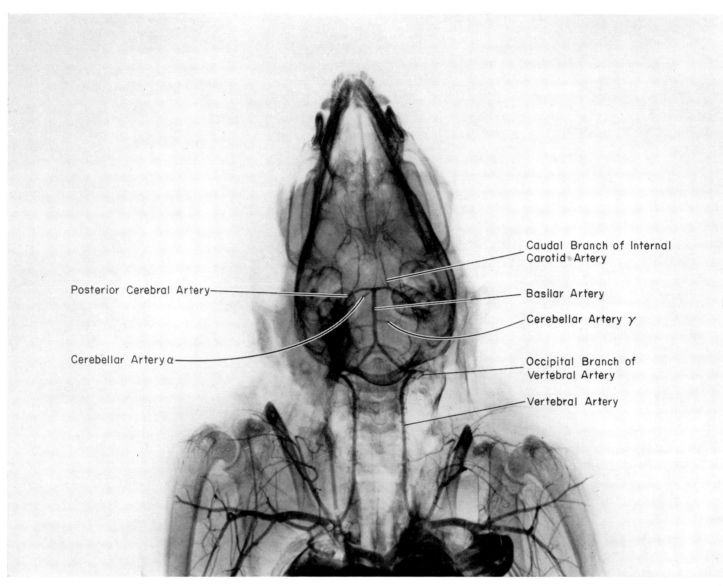

Posterior Cerebral Artery

Cerebellar Artery α

Caudal Branch of Internal Carotid Artery

Basilar Artery

Cerebellar Artery γ

Occipital Branch of Vertebral Artery

Vertebral Artery

× 3·5

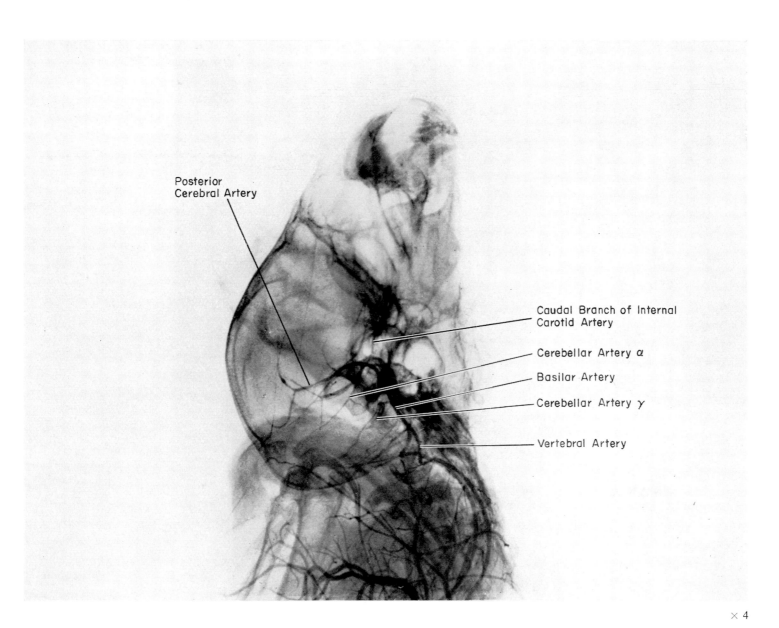

Posterior
Cerebral Artery

Caudal Branch of Internal
Carotid Artery

Cerebellar Artery α

Basilar Artery

Cerebellar Artery γ

Vertebral Artery

× 4

The importance of the vertebral arteries is shown clearly.

Primates

There are many minor species differences but in general the arterial system resembles man. Only major variations from man will therefore be described.

In general a single midline anterior cerebral over part of the pericallosal course is the rule.

The cerebellar artery ε (posterior inferior cerebellar artery) has been said (Hofmann, 1900) to be absent; but a small artery in this position is not particularly uncommon. Gillilan describes the cerebellar arteries in human terminology (1969).

Prosimii

In the lemurs and the *Daubentonia* (lorises and bush-babies), the aortic arch generally gives off only two main vessels towards the head, the brachycephalic (which then divides into innominate and left common carotid) and the left subclavian, though there may be exceptions.

The external carotid in the *Lorisdae* and *Tarsidae* generally gives off lingual, facial and a combined occipital-posterior auricular artery. The internal maxillary divides as in man with the exception of the middle meningeal which may arise from a recurrent branch of the ophthalmic (Davies, 1947, on the slow loris).

In the *Lemuridae* and *Tarsidae* the middle meningeal may arise from a large stapedial artery.

The internal carotid differs radically between *Lorisidae* and *Lemuridae*. In the lemurs the internal carotid enters the carotid canal in the temporal bone where it gives off a stapedial artery. In *Lorisidae* there is disagreement in the literature. Osman Hill (1953) states in general that a stapedial artery is given off outside the skull and enters the head by a separate foramen in the posterior wall of the tympanic bulla, while the internal carotid takes a short cut into the cranial cavity by way of foramen lacerum medium. It has been suggested, however (Adams, 1957), that at least in some *Lorisidae* the cervical internal carotid has atrophied and the main supply to the cerebral carotid comes by way of an hypertrophied ascending pharyngeal artery which may be mistaken for the internal carotid. This breaks up on the external surface of the skull base if not actually in the foramen into several small branches forming a rete, which re-unite still within the thickness of the bone as the cerebral carotid. The authors have confirmed the existence of this rete in five species.

Anthropoidea

Although the origins of great vessels from the aorta is frequently as in man, and particularly so in Hominoidea such as the gorilla, there are also frequent examples of families and individuals in whom there are two branches only, brachycephalic and left subclavian.

In general, the plan of external and internal carotid branches resembles that of man, but with some exceptions as mentioned below.

Among *Cebidae* (New World monkeys) there are great variations. The basilar is reduplicated for part of its course in *Atelinae* (Spider monkeys and Woolly monkeys) (Decerisy, 1950, 1951) Elge, 1910. In squirrel monkeys (*Saimiri*) the external carotid is short and divides into ventral and dorsal branches, the ventral branch going off at right-angles as a common origin for the superior thyroid and the lingual-facial trunks. The dorsal trunk supplies the remainder of the branches including both an occipital and a posterior auricular. The two anterior cerebrals unite and remain as a common vessel over the rostral half of the corpus callosum. In capuchins (members of the *Cebinae*) the posterior auricular may arise from the superficial temporal. *Alouattinae* (howler monkeys) show very close branching from a very short external carotid. In spider monkeys as in *Cebinae*, the lingual and facial arteries arise by a common trunk; but in another species from the *Atelinae* (*Brachyteles arachnoides*) the lingual and facial are said to arise separately (Osman Hill). The face is largely supplied by a transverse facial given off by the superficial temporal and the latter also sends a branch to anastomose with branches of the lachrymal artery emerging from the malar foramen. The middle meningeal derives its supply from the lachrymal branch of the ophthalmic and there is often a large anterior meningeal derived from ethmoidal branches of the ophthalmic. The two anterior cerebrals unite as far as the genu; but separate again.

Cercopithecoidea (Old World monkeys) show many of the same features, often only two branches from the aorta for cranial vessels and a linguo-facial trunk. The occipital artery, however, may sometimes be missing. The middle meningeal arises from the internal maxillary and enters the head via foramen ovale.

In some members of the family the external carotid artery is so short that it scarcely exists; but the external carotid branches arise from two short trunks. The baboon shows a better developed external carotid.

The anterior cerebrals unite for a short distance at the midline and the pericallosal artery is usually unpaired.

Tupaia glis
Common Tree Shrew

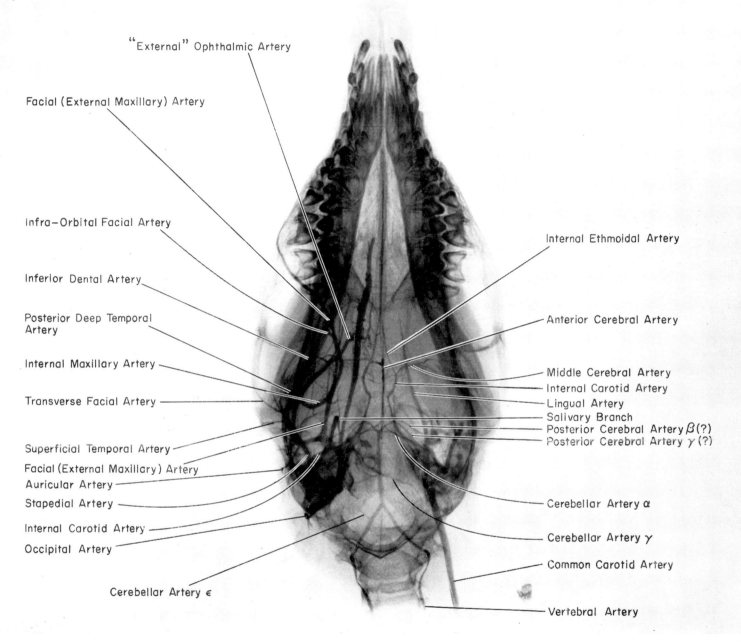

"External" Ophthalmic Artery

Facial (External Maxillary) Artery

Infra−Orbital Facial Artery

Inferior Dental Artery

Posterior Deep Temporal Artery

Internal Maxillary Artery

Transverse Facial Artery

Superficial Temporal Artery

Facial (External Maxillary) Artery

Auricular Artery

Stapedial Artery

Internal Carotid Artery

Occipital Artery

Cerebellar Artery ε

Internal Ethmoidal Artery

Anterior Cerebral Artery

Middle Cerebral Artery

Internal Carotid Artery

Lingual Artery

Salivary Branch

Posterior Cerebral Artery β(?)

Posterior Cerebral Artery γ (?)

Cerebellar Artery α

Cerebellar Artery γ

Common Carotid Artery

Vertebral Artery

× 2·5

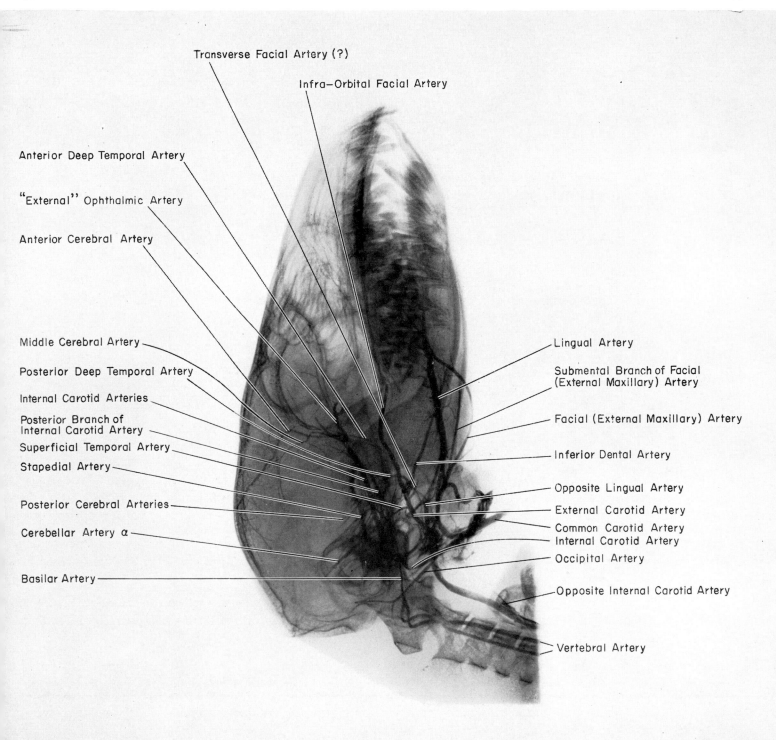

Transverse Facial Artery (?)

Infra–Orbital Facial Artery

Anterior Deep Temporal Artery

"External" Ophthalmic Artery

Anterior Cerebral Artery

Middle Cerebral Artery

Posterior Deep Temporal Artery

Internal Carotid Arteries

Posterior Branch of Internal Carotid Artery

Superficial Temporal Artery

Stapedial Artery

Posterior Cerebral Arteries

Cerebellar Artery α

Basilar Artery

Lingual Artery

Submental Branch of Facial (External Maxillary) Artery

Facial (External Maxillary) Artery

Inferior Dental Artery

Opposite Lingual Artery

External Carotid Artery

Common Carotid Artery

Internal Carotid Artery

Occipital Artery

Opposite Internal Carotid Artery

Vertebral Artery

× 2·5

In many ways the arrangement of the cranial arteries resembles higher primates. For instance, the posterior fossa arteries appear to be a superior cerebellar (cerebellar artery α), an anterior-inferior cerebellar (cerebellar artery γ) and a posterior inferior (cerebellar artery ε).

On the other hand, there are two posterior cerebral arteries on each side.

The striking difference from most primates is in Tupaia's possession of a large stapedial artery running over the lateral aspect and floor of the middle fossa to enter the orbit as the external ophthalmic artery. In this it has a close resemblance to the insectivores.

In this specimen part of the facial (external maxillary) is superimposed upon the internal maxillary artery in the ventro-dorsal view. There is some distortion close to the point of injection on the better filled side.

Note the asymmetry of the anterior part of the Circle of Willis; the pericallosal part of the anterior cerebral comes exclusively from one side.

Steuerwald (1969) should be consulted.

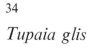

Tupaia glis

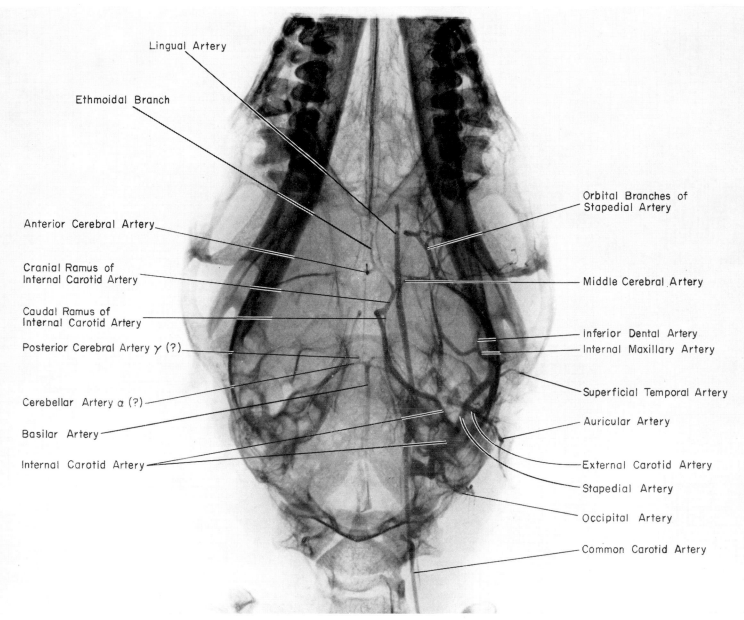

Lingual Artery

Ethmoidal Branch

Orbital Branches of
Stapedial Artery

Anterior Cerebral Artery

Cranial Ramus of
Internal Carotid Artery

Middle Cerebral Artery

Caudal Ramus of
Internal Carotid Artery

Posterior Cerebral Artery γ (?)

Inferior Dental Artery

Internal Maxillary Artery

Cerebellar Artery α (?)

Superficial Temporal Artery

Auricular Artery

Basilar Artery

External Carotid Artery

Internal Carotid Artery

Stapedial Artery

Occipital Artery

Common Carotid Artery

× 3·3

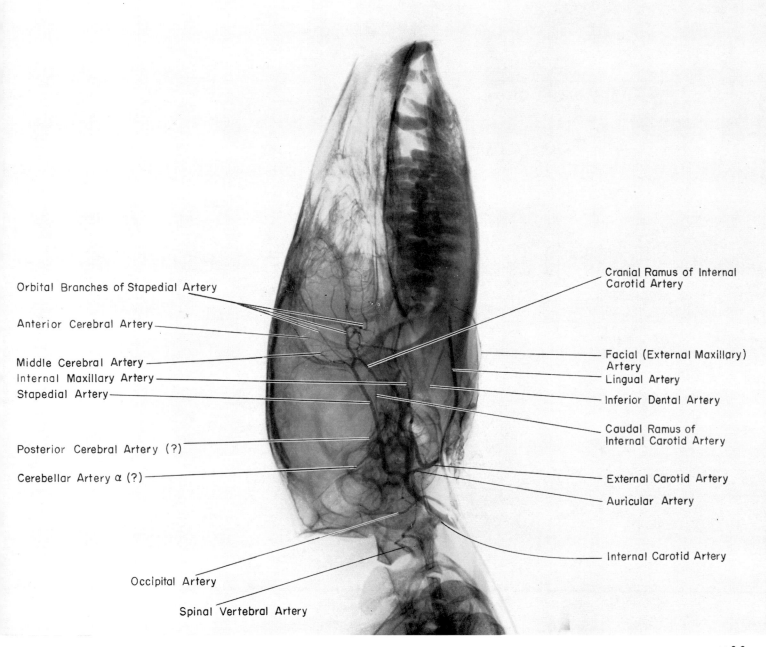

Orbital Branches of Stapedial Artery

Anterior Cerebral Artery

Middle Cerebral Artery

Internal Maxillary Artery

Stapedial Artery

Posterior Cerebral Artery (?)

Cerebellar Artery α (?)

Occipital Artery

Spinal Vertebral Artery

Cranial Ramus of Internal Carotid Artery

Facial (External Maxillary) Artery

Lingual Artery

Inferior Dental Artery

Caudal Ramus of Internal Carotid Artery

External Carotid Artery

Auricular Artery

Internal Carotid Artery

× 2·2

Lemur catta
Ring-tailed Lemur

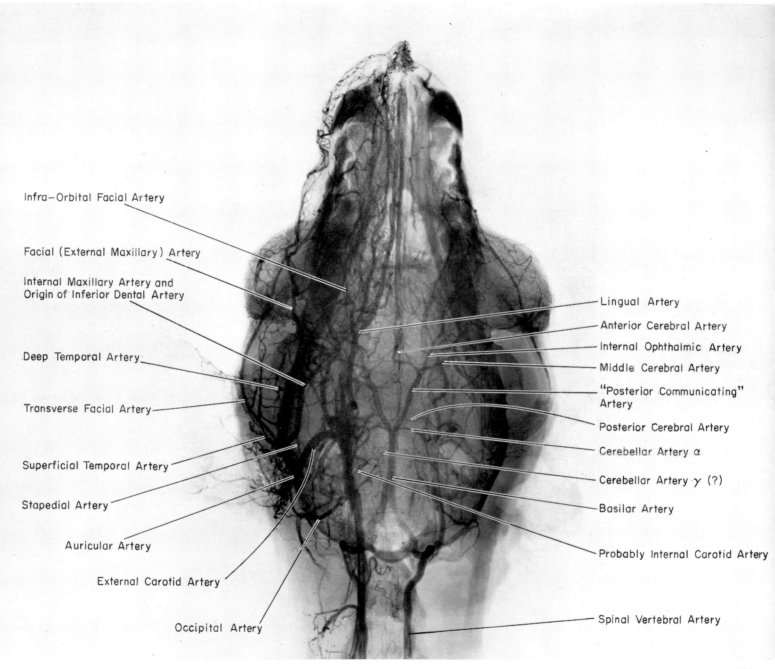

Infra-Orbital Facial Artery

Facial (External Maxillary) Artery

Internal Maxillary Artery and
Origin of Inferior Dental Artery

Deep Temporal Artery

Transverse Facial Artery

Superficial Temporal Artery

Stapedial Artery

Auricular Artery

External Carotid Artery

Occipital Artery

Lingual Artery

Anterior Cerebral Artery

Internal Ophthalmic Artery

Middle Cerebral Artery

"Posterior Communicating"
Artery

Posterior Cerebral Artery

Cerebellar Artery α

Cerebellar Artery γ (?)

Basilar Artery

Probably Internal Carotid Artery

Spinal Vertebral Artery

× 2·0

Tandler has a description of *Lemur varius* which in the general distribution of the internal carotid, the stapedial artery and the internal maxillary closely resembles this specimen of *Lemur catta*. Osman Hill (1953) also describes a moderately well-developed stapedial artery in Lemuroids. The internal carotid in this specimen is so small as to be identified with great difficulty. The cerebral arteries derive almost all their blood supply from the vertebrals.

Tandler also mentions a large ascending pharyngeal artery which we have not been able to identify, which he says forms one of a trio of branches including the occipital and the internal carotid, arising simultaneously from the common carotid.

The stapedial artery terminates as a superior ramus which anastomoses within the orbit with the internal ophthalmic branch of the internal carotid and the orbital (external ophthalmic) branch at the internal maxillary, thus providing a very large blood supply to this area.

In this specimen a feature is seen which seems to be unique

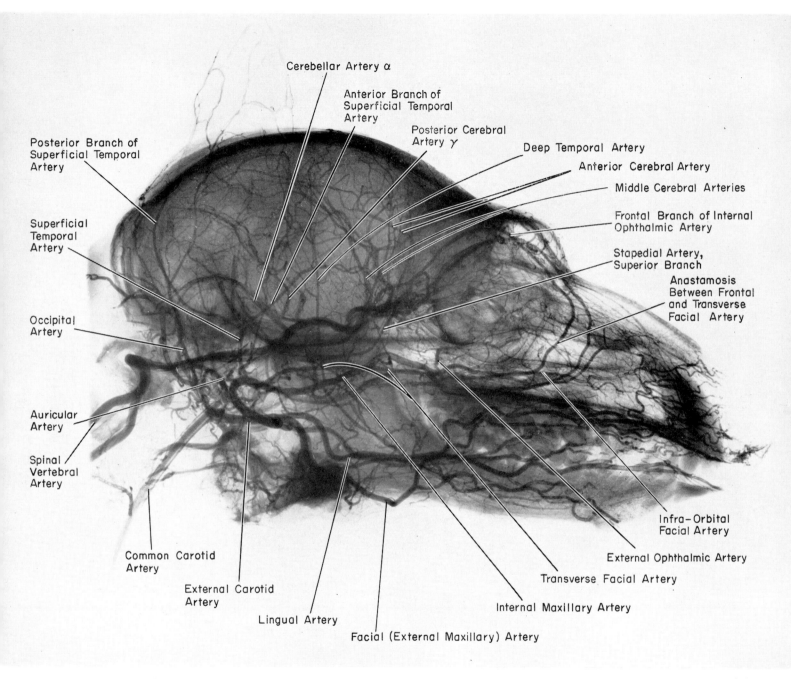

Cerebellar Artery α

Anterior Branch of
Superficial Temporal
Artery

Posterior Cerebral
Artery γ

Deep Temporal Artery

Anterior Cerebral Artery

Middle Cerebral Arteries

Posterior Branch of
Superficial Temporal
Artery

Frontal Branch of Internal
Ophthalmic Artery

Superficial
Temporal
Artery

Stapedial Artery,
Superior Branch

Anastamosis
Between Frontal
and Transverse
Facial Artery

Occipital
Artery

Auricular
Artery

Spinal
Vertebral
Artery

Infra–Orbital
Facial Artery

External Ophthalmic Artery

Common Carotid
Artery

Transverse Facial Artery

External Carotid
Artery

Internal Maxillary Artery

Lingual Artery

Facial (External Maxillary) Artery

× 1·6

among primates. The transverse facial artery is very large
and is in direct communication with the frontal branch of the
internal ophthalmic artery.

Loris tardigradus
Slender Loris

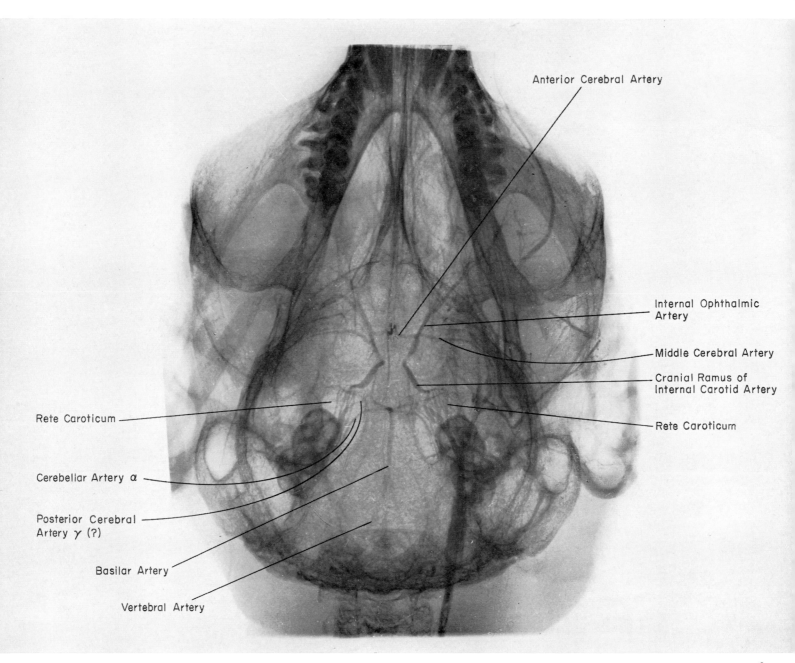

Anterior Cerebral Artery

Internal Ophthalmic Artery

Middle Cerebral Artery

Cranial Ramus of Internal Carotid Artery

Rete Caroticum

Rete Caroticum

Cerebellar Artery α

Posterior Cerebral Artery γ (?)

Basilar Artery

Vertebral Artery

× 3

The rete caroticum is quite an elaborate one with six or more parallel channels.

The internal ophthalmic artery is very large.

The recurrent meningeal cannot be distinguished.

Nycticebus coucang
Slow Loris

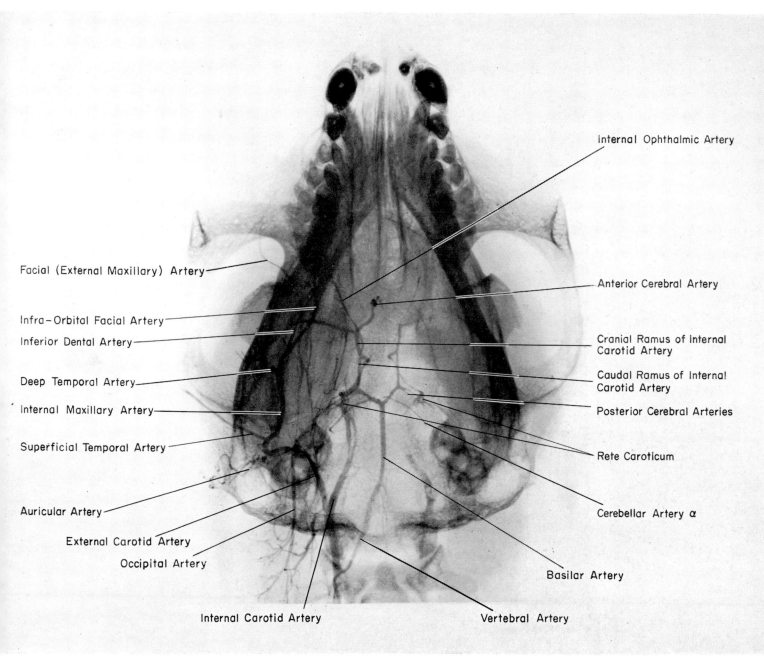

Internal Ophthalmic Artery

Facial (External Maxillary) Artery

Anterior Cerebral Artery

Infra-Orbital Facial Artery

Inferior Dental Artery

Cranial Ramus of Internal Carotid Artery

Deep Temporal Artery

Caudal Ramus of Internal Carotid Artery

Internal Maxillary Artery

Posterior Cerebral Arteries

Superficial Temporal Artery

Rete Caroticum

Auricular Artery

Cerebellar Artery α

External Carotid Artery

Occipital Artery

Basilar Artery

Internal Carotid Artery

Vertebral Artery

× 2·3

Only the major branches have been shown. The rete caroticum is a fairly simple structure of about three parallel channels. It has been described in detail by Adams (1957). Beddard drew the Circle of Willis in 1904.

Arctocebus calabarensis
Angwantibo

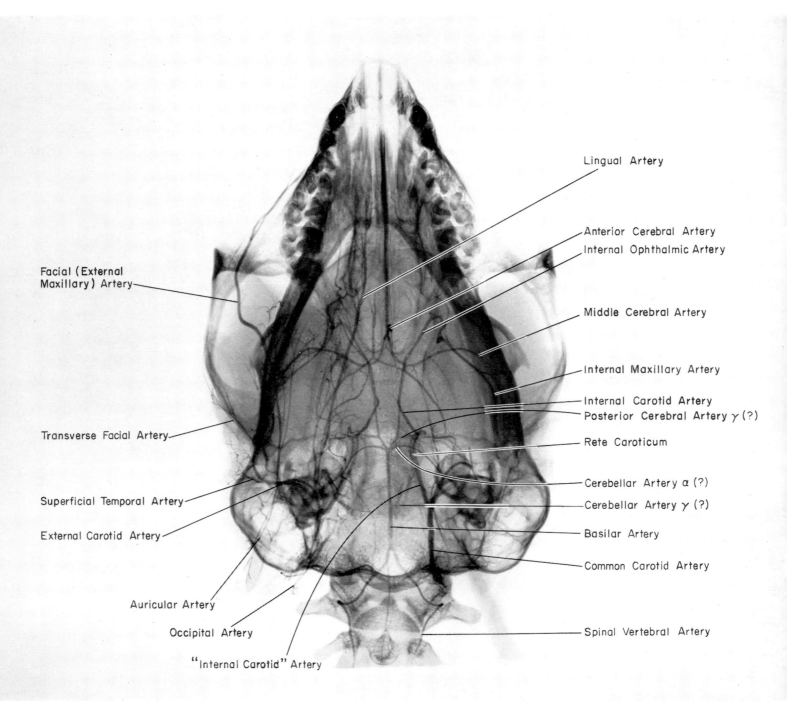

Lingual Artery

Anterior Cerebral Artery

Internal Ophthalmic Artery

Middle Cerebral Artery

Internal Maxillary Artery

Internal Carotid Artery

Posterior Cerebral Artery γ (?)

Rete Caroticum

Cerebellar Artery α (?)

Cerebellar Artery γ (?)

Basilar Artery

Common Carotid Artery

Spinal Vertebral Artery

Facial (External Maxillary) Artery

Transverse Facial Artery

Superficial Temporal Artery

External Carotid Artery

Auricular Artery

Occipital Artery

"Internal Carotid" Artery

× 2·45

Filling of the external carotid vessels is very incomplete; but in the lateral view the first few branches of the two sides are superimposed. The internal carotid system, on the other hand, is well filled and thus the anastomosis in the orbit between the internal ophthalmic artery and the internal maxillary has carried barium from the former to the latter. It seems unlikely that this should be the normal direction for the flow of blood.

The Angwantibo has a very simple rete caroticum, merely a reduplication of the main artery as it enters the skull base in front of and medial to the mastoid bulla.

The positive classification of posterior cerebral and cerebellar arteries by Hofmann's terminology is speculative as so often with these injection radiographs.

An "arch" formed by one vessel from each side in the floor of the mouth or the upper part of the neck has not been

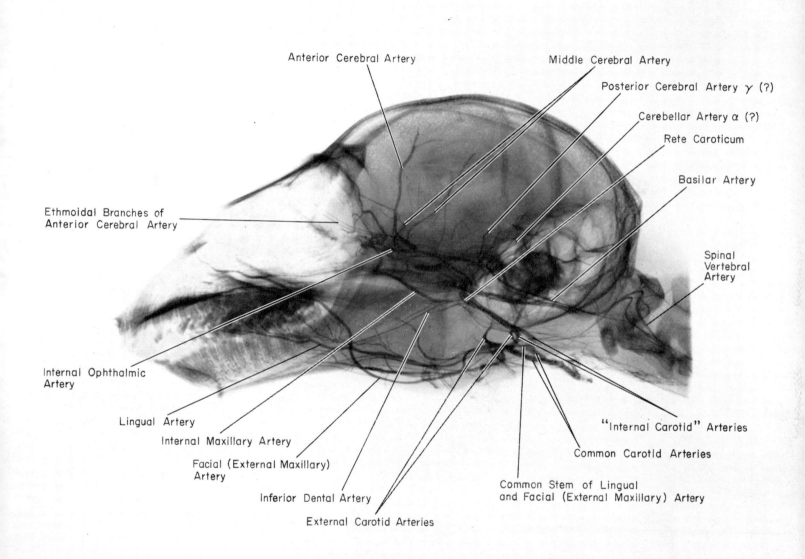

Anterior Cerebral Artery

Middle Cerebral Artery

Posterior Cerebral Artery γ (?)

Cerebellar Artery α (?)

Rete Caroticum

Basilar Artery

Ethmoidal Branches of
Anterior Cerebral Artery

Spinal
Vertebral
Artery

Internal Ophthalmic
Artery

Lingual Artery

Internal Maxillary Artery

Facial (External Maxillary)
Artery

Inferior Dental Artery

External Carotid Arteries

"Internal Carotid" Arteries

Common Carotid Arteries

Common Stem of Lingual
and Facial (External Maxillary) Artery

× 2·7

named although clearly seen in the ventro-dorsal view. This
is because its exact origins and positions cannot be confirmed
in the lateral view.

No sign can be seen of the stapedial artery expected to be
present in *Lorisidae* (Osman Hill, 1953). Presumably it is too
small to be visualised.

Galago crassicaudatus
Thick-tailed Bushbaby

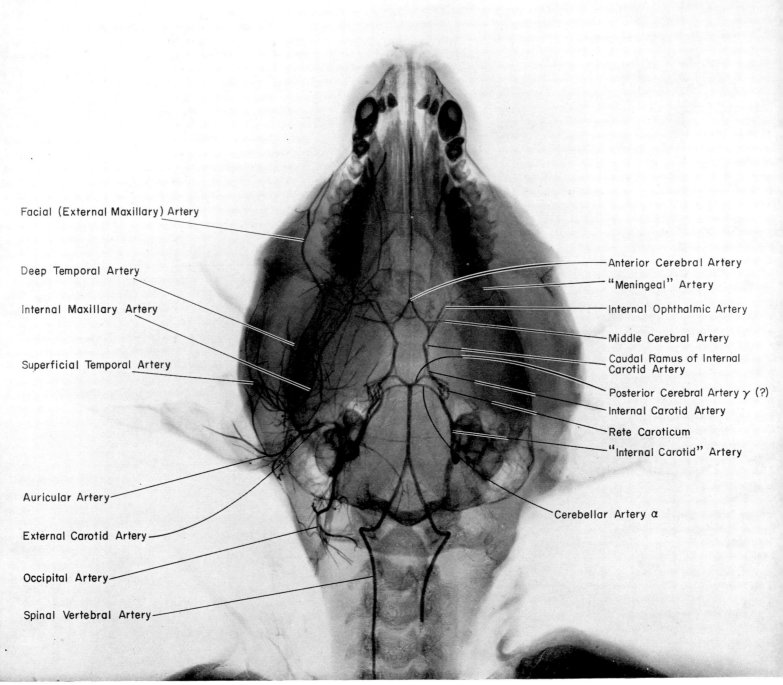

Facial (External Maxillary) Artery

Deep Temporal Artery

Internal Maxillary Artery

Superficial Temporal Artery

Auricular Artery

External Carotid Artery

Occipital Artery

Spinal Vertebral Artery

Anterior Cerebral Artery

"Meningeal" Artery

Internal Ophthalmic Artery

Middle Cerebral Artery

Caudal Ramus of Internal Carotid Artery

Posterior Cerebral Artery γ (?)

Internal Carotid Artery

Rete Caroticum

"Internal Carotid" Artery

Cerebellar Artery α

× 2·15

The rete caroticum is very easily seen. It consists of about four channels.

The first intracranial branch of the internal carotid is an artery with a course forwards then laterally around the middle fossa. This in the genus *Nycticebus* has been described as the recurrent meningeal, representing the middle meningeal of higher forms (Osman Hill, 1953; Davies, 1947).

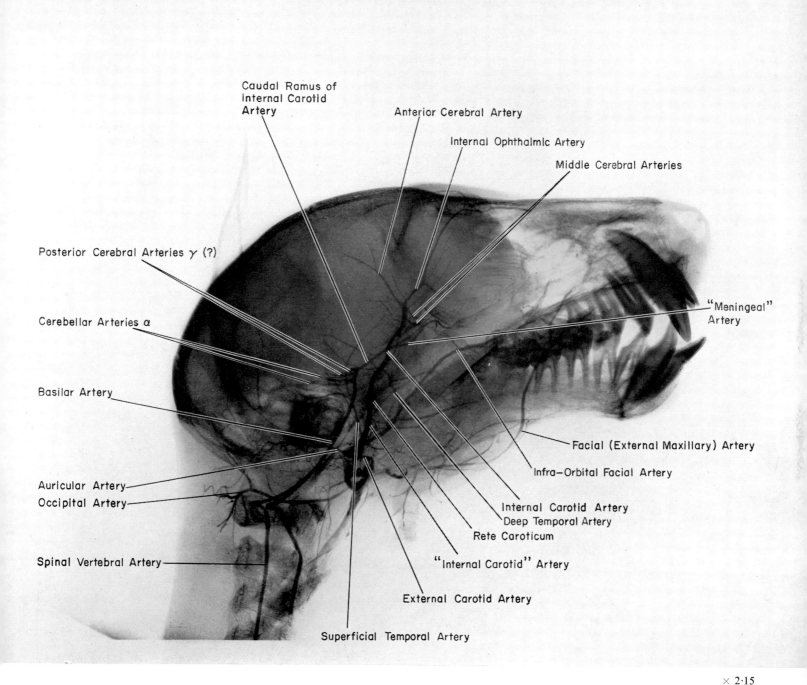

Caudal Ramus of
Internal Carotid
Artery

Anterior Cerebral Artery

Internal Ophthalmic Artery

Middle Cerebral Arteries

Posterior Cerebral Arteries γ (?)

Cerebellar Arteries α

Basilar Artery

Auricular Artery

Occipital Artery

Spinal Vertebral Artery

"Meningeal" Artery

Facial (External Maxillary) Artery

Infra–Orbital Facial Artery

Internal Carotid Artery

Deep Temporal Artery

Rete Caroticum

"Internal Carotid" Artery

External Carotid Artery

Superficial Temporal Artery

× 2·15

Galago senegalensis
Senegal Bushbaby

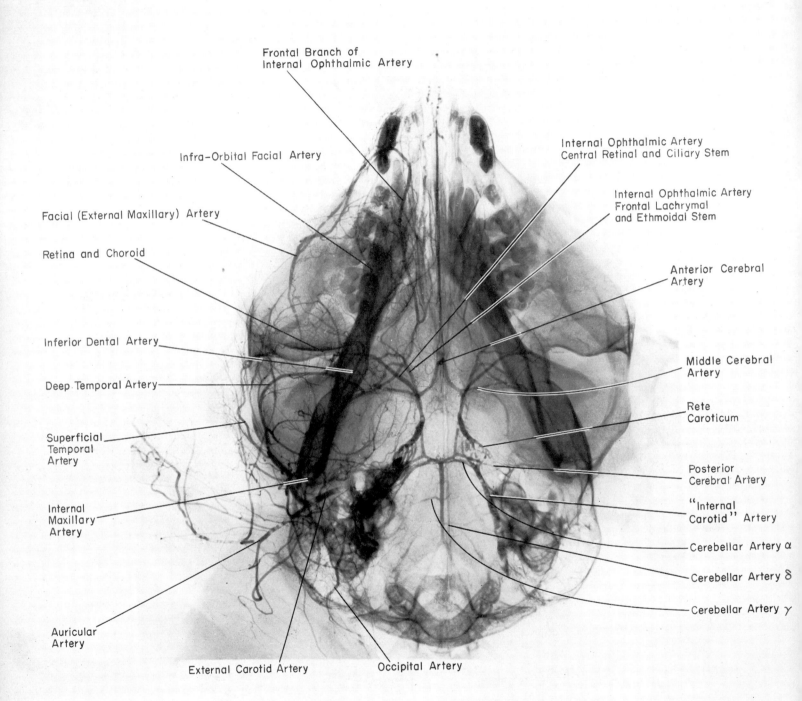

Frontal Branch of
Internal Ophthalmic Artery

Infra-Orbital Facial Artery

Facial (External Maxillary) Artery

Retina and Choroid

Inferior Dental Artery

Deep Temporal Artery

Superficial
Temporal
Artery

Internal
Maxillary
Artery

Auricular
Artery

External Carotid Artery

Occipital Artery

Internal Ophthalmic Artery
Central Retinal and Ciliary Stem

Internal Ophthalmic Artery
Frontal Lachrymal
and Ethmoidal Stem

Anterior Cerebral
Artery

Middle Cerebral
Artery

Rete
Caroticum

Posterior
Cerebral Artery

"Internal
Carotid" Artery

Cerebellar Artery α

Cerebellar Artery δ

Cerebellar Artery γ

× 3·2

Ga

Al

Midd

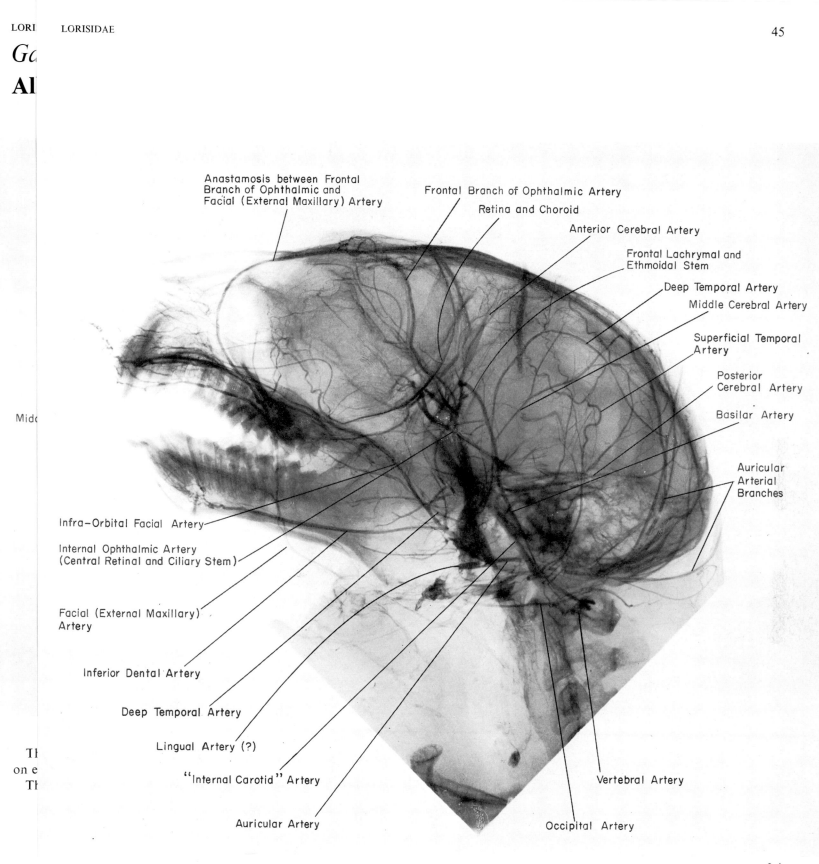

Anastamosis between Frontal Branch of Ophthalmic and Facial (External Maxillary) Artery

Frontal Branch of Ophthalmic Artery

Retina and Choroid

Anterior Cerebral Artery

Frontal Lachrymal and Ethmoidal Stem

Deep Temporal Artery

Middle Cerebral Artery

Superficial Temporal Artery

Posterior Cerebral Artery

Basilar Artery

Auricular Arterial Branches

Infra–Orbital Facial Artery

Internal Ophthalmic Artery (Central Retinal and Ciliary Stem)

Facial (External Maxillary) Artery

Inferior Dental Artery

Deep Temporal Artery

Lingual Artery (?)

"Internal Carotid" Artery

Auricular Artery

Vertebral Artery

Occipital Artery

× 3·4

Th
on e
Th

Two specimens are illustrated. In one the main trunks of the common, external and "internal" carotid arteries are poorly filled; but this specimen shows the enormous proportions of the blood supply to the eye.

There is a well-developed anastomosis between the lachrymal, frontal and ethmoidal stem of the internal ophthalmic artery and the internal maxillary artery.

The deep temporal artery is an unusually large vessel.

The rete caroticum has a relatively complex form, consisting of at least eight channels.

In the second specimen the main trunks alone have been filled. In this animal the rete was less elaborate on one side and, indeed, there does not seem to be much constancy about the number of small channels.

See Kanagasuntherami and Krichnamarti (1965).

Galago demidovii
Demidoff's Bushbaby

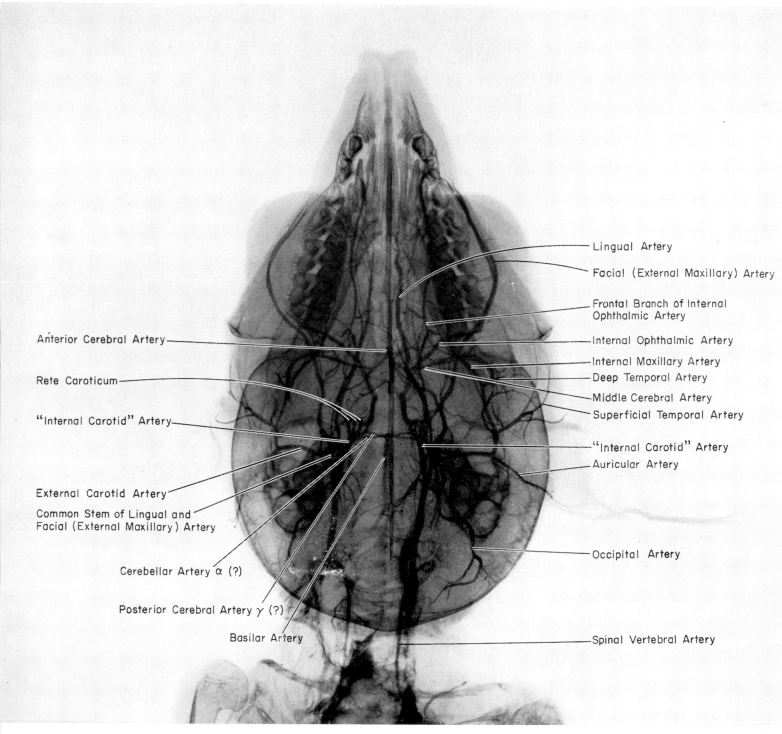

Lingual Artery

Facial (External Maxillary) Artery

Frontal Branch of Internal Ophthalmic Artery

Anterior Cerebral Artery

Internal Ophthalmic Artery

Internal Maxillary Artery

Deep Temporal Artery

Rete Caroticum

Middle Cerebral Artery

Superficial Temporal Artery

"Internal Carotid" Artery

"Internal Carotid" Artery

Auricular Artery

External Carotid Artery

Common Stem of Lingual and Facial (External Maxillary) Artery

Occipital Artery

Cerebellar Artery α (?)

Posterior Cerebral Artery γ (?)

Basilar Artery

Spinal Vertebral Artery

× 4·2

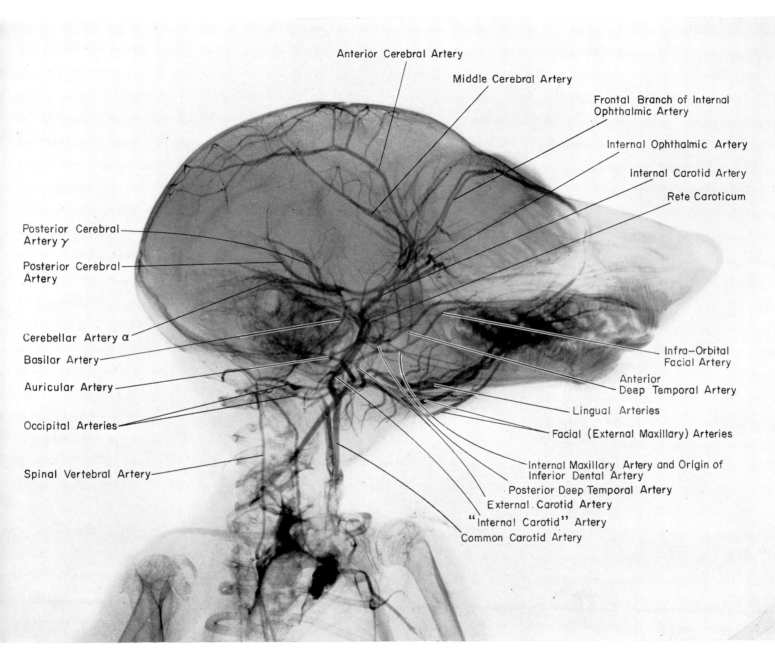

Anterior Cerebral Artery

Middle Cerebral Artery

Frontal Branch of Internal Ophthalmic Artery

Internal Ophthalmic Artery

Internal Carotid Artery

Rete Caroticum

Posterior Cerebral Artery γ

Posterior Cerebral Artery

Cerebellar Artery α

Basilar Artery

Auricular Artery

Occipital Arteries

Spinal Vertebral Artery

Infra–Orbital Facial Artery

Anterior Deep Temporal Artery

Lingual Arteries

Facial (External Maxillary) Arteries

Internal Maxillary Artery and Origin of Inferior Dental Artery

Posterior Deep Temporal Artery

External Carotid Artery

"Internal Carotid" Artery

Common Carotid Artery

× 4·2

The injection of one specimen is so complete that the radiograph of a half-injected specimen is also reproduced in order to show the main branches of the common and external carotid arteries. The rete caroticum, in the usual semi-extra-cranial situation, consists of three large branches.

It seems probable that the posterior cerebral δ (Hofmann) corresponding to man's lateral posterior choroidal artery is a branch of the posterior cerebral γ in this animal.

There is no sign of a stapedial artery, though it is expected in *Lorisidae* (Osman Hill, 1953). Presumably it is too small to be visualised.

Galago demidovii

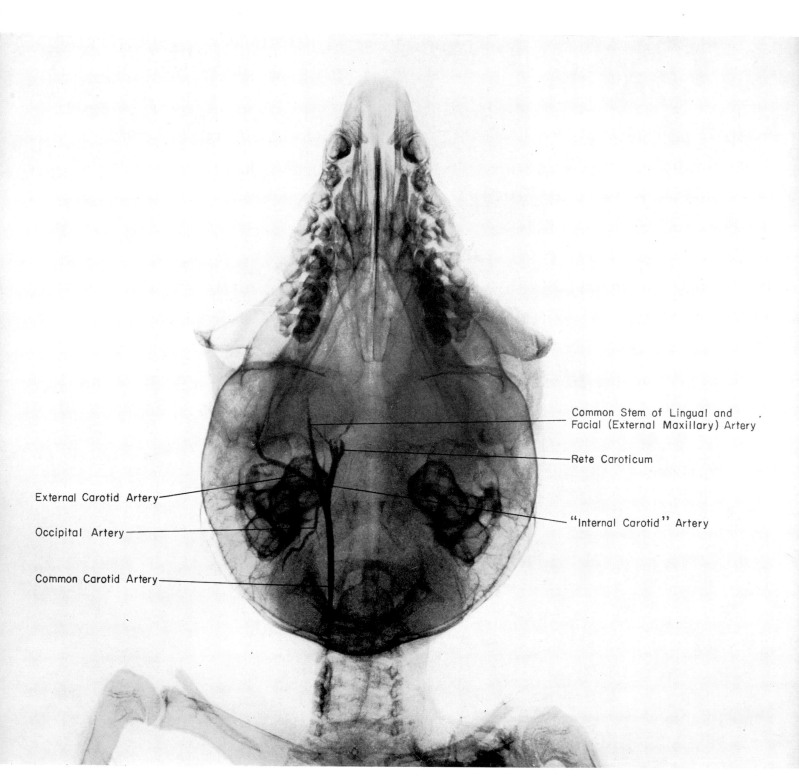

Common Stem of Lingual and
Facial (External Maxillary) Artery

Rete Caroticum

External Carotid Artery

"Internal Carotid" Artery

Occipital Artery

Common Carotid Artery

× 4·2

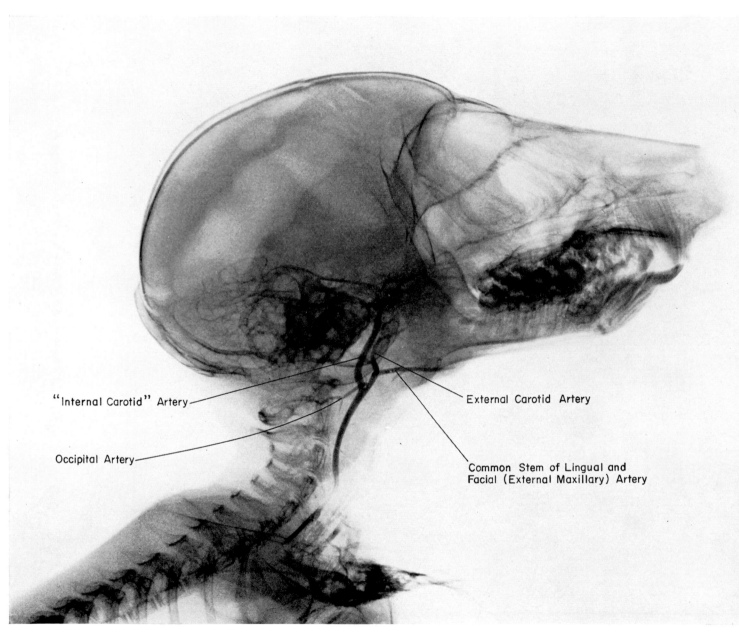

"Internal Carotid" Artery

Occipital Artery

External Carotid Artery

Common Stem of Lingual and
Facial (External Maxillary) Artery

× 4·2

Lagothrix
Woolly Monkey

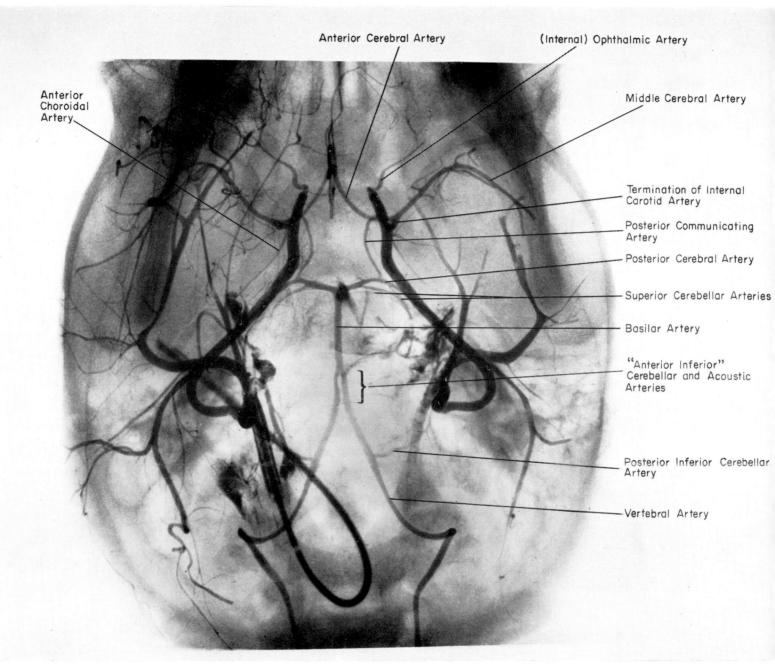

Anterior Cerebral Artery

(Internal) Ophthalmic Artery

Anterior Choroidal Artery

Middle Cerebral Artery

Termination of Internal Carotid Artery

Posterior Communicating Artery

Posterior Cerebral Artery

Superior Cerebellar Arteries

Basilar Artery

"Anterior Inferior" Cerebellar and Acoustic Arteries

Posterior Inferior Cerebellar Artery

Vertebral Artery

× 2·25

Only the internal carotid and vertebral artery branches have been labelled; but note that the occipital and auricular arteries have a common stem.

The anterior choroidal artery arises from the internal carotid.

There is a second much smaller pair of superior cerebellar arteries, corresponding presumably to Hofmann's cerebellar artery β.

The "anterior inferior" cerebellar arteries spring from the vertebrals near their junction with the basilar artery. On the

original radiograph it is possible to see a pair of what are probably acoustic arteries. Presumably the cranial ends of the vertebrals constitute a paired basilar artery.

There are very well developed posterior inferior cerebellar arteries.

Macaca nemestrina
Pig-tailed Macaque

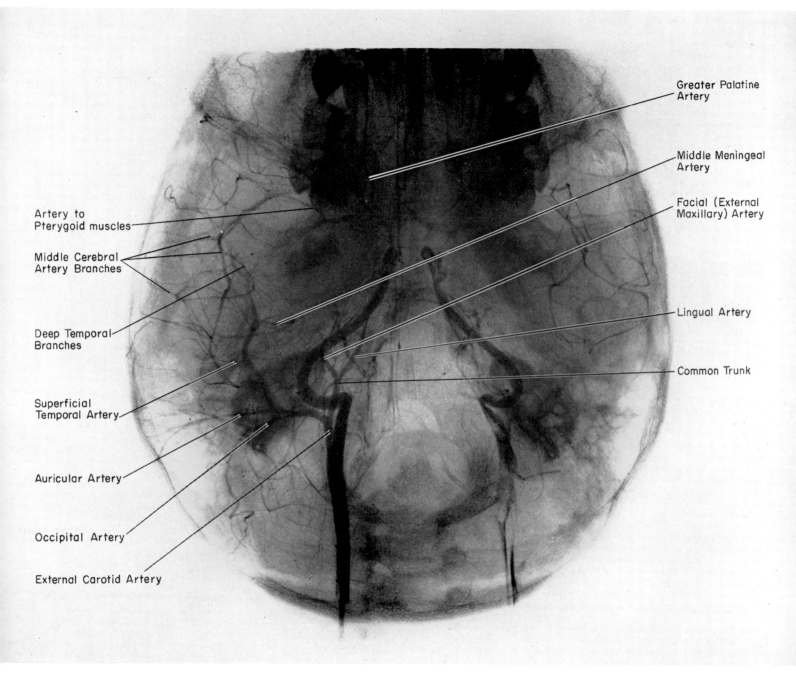

Greater Palatine Artery

Middle Meningeal Artery

Facial (External Maxillary) Artery

Artery to Pterygoid muscles

Middle Cerebral Artery Branches

Deep Temporal Branches

Lingual Artery

Common Trunk

Superficial Temporal Artery

Auricular Artery

Occipital Artery

External Carotid Artery

× 2·25

In this rather poor specimen the external carotid branches are superimposed upon the middle cerebral artery and its branches.

Macaca mulatta
Rhesus Monkey

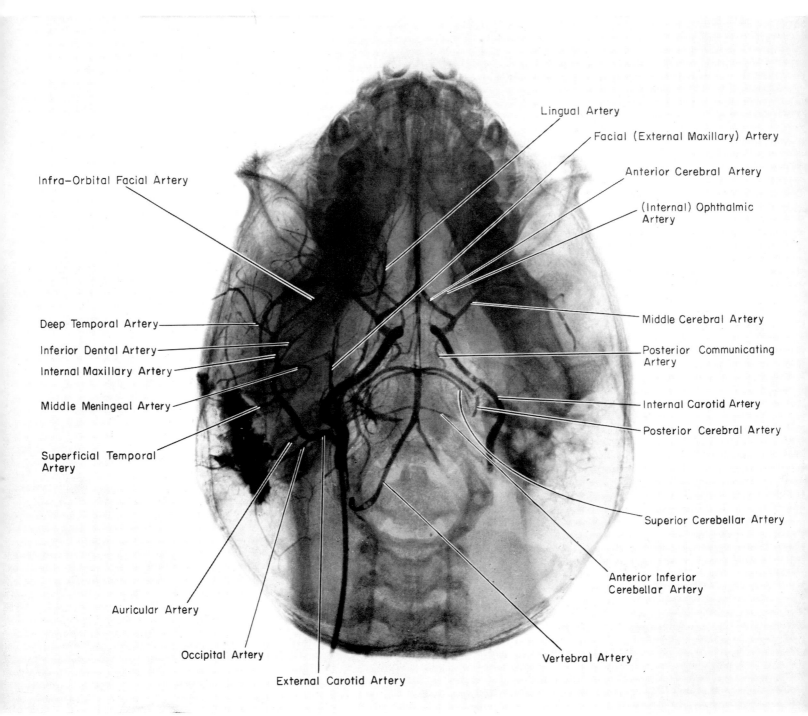

Infra–Orbital Facial Artery

Deep Temporal Artery

Inferior Dental Artery

Internal Maxillary Artery

Middle Meningeal Artery

Superficial Temporal
Artery

Auricular Artery

Occipital Artery

External Carotid Artery

Lingual Artery

Facial (External Maxillary) Artery

Anterior Cerebral Artery

(Internal) Ophthalmic
Artery

Middle Cerebral Artery

Posterior Communicating
Artery

Internal Carotid Artery

Posterior Cerebral Artery

Superior Cerebellar Artery

Anterior Inferior
Cerebellar Artery

Vertebral Artery

$\times$ 2·2

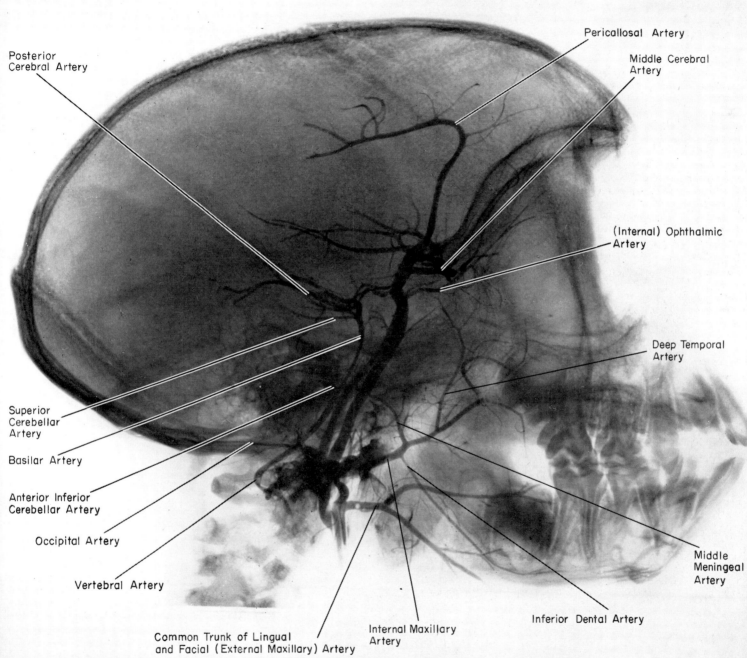

Posterior
Cerebral Artery

Pericallosal Artery

Middle Cerebral
Artery

(Internal) Ophthalmic
Artery

Deep Temporal
Artery

Superior
Cerebellar
Artery

Basilar Artery

Anterior Inferior
Cerebellar Artery

Occipital Artery

Vertebral Artery

Middle
Meningeal
Artery

Inferior Dental Artery

Common Trunk of Lingual
and Facial (External Maxillary) Artery

Internal Maxillary
Artery

× 2·0

The branching of the internal maxillary artery is well seen in the ventro-dorsal view. Though very similar it is not identical to man. See the papers of Castelli and Huelke (1965), Dyrud (1944), Kassell and Langfitt (1965), Linebach (1933) McCoy et al (1967).

The anterior inferior cerebellar arteries are large. There is no posterior inferior cerebellar artery.

Macaca sylvana
Barbary Ape

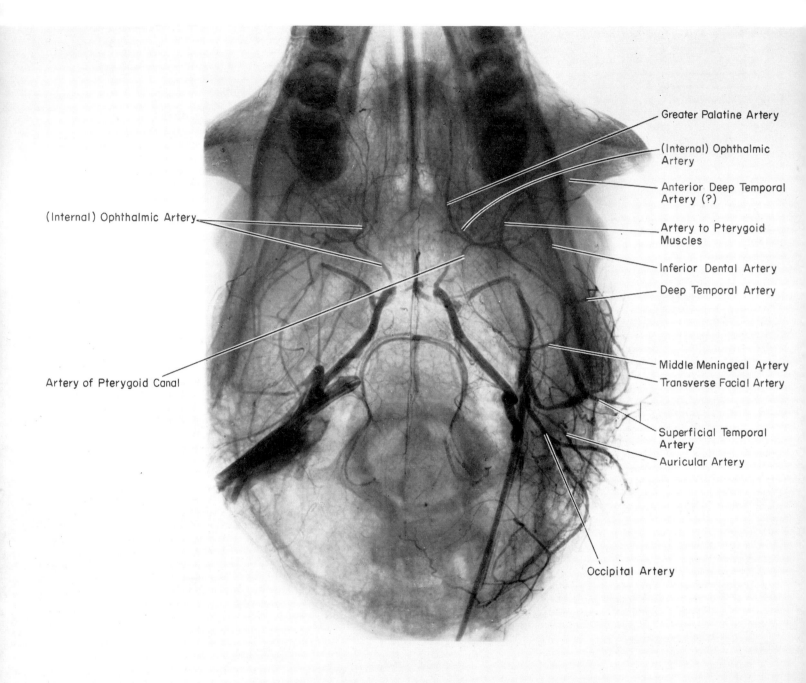

Greater Palatine Artery

(Internal) Ophthalmic Artery

Anterior Deep Temporal Artery (?)

Artery to Pterygoid Muscles

Inferior Dental Artery

Deep Temporal Artery

Middle Meningeal Artery

Transverse Facial Artery

Superficial Temporal Artery

Auricular Artery

Occipital Artery

(Internal) Ophthalmic Artery

Artery of Pterygoid Canal

× 1·5

The branches of the internal maxillary are of great interest, revealing some of their embryological history and the common basic pattern of the mammalian cranial arterial tree.

On one side the pattern is more or less usual. The internal ophthalmic artery is large and has but a narrow connection with orbital branches of the internal maxillary artery. The middle meningeal artery is small and distributed as far as can be seen in the usual way.

On the other side, there is a fairly large link between the middle meningeal and the internal maxillary close to the orbit by way of the artery of the pterygoid canal and the greater palatine artery. This is a remnant of the inferior division of the stapedial artery and also the homologue of the ramus anastomoticus of canidae and some other mammals. The ophthalmic arteries have filled reasonably well by round-about ways, as though by an external ophthalmic as in many

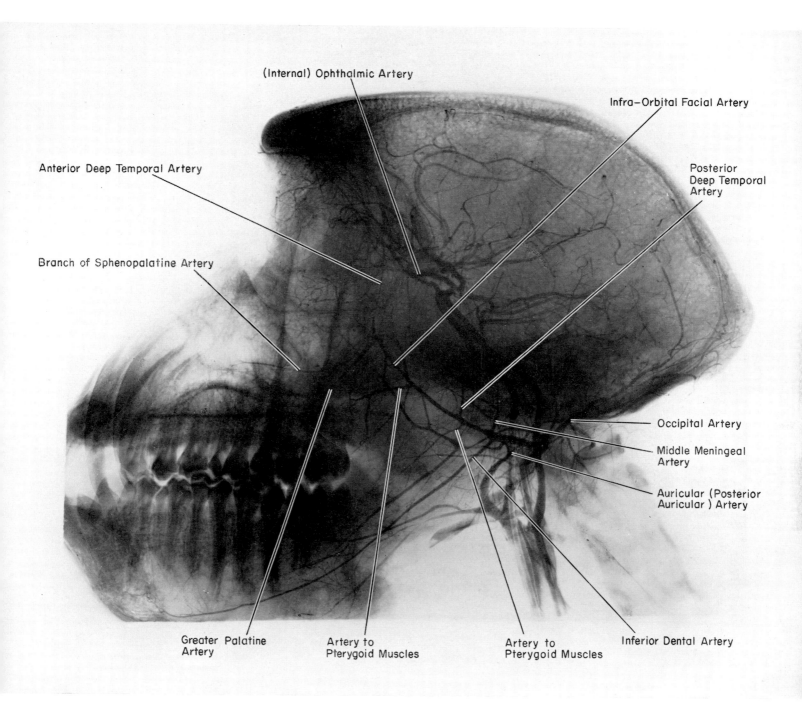

(Internal) Ophthalmic Artery

Infra–Orbital Facial Artery

Anterior Deep Temporal Artery

Posterior Deep Temporal Artery

Branch of Sphenopalatine Artery

Occipital Artery

Middle Meningeal Artery

Auricular (Posterior Auricular) Artery

Greater Palatine Artery

Artery to Pterygoid Muscles

Artery to Pterygoid Muscles

Inferior Dental Artery

× 1·8

other mammals. In this case, however, the internal ophthalmic is large and it is only an adventitious block to the injection-material which has revealed the existence of another route.

Cynopithecus niger
Celebes Black Ape

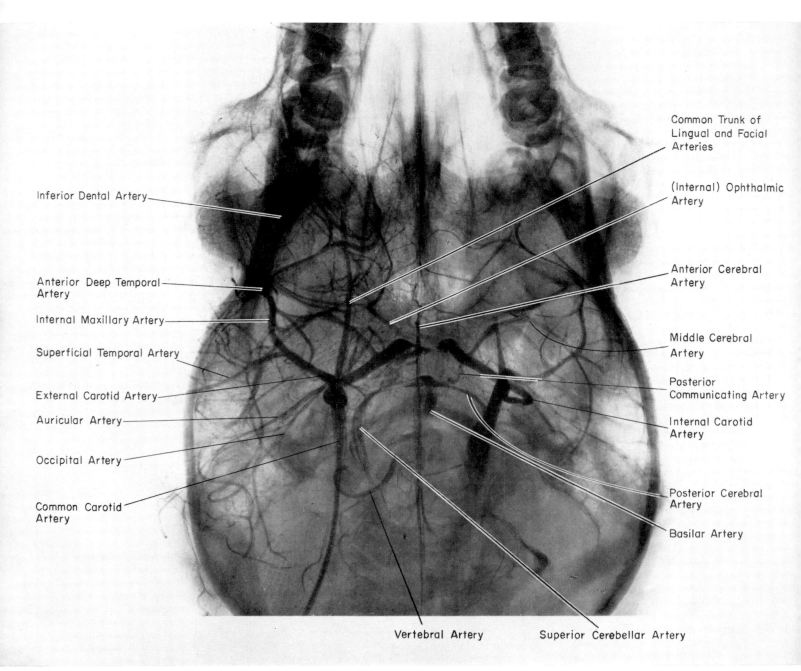

Inferior Dental Artery

Anterior Deep Temporal Artery

Internal Maxillary Artery

Superficial Temporal Artery

External Carotid Artery

Auricular Artery

Occipital Artery

Common Carotid Artery

Common Trunk of Lingual and Facial Arteries

(Internal) Ophthalmic Artery

Anterior Cerebral Artery

Middle Cerebral Artery

Posterior Communicating Artery

Internal Carotid Artery

Posterior Cerebral Artery

Basilar Artery

Vertebral Artery

Superior Cerebellar Artery

× 1·75

The arterial anatomy is very similar to man except that the pericallosal artery is unpaired and the internal ophthalmic is larger in the ape.

In the lateral view the superficial temporal and auricular arteries have not been labelled because they are so much obscured by the superimposition of other structures.

It is possible to recognise more branches of the internal maxillary and ophthalmic arteries than have actually been indicated.

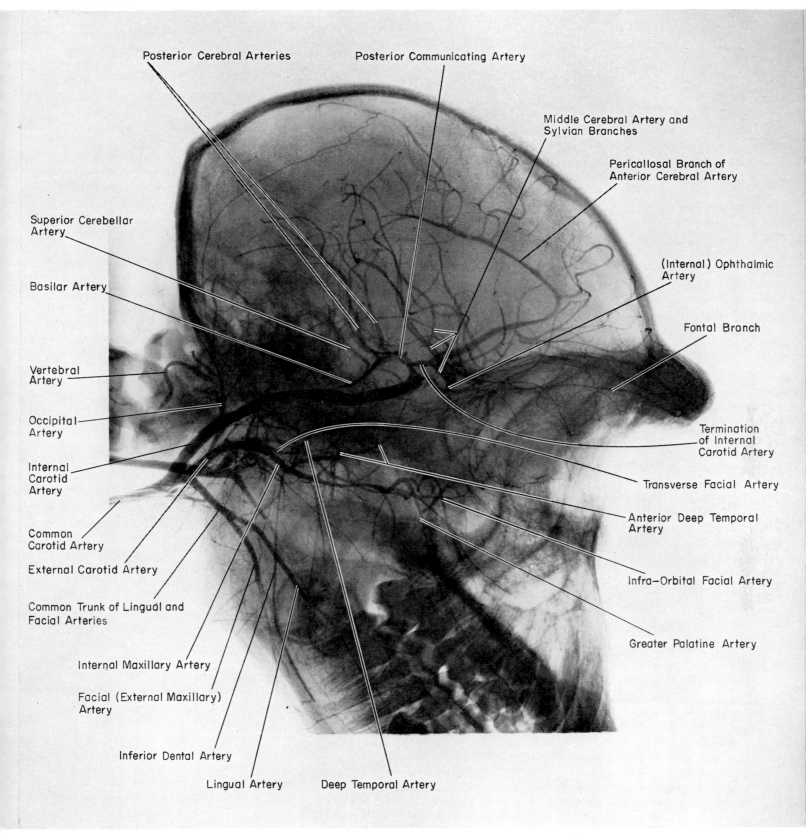

Posterior Cerebral Arteries

Posterior Communicating Artery

Middle Cerebral Artery and
Sylvian Branches

Pericallosal Branch of
Anterior Cerebral Artery

Superior Cerebellar
Artery

Basilar Artery

(Internal) Ophthalmic
Artery

Fontal Branch

Vertebral
Artery

Occipital
Artery

Termination
of Internal
Carotid Artery

Internal
Carotid
Artery

Transverse Facial Artery

Common
Carotid Artery

Anterior Deep Temporal
Artery

External Carotid Artery

Infra—Orbital Facial Artery

Common Trunk of Lingual and
Facial Arteries

Greater Palatine Artery

Internal Maxillary Artery

Facial (External Maxillary)
Artery

Inferior Dental Artery

Lingual Artery

Deep Temporal Artery

× 2·0

Cercopithecus aethiops
Vervet Monkey

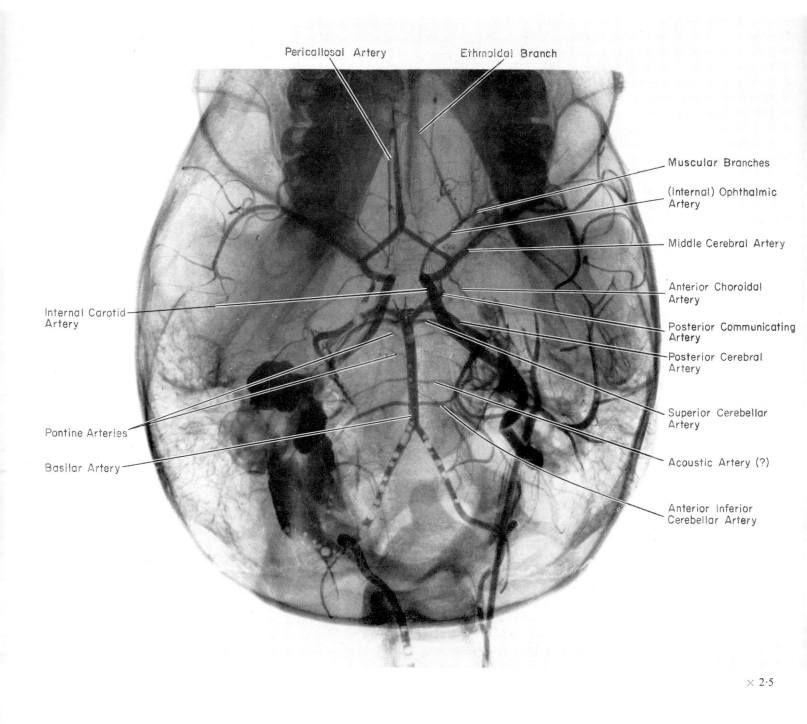

Pericallosal Artery

Ethmoidal Branch

Muscular Branches

(Internal) Ophthalmic Artery

Middle Cerebral Artery

Anterior Choroidal Artery

Internal Carotid Artery

Posterior Communicating Artery

Posterior Cerebral Artery

Superior Cerebellar Artery

Pontine Arteries

Basilar Artery

Acoustic Artery (?)

Anterior Inferior Cerebellar Artery

× 2·5

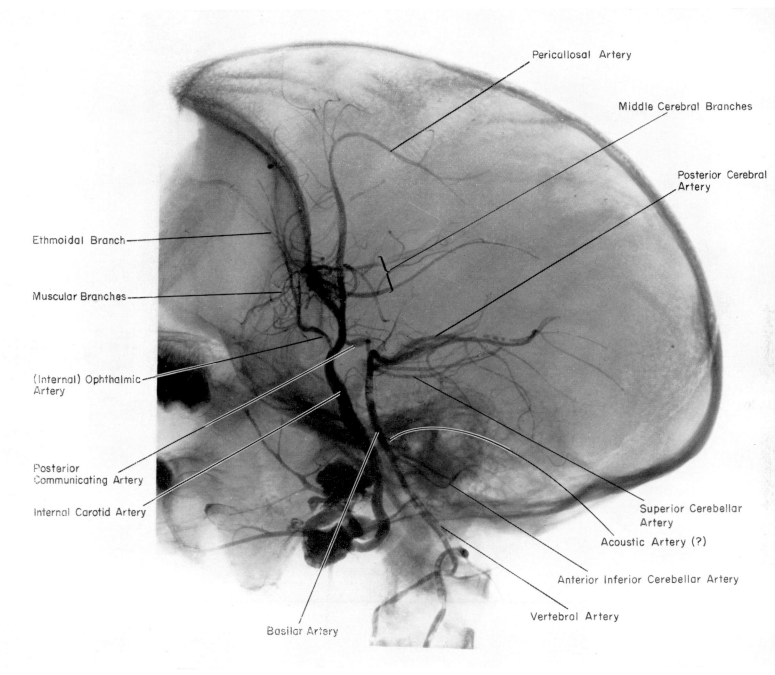

Pericallosal Artery

Middle Cerebral Branches

Posterior Cerebral Artery

Ethmoidal Branch

Muscular Branches

(Internal) Ophthalmic Artery

Posterior Communicating Artery

Internal Carotid Artery

Superior Cerebellar Artery

Acoustic Artery (?)

Anterior Inferior Cerebellar Artery

Vertebral Artery

Basilar Artery

× 2·25

External carotid branches have not been named.

The cerebellar and pontine arteries are remarkably large. They appear to be the superior cerebellar, pontine (two pairs), acoustic and anterior inferior cerebellar vessels, corresponding perhaps in this animal to Hofmann's cerebellar arteries α, β, γ and δ.

There is no posterior inferior cerebellar artery.

The anterior choroidal arises from the internal carotid artery as in man.

Colobus abyssinicus kikuyuensis
Kenya Colobos Monkey

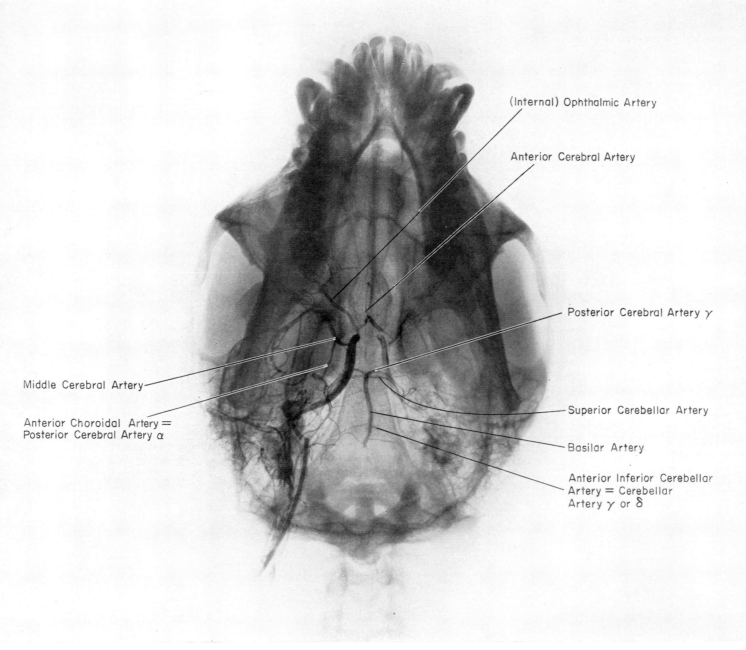

(Internal) Ophthalmic Artery

Anterior Cerebral Artery

Posterior Cerebral Artery γ

Middle Cerebral Artery

Anterior Choroidal Artery =
Posterior Cerebral Artery α

Superior Cerebellar Artery

Basilar Artery

Anterior Inferior Cerebellar
Artery = Cerebellar
Artery γ or δ

× 1·3

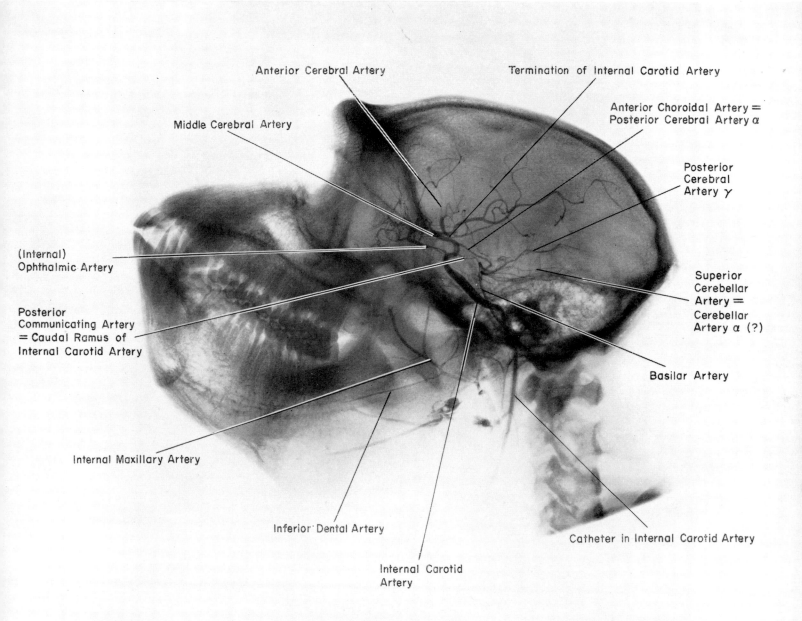

Anterior Cerebral Artery

Termination of Internal Carotid Artery

Middle Cerebral Artery

Anterior Choroidal Artery =
Posterior Cerebral Artery α

Posterior
Cerebral
Artery γ

(Internal)
Ophthalmic Artery

Superior
Cerebellar
Artery =
Cerebellar
Artery α (?)

Posterior
Communicating Artery
= Caudal Ramus of
Internal Carotid Artery

Basilar Artery

Internal Maxillary Artery

Catheter in Internal Carotid Artery

Inferior Dental Artery

Internal Carotid
Artery

× 1·2

Only the internal carotid system and the basilar have been satisfactorily outlined. These show resemblance both to man and to certain non-primates. An attempt has been made to draw comparisons by using a dual terminology, that commonly applied to man alongside terms derived largely from Hofmann.

In particular the huge anterior choroidal arising from the middle cerebral artery should be noted. This is a version of Hofmann's posterior cerebral artery α.

Edentata

Many of the edentates possess large and highly specialised tongues. This is reflected in the development of the lingual artery.

Another feature common, but not universal, in the order is the relatively small size of the internal maxillary artery.

Individual features are described as captions.

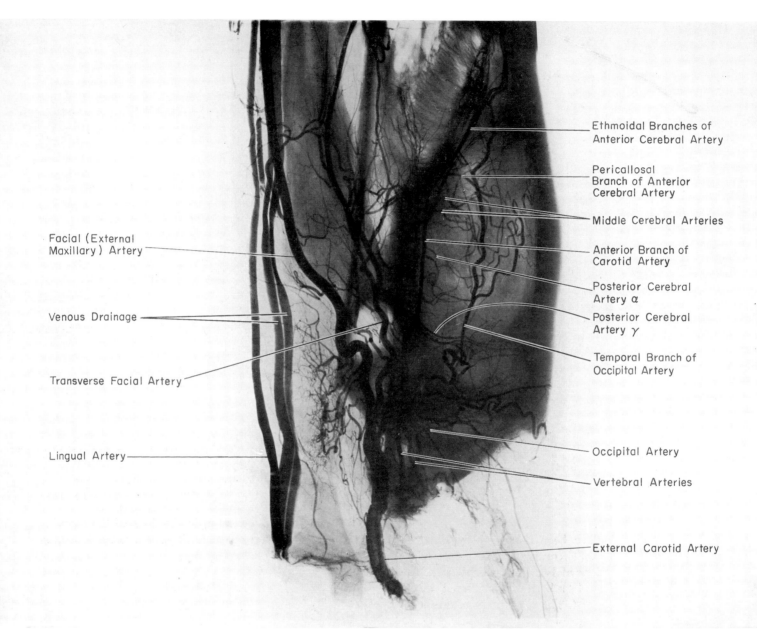

Ethmoidal Branches of
Anterior Cerebral Artery

Pericallosal
Branch of Anterior
Cerebral Artery

Middle Cerebral Arteries

Facial (External
Maxillary) Artery

Anterior Branch of
Carotid Artery

Posterior Cerebral
Artery α

Venous Drainage

Posterior Cerebral
Artery γ

Temporal Branch of
Occipital Artery

Transverse Facial Artery

Occipital Artery

Lingual Artery

Vertebral Arteries

External Carotid Artery

× 1·0

Tamandua tetradactyla
Tamandua

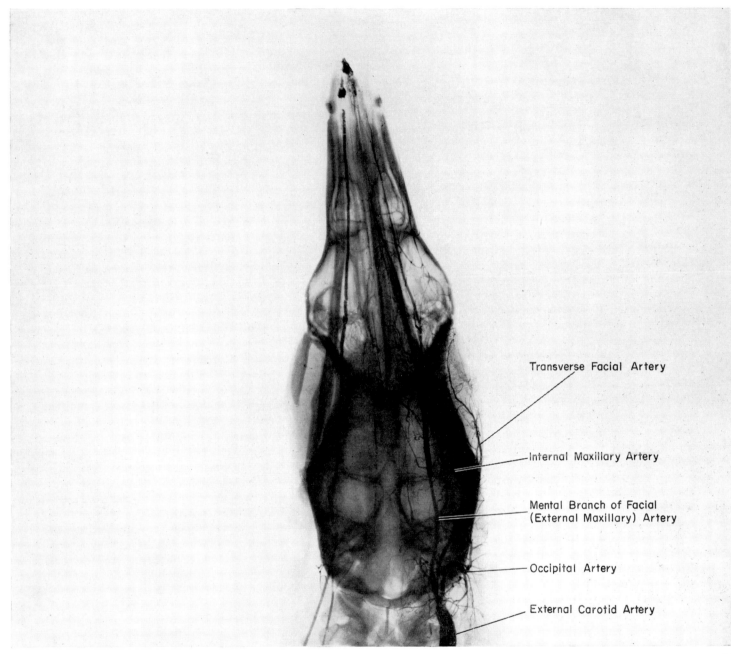

Transverse Facial Artery

Internal Maxillary Artery

Mental Branch of Facial
(External Maxillary) Artery

Occipital Artery

External Carotid Artery

× 1·0

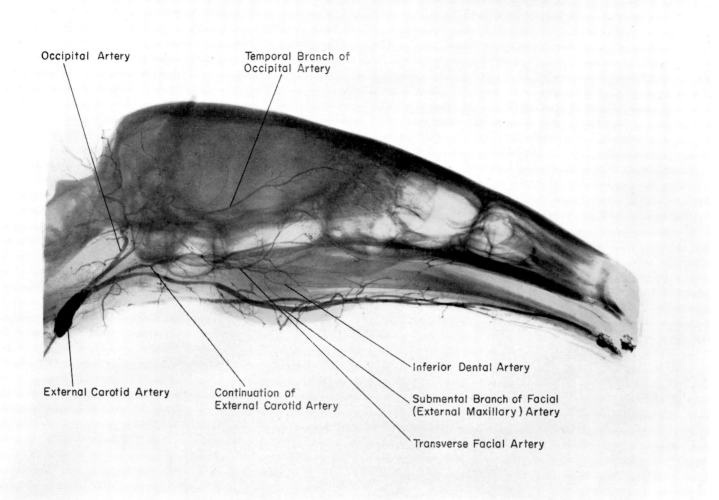

Occipital Artery

Temporal Branch of Occipital Artery

External Carotid Artery

Continuation of External Carotid Artery

Inferior Dental Artery

Submental Branch of Facial (External Maxillary) Artery

Transverse Facial Artery

× 1·0

Only the external carotid and its larger branches show good filling and the lingual artery has not filled at all.

The external carotid gives rise to a large occipital artery which has occipital, auricular and superficial temporal branches. There appear to be communications between the occipital artery and a large artery within the spinal canal (the anterior spinal or the cervical origin of the basilar artery).

At the point of origin of the occipital artery, the external carotid supplies a large facial (external maxillary) artery whose main branch is submental. The external carotid then continues as a fairly small artery and after supplying a transverse facial, becomes the internal maxillary artery.

The internal maxillary gives rise to a substantial inferior dental and a small buccal artery and continues as the infra-orbital facial.

Hyrtl (1854) has described the vessels of the whole head and so has Beddard (1909). From their descriptions the intracranial arteries seem very like those of *Manis tricuspis* although there is no relationship between them. The intracranial arteries are also said to resemble those of *Myrmecophaga tridactyla* the giant ant-eater. Strangely enough the intracranial arteries of our own specimen of *Myrmecophaga tridactyla* are quite different from Beddard's.

Cabassous centralis
Naked-tailed Armadillo

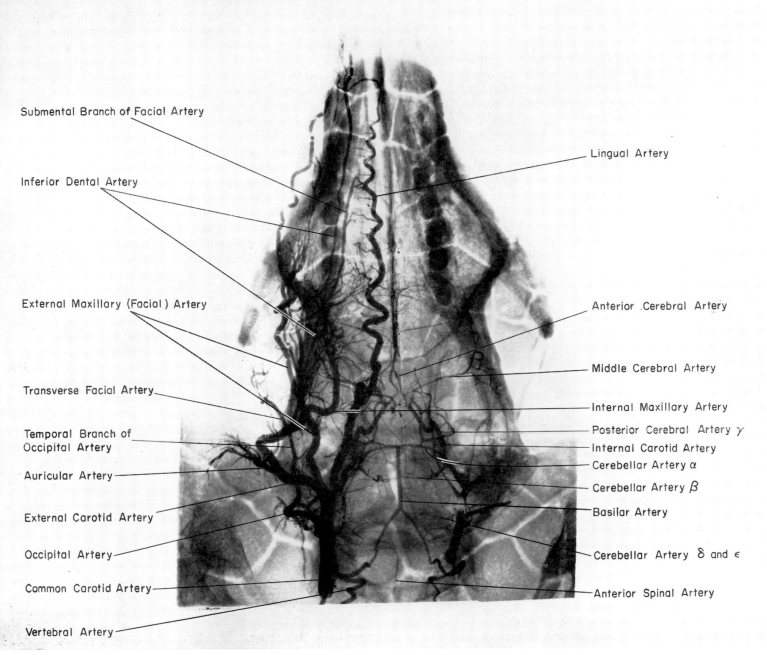

Submental Branch of Facial Artery

Lingual Artery

Inferior Dental Artery

External Maxillary (Facial) Artery

Anterior Cerebral Artery

Middle Cerebral Artery

Transverse Facial Artery

Internal Maxillary Artery

Posterior Cerebral Artery γ

Temporal Branch of
Occipital Artery

Internal Carotid Artery

Cerebellar Artery α

Auricular Artery

Cerebellar Artery β

External Carotid Artery

Basilar Artery

Occipital Artery

Cerebellar Artery δ and ε

Common Carotid Artery

Anterior Spinal Artery

Vertebral Artery

× 1·7

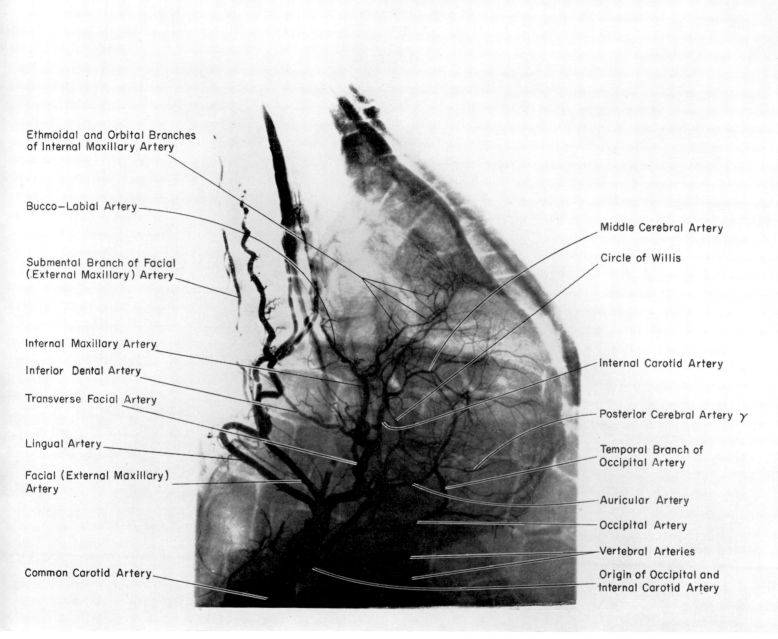

Ethmoidal and Orbital Branches
of Internal Maxillary Artery

Bucco—Labial Artery

Submental Branch of Facial
(External Maxillary) Artery

Internal Maxillary Artery

Inferior Dental Artery

Transverse Facial Artery

Lingual Artery

Facial (External Maxillary)
Artery

Common Carotid Artery

Middle Cerebral Artery

Circle of Willis

Internal Carotid Artery

Posterior Cerebral Artery γ

Temporal Branch of
Occipital Artery

Auricular Artery

Occipital Artery

Vertebral Arteries

Origin of Occipital and
Internal Carotid Artery

× 1·7

In the same way as in other edentates, the occipital artery supplies a temporal branch.

The internal carotid and occipital arteries may possibly have a common stem.

The Circle of Willis is supplied by the internal carotid and the vertebral arteries.

The anterior cerebral appears to come from the internal carotid before its division into cranial and caudal rami. The posterior branch continues as the posterior cerebral (γ perhaps)

but has a narrow connecting piece with the large cerebellar artery (α?). There is a row of four or five cerebellar arteries on each side.

Pholidota

The literature contains only very limited information about the cerebral arteries of Pangolins. Sonntag (1925) summarised the position, relying heavily upon Hyrtl for the names and branching of the common and external carotid arteries. There are no accounts of the intracranial arteries.

Unfortunately, Sonntag and Hyrtl do not accord well with a system of names which seems logical by analogy with other mammals. For instance, the external maxillary in *Manis*, according to Hyrtl, gives rise to a buccal and transverse facial arteries.

We have, therefore, not found it possible to follow previous accounts in all respects.

The common carotid evidently divides into a large external and a small internal carotid artery.

The external carotid then divides again into two equal portions, the lingual taking fully one-half of the blood. The continuation of the external carotid supplies an occipital artery which also gives rise to auricular branches and then a facial (external maxillary) artery whose largest branch is the submental.

Next, there is a very narrow superficial temporal artery and a large internal maxillary.

The internal maxillary supplies in turn a large "inferior dental" which runs through the mandible to the region of the lower lip, a buccal and a pharyngeal artery. The internal maxillary continues as the infra-orbital facial, supplying ethmoidal, nasal and external ophthalmic arteries.

The Circle of Willis is remarkable, deriving its blood both from internal carotid and spinal vertebral arteries; the latter forming a five- or six-fold rete on each side, singling down at the level of C.1.

The basilar is short by comparison with the Circle of Willis so that cerebellar arteries (perhaps α and β) arise from the posterior branches of the internal carotid.

Manis tricuspis
Tree Pangolin

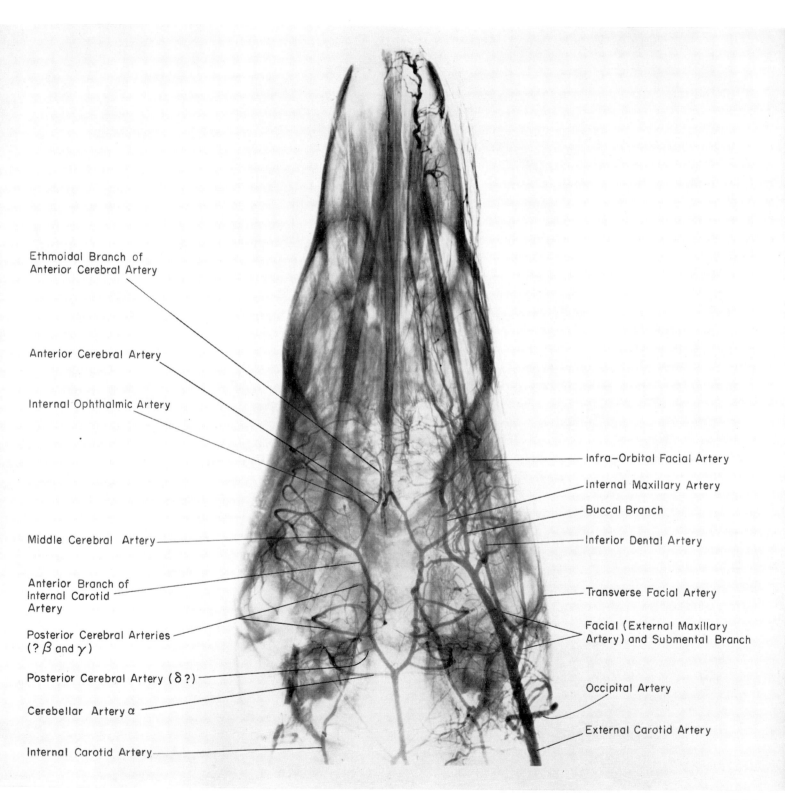

Ethmoidal Branch of
Anterior Cerebral Artery

Anterior Cerebral Artery

Internal Ophthalmic Artery

Middle Cerebral Artery

Anterior Branch of
Internal Carotid
Artery

Posterior Cerebral Arteries
(? β and γ)

Posterior Cerebral Artery (δ?)

Cerebellar Artery α

Internal Carotid Artery

Infra-Orbital Facial Artery

Internal Maxillary Artery

Buccal Branch

Inferior Dental Artery

Transverse Facial Artery

Facial (External Maxillary
Artery) and Submental Branch

Occipital Artery

External Carotid Artery

× 2·6

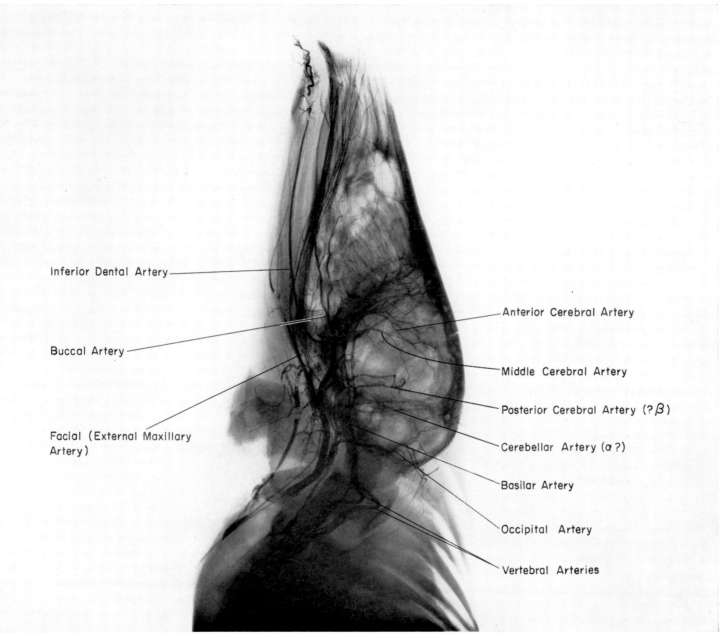

Inferior Dental Artery——————

Buccal Artery————

Facial (External Maxillary Artery)

Anterior Cerebral Artery

Middle Cerebral Artery

Posterior Cerebral Artery (?β)

Cerebellar Artery (α?)

Basilar Artery

Occipital Artery

Vertebral Arteries

$\times$ 1·5

The lingual artery has not filled.

Note the ethmoidal branches of the anterior cerebral, the internal ophthalmic artery, the posterior cerebrals (α and γ?) and the cerebellar arteries which are presumed to be α, β, γ and δ.

Manis tricuspis

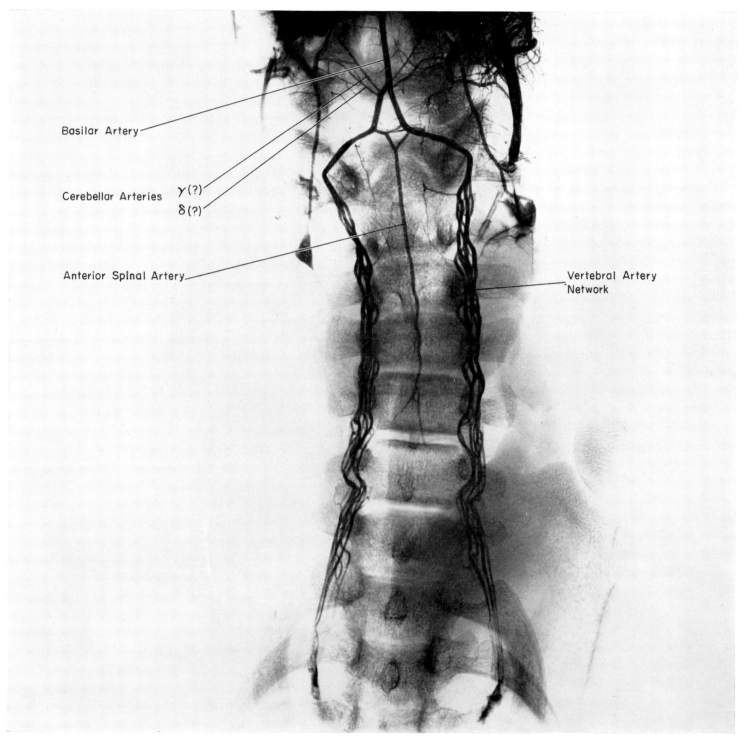

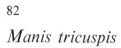

Basilar Artery

Cerebellar Arteries   γ (?)
                       δ (?)

Anterior Spinal Artery

Vertebral Artery
Network

× 2·2

Manis pentadactyla
Chinese Pangolin

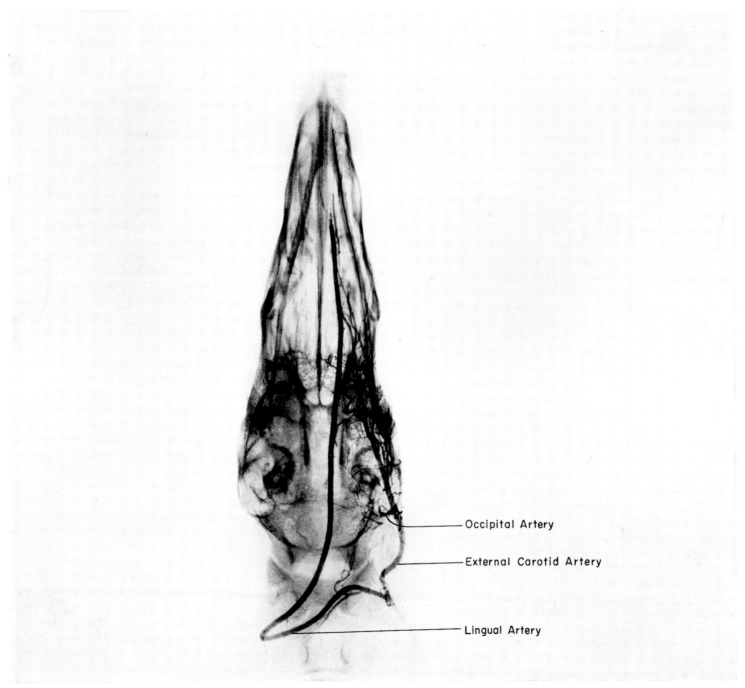

Occipital Artery

External Carotid Artery

Lingual Artery

× 1·3

Only the branches of the external carotid have been outlined.

Lagomorpha

The following description follows Tandler (1899). There have been points of dispute about the naming of certain vessels; but the description here seems logical and in step with the nomenclature applied to rodentia and insectivora.

Readers requiring more detail are referred to Bugge (1967, 1968, 1969) and Wiland (1968).

The common carotid artery divides into internal and external carotids after giving off the thyroid branch.

The external carotid bends medially and usually gives origin to the occipital artery (but this may also arise from the common carotid). It then continues upwards and supplies the external maxillary (facial) and the lingual arteries in turn or by a common stem. The external carotid then gives off a major branch which bends dorsally between the tympanic bulla and the mandible providing the anterior and posterior auricular arteries and terminates at the zygomatic arch by dividing into the superficial temporal and the transverse facial artery.

The external carotid continues in a cranial direction, medial to the pterygoid muscle and its main continuation reaches the pterygoid canal. Prior to disappearing into this canal it gives origin to the inferior alveolar (inferior dental) artery and a branch, the middle meningeal, running back through the medial end of the Glaserian fissure. This apparently recurrent branch must be, developmentally, the distal part of the lower branch of the stapedial artery. (These arrangements are very similar in the guinea pig). Beyond the pterygoid canal the artery flows into the face; but it gives off a very large branch in the posterior part of the orbit, the orbital ramus or external ophthalmic artery, which divides above the optic nerve into lachrymal and frontal branches and then unites with the small internal ophthalmic artery.

From the continuation of the internal maxillary, close to its attachment to the derivative of the inferior branch of the stapedial coming through the Glaserian fissure, another branch is given off and this runs upwards and perforates the orbital wall through the suture between greater and lesser wings of the sphenoid to reach the subdural space. This may be called the anterior meningeal artery.

Cerebral Vessels

The following account is based upon Hofmann (1900).

The relatively narrow internal carotid, after passing through the dura, immediately gives rise to a somewhat variable, usually rather small, ophthalmic artery and then divides into a cranial and a caudal ramus.

The cranial ramus runs anterior to the uncus and after losing one or two little arteries, possibly the anterior choroidal and also the middle cerebral trunk, arrives in front of the optic chiasm. It joins its opposite number to form a common anterior cerebral trunk; but soon separates again into two arteries of the corpus callosum which supply the medial surfaces of the hemispheres and anastomose on the splenium with branches of the posterior cerebral artery.

The common stem of the anterior cerebral gives rise to the lateral artery of the olfactory bulb. This artery supplies not only the lateral but the medial part of the olfactory bulb as well and sends a branch to the subdural ethmoidal rete on the cribriform plate, which is further connected to the olfactory bulb through its own short twigs and to the nasal cavity by branches running with the olfactory fibres. The anterior olfactory artery may also arise from the anterior cerebral.

The middle cerebral gives origin to the following branches, though some may alternatively arise directly from the cranial ramus of the cerebral carotid.

(1) A posterior olfactory artery.
(2) A large posterior Sylvian branch to the caudal part of the upper surface of the cerebral hemisphere, posterior to a line between the anterior end of the Sylvian fissure and the occipital protuberance.
(3) Another large branch which soon divides into two (anterior and middle) Sylvian arteries which supply the surface of the hemisphere anterior to the line mentioned above.
(4) Further, small branches to the olfactory lobe.

The caudal ramus of the cerebral carotid is narrow anterior to the origin of the posterior cerebral γ and may be thought of as a posterior communicating artery.

It sends small branches medially to the bulb of the fornix and the infundibulum and laterally to the cerebral peduncle and may provide an alternative origin for the anterior choroidal artery.

The posterior cerebral artery γ must obtain most of its blood from the basilar artery. It runs laterally, then around the brainstem, passing in front of the medial geniculate body to reach the medial surface of the cerebral hemisphere. It supplies the following branches:

(1) From the root close to the posterior communicating artery there are twigs to the infundibulum and the posterior perforated substance.
(2) Small branches to the optic thalamus and the medial geniculate body.
(3) A very large artery which sends a series of branches to the anterior corpus quadrigeminum and one which forms the medial posterior choroidal artery.
(4) Terminal branches, three to five in number, which supply the posterior part of the uncus and the medial and inferior surfaces of the hemisphere posteriorly and anastomose on the splenium with the artery of the corpus callosum.

A cerebellar artery α springs either from the caudal ramus of the carotid or from the cranial end of the basilar artery. It runs laterally over the pons and sends end vessels up to the midline to supply the superior vermis and the upper part of the cerebellar hemisphere. One of the terminal branches runs in the groove between the flocculus and the lateral part of the antero-superior lobe to anastomose with the cerebellar artery γ and may sometimes form the major pathway for blood from the cerebellar artery γ to the distribution of the cerebellar artery α.

There may also be an artery to the posterior corpus quadrigeminum arising either from the cerebellar artery α or the cerebral carotid.

The basilar is, for the most part, an unpaired vessel in the midline deriving its origin from the ventral rami of the large, first spinal nerve arteries. Over the ventral surface of the corpus trapezoideum it divides into two, which again unite at the upper border of the pons.

The basilar artery gives off:

(1) Three or four pontine branches running laterally.

(2) Either a superior and inferior artery to the trigeminal nerve or an inferior artery alone, the superior being vestigial.

(3) A little vessel which runs in the groove between the pons and the corpus trapezoideum and may supply the internal auditory artery.

(4) Small branches to the corpus trapezoideum.

(5) A cerebellar artery γ. This runs in the groove between the corpus trapezoideum and the medulla, usually gives origin to internal auditory artery and supplies the inferior vermis and the caudal part of the cerebellar hemisphere and the choroid plexus of the 4th ventricle.

(6) The anastomotic branch to the cerebellar artery α (described above) which may sometimes form the main supply for all the branches of the cerebellar artery γ.

(7) Lateral branches to the medulla.

(8) A series of central perforating arteries to the brainstem.

Lepus europaeus
European Hare

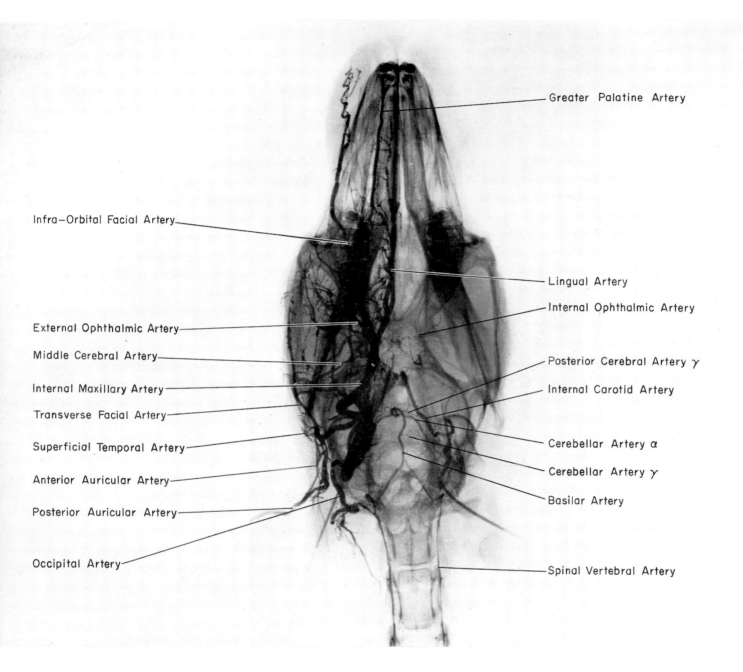

Greater Palatine Artery

Infra–Orbital Facial Artery

Lingual Artery

Internal Ophthalmic Artery

External Ophthalmic Artery

Middle Cerebral Artery

Posterior Cerebral Artery γ

Internal Maxillary Artery

Internal Carotid Artery

Transverse Facial Artery

Superficial Temporal Artery

Cerebellar Artery α

Anterior Auricular Artery

Cerebellar Artery γ

Posterior Auricular Artery

Basilar Artery

Occipital Artery

Spinal Vertebral Artery

× 1·2

The arrangement of the vessels is very similar to the rabbit.
Identification of the individual branches of the external ophthalmic is somewhat speculative.

The superficial temporal artery seems to be very small and arises from the anterior auricular. Anterior and posterior auricular and transverse facial artery all come from a common trunk. The transverse facial has a superficial as well as a deep branch, the former behaving very much like a superficial temporal artery placed somewhat ventrally.

The lingual and facial (external maxillary) arteries also derive from a common stem.

The origin of the internal carotid artery is unfortunately obscured.

The anterior cerebral artery is poorly filled in this specimen.

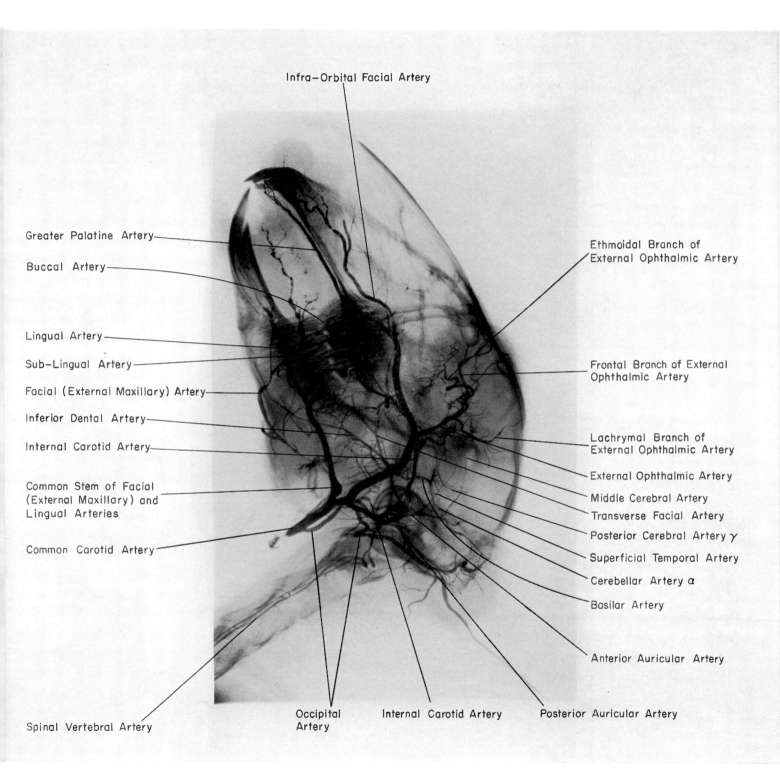

Infra–Orbital Facial Artery

Greater Palatine Artery

Buccal Artery

Lingual Artery

Sub–Lingual Artery

Facial (External Maxillary) Artery

Inferior Dental Artery

Internal Carotid Artery

Common Stem of Facial
(External Maxillary) and
Lingual Arteries

Common Carotid Artery

Spinal Vertebral Artery

Occipital
Artery

Internal Carotid Artery

Ethmoidal Branch of
External Ophthalmic Artery

Frontal Branch of External
Ophthalmic Artery

Lachrymal Branch of
External Ophthalmic Artery

External Ophthalmic Artery

Middle Cerebral Artery

Transverse Facial Artery

Posterior Cerebral Artery γ

Superficial Temporal Artery

Cerebellar Artery α

Basilar Artery

Anterior Auricular Artery

Posterior Auricular Artery

× 1·3

Oryctolagus cuniculus
European Rabbit

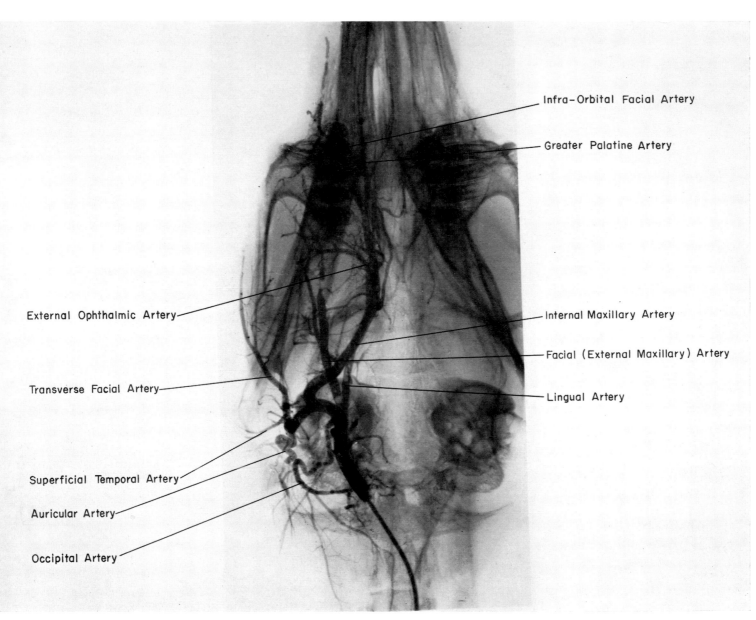

Infra-Orbital Facial Artery

Greater Palatine Artery

External Ophthalmic Artery

Internal Maxillary Artery

Facial (External Maxillary) Artery

Transverse Facial Artery

Lingual Artery

Superficial Temporal Artery

Auricular Artery

Occipital Artery

× 1·1

Most of the contrast medium lies in the external carotid branches. The origin of the inferior dental artery from the internal maxillary is superimposed upon the transverse facial artery.

Oryctolagus cuniculus
New Zealand White Rabbit

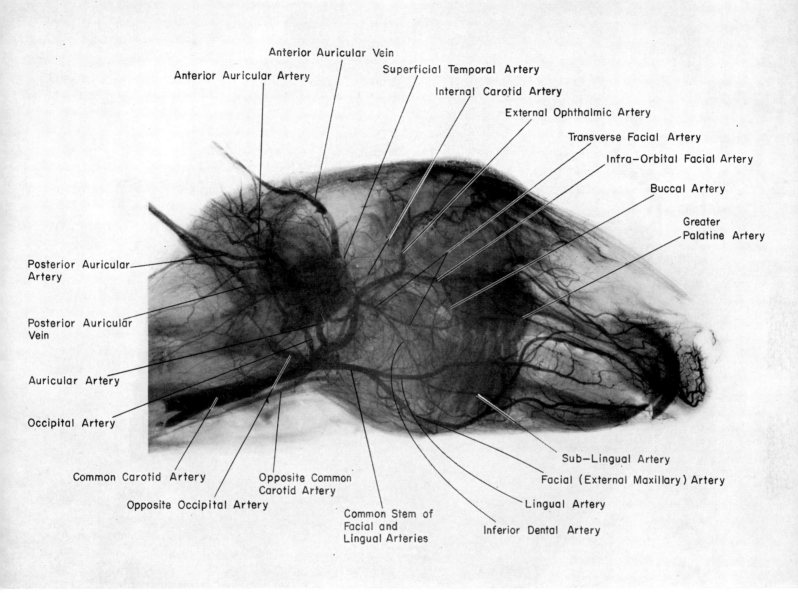

Anterior Auricular Vein

Anterior Auricular Artery

Superficial Temporal Artery

Internal Carotid Artery

External Ophthalmic Artery

Transverse Facial Artery

Infra–Orbital Facial Artery

Buccal Artery

Greater Palatine Artery

Posterior Auricular Artery

Posterior Auricular Vein

Auricular Artery

Occipital Artery

Common Carotid Artery

Opposite Occipital Artery

Opposite Common Carotid Artery

Common Stem of Facial and Lingual Arteries

Inferior Dental Artery

Lingual Artery

Sub–Lingual Artery

Facial (External Maxillary) Artery

× 1·1

Only the external carotid branches have been outlined.

Rodentia

The division of rodents into the suborders Sciuromorpha, Myomorpha and Hystricomorpha seems, from a limited survey, to be reflected in the general pattern of their cranial arteries. Tandler (1899) described the cranial arteries of some half-dozen rodents, examples from all three suborders (though he did not characterise them as such), pointing out the major differences and tracing the embryological events which might transform one system into another. His examples include the common squirrel (*Sciurus vulgaris*), *Sciurus aureogaster*, the American squirrel now *Tamios striatus striatus* (Eastern chipmunk), *Arctomys* now *Marmota monax* (all Sciuromorpha) and springhaas which is sometimes so classified, the rat (his only example from the Myomorpha) and the guinea pig (*Cavia cobaya*) (one of the Hystricomorpha).

Simplified descriptions of the characteristic features of each of the three suborders are given here based upon Tandler (1899), Hofmann (1900), Daniel et al. (1953), Bugge (1970, 1971) and our own studies to reveal the general pattern of a somewhat confused subject. Guthrie (1963) has described the carotid circulation.

Sciuromorpha

The external carotid artery is much larger than the internal and appears to be the direct continuation of the common carotid.

It gives rise in turn to a medium-sized occipital artery, a lingual and facial (external maxillary) which may in some species come from a common trunk, a medium-sized auricular artery and a large internal maxillary.

The origin and distribution of the anterior auricular branch of the auricular artery, the superficial temporal and the transverse facial vary greatly from species to species.

The internal maxillary gives origin in one way or another to a deep temporal artery and then goes on to supply an inferior dental (or both may come from a common stem). The internal maxillary has as its terminal branches, the infraorbital and bucco-labial vessels. Prior to this, in the region of the orbital fissure, the internal maxillary may supply a ramus anastomoticus and/or arteria anastomotica to the intracranial circulation. One or other of these branches when present pick up and are continued as the intracranial internal carotid. Thus, blood from the internal maxillary artery is passed to the Circle of Willis.

The Internal Carotid Artery

Beyond the origin of the stapedial artery at or near the skull base, the internal carotid often disappears or becomes very narrow. It sometimes reappears as described above, as the intra-cranial continuation of one of the two possible anastomotic branches of the internal maxillary artery.

The Stapedial Artery

The stapedial artery is present but only connected with the brain's blood supply through anastomoses in the region of the orbit. It may, however, give origin to a large meningeal branch as it emerges from the temporal bone. It finally forms the main supply for lachrymal, frontal and ethmoidal twigs.

The Vertebral Arteries

In the majority of Sciuromorpha examined, the vertebral arteries contribute the major blood supply to the brain. They in turn receive their blood both from the occipital arteries and from the spinal vertebral arteries. Thus, much of the blood supply to the brain passes through external carotid vessels.

The Circle of Willis

In spite of the attachment of the anastomosis between the internal maxillary artery and the persisting end of the internal carotid, the caudal and cranial branches of the internal carotid usually appear to constitute a forwardly directed pathway for the passage of blood from the basilar towards the middle and anterior cerebral arteries.

Without careful dissection it is not possible to name the various posterior cerebral vessels with certainty; but from their positions we would judge them usually to be posterior cerebrals γ and δ (Hofmann).

* * *

There are many minor variations of this overall pattern among the Sciuromorpha apart from those already mentioned. Some of these are apparent from the illustrated injection studies. Details of the distal connections between the stapedial artery and the internal maxillary differ, for instance, from species to species.

Variations in the communications between the internal maxillary artery and the Circle of Willis are disputed. In the common squirrel, according to Tandler (1899), and in our specimen of *Cynomys ludovicianus* at one end of the spectrum there is no arteria anastomotica and no anastomotic ramus. The ophthalmic artery arising from the termination of the internal carotid may either be very small or, as in *Cynomys*, large. At the other end of the spectrum many Sciuromorphae have a large ramus anastomoticus and may have free communications between internal maxillary and cerebral vessels via orbital branches of the internal maxillary and of the anterior cerebral artery.

In the "common squirrel" (Tandler) the upper branch of the stapedial artery is said to provide the lachrymal, frontal and ethmoidal arteries in the orbit after it has anastomosed with the upper division of the orbital branch of the internal maxillary. The lower branch of the stapedial artery unites with the internal maxillary as it enters the pterygoid canal. The orbital branches of the internal maxillary are two in number. One has been mentioned above as uniting with the upper branch of the stapedial, the other, the inferior orbital ramus, supplies the lower muscles of the eye.

Sciurus aureogaster (according to Tandler), while resembling the common squirrel in most respects, does have an anastomotic connection between the internal maxillary artery and the terminal internal carotid. The ophthalmic artery is said to be larger than in the common squirrel.

Sciurus americanus, Tandler says, has an even larger anastomotic ramus than the *Sciurus aurogaster*.

There is confusion about *Cynomys ludovicianus*. Tandler describes a different kind of cerebral circulation for *Arctomys marmota*. According to him the anastomotic connection of the internal carotid divides in the orbit and has a double attachment, the larger part of the internal maxillary and the smaller to the lower branch of the orbital end of the stapedial artery. As can be seen, however, from the injected specimen, the "anastomotic" supply to the Circle of Willis is absent.

The variation which Tandler described as occurring in the springhaas is sufficiently interesting to be dealt with more fully, though we have not ourselves seen a specimen. The vertebral arterial supply to the Circle of Willis is of lesser importance to the cerebral hemispheres than in many rodents and the main supplying vessel is the internal carotid which is well preserved through its whole course. The main trunk of the internal maxillary has disappeared and so has the main trunk and divisions of the stapedial artery. A subdural arteria anastomotica arising from the internal carotid is nevertheless found; but instead of conducting blood towards the brain from the internal maxillary and stapedial arteries, blood must pass in an opposite direction from internal carotid outward, for this anastomotic artery has preserved its upper connection with the persisting, distal lachrymal, frontal and ethmoidal twigs of the stapedial and its lower connection with the infra-orbital termination of the internal maxillary. Blood, in fact, must also flow back along that part of the internal maxillary artery which passes through the pterygoid canal, for at its posterior end are given off the deep temporal arteries and the inferior dental. Thus, whatever advantages Sciuromorpha derive from passing their cerebral blood through external carotid branches have been dispensed with in this animal. Instead there is a diametrically opposite system; much of the blood to the face and jaw being drawn from the internal carotid artery.

Myomorpha

The common carotid artery divides at about the level of the larynx into two equally large vessels—the external and internal carotids.

The External Carotid

The external carotid almost immediately supplies a thyroid branch and then an occipital of variable proportions. Subsequently, the external carotid appears to divide into three more or less equal stems; one is the lingual, one the facial (external maxillary) and one the continuation of the external carotid itself.

This continuation bends posteriorly then again anteriorly and laterally. It gives origin to the auricular artery or arteries, and in a variable manner, the superficial temporal. It terminates as the transverse facial artery.

Close to the origin of the superficial temporal, a small medially directed vessel supplies both a pterygoid muscular and an inferior dental branch. This vessel is the rudimentary internal maxillary.

The Internal Carotid

This divides just below the mastoid bulla into two, a more dorsal stapedial artery and a more ventral internal carotid continuation.

The internal carotid passes in a typical fashion through a bony carotid canal to emerge in the subdural space where it runs for a considerable distance as dictated by the long sella turcica. It then perforates the dura and divides into cranial and caudal (posterior communicating) branches.

The Stapedial Artery

The stapedial artery is larger than in the Sciuromorpha. It enters the bulla wall in a typical fashion separately from the internal carotid, above and behind it. On the wall of the middle ear, reaching the promontary, it crosses foramen ovale between the crura of the stapes. It then enters a bony canal and leaves the tympanic cavity via the Glasserian fissure. From here it passes to the pterygoid canal and after traversing the canal gives rise to a pterygoid branch and then the deep temporal artery. It continues as the infra-orbital facial artery. As the infra-orbital facial passes below the fibrous floor of the orbit it gives rise to an orbital branch which pierces the floor and breaks up into supra-orbital, lachrymal and ethmoidal branches.

More distally the infra-orbital facial gives rise to the bucco-labial.

Thus many branches which in a typical Sciuromorph would be supplied by the internal maxillary alone or in combination with the stapedial artery, are supplied in Myomorpha by the stapedial alone.

The Circle of Willis

The basilar artery derives its origin from the two large cranial vertebral arteries which themselves are the direct continuations of the spinal vertebral arteries, only a little reinforced by branches of the occipital artery.

The posterior cerebral arteries (probably γ by Hofmann's classification) and the cerebellar arteries (probably α) are terminal branches of the basilar. The posterior communicating arteries (caudal branches of internal carotid) are moderately well-developed; but are not so large as the cranial branches of the internal carotid. From the cranial branch arises a fairly large ophthalmic artery (supplying ciliary branches), a middle cerebral and an anterior cerebral. The anterior cerebral divides into two almost equal parts, the ethmoidal branch running directly forwards, the other to join its opposite number in the midline and form the pericallosal artery.

Hystricomorpha

With certain exceptions, mentioned in the descriptions of individual specimens, the Hystricomorph arterial tree follows a characteristic pattern first described by Tandler in the guinea pig. Bugge (1971) has added greatly to our knowledge.

The external carotid artery is the direct continuation of the common carotid, the internal having almost or completely disappeared.

The occipital artery, which is often fairly small, springs from the external carotid close to the origin of the ascending pharyngeal. Both branches behave in a normal way. The external carotid then continues upwards under the digastric muscle, providing a main and a subsidiary branch at the upper edge of this muscle. The main branch is the common trunk of the lingual and facial (external maxillary) arteries, the smaller branch runs backwards.

This, the external carotid, then runs lateral to the mandibular muscles, continuing obliquely backwards and upwards to the retro-mandibular fossa. Here it gives off the large posterior auricular artery and ends as the narrow superficial temporal artery.

In some animals a narrow tributary arises close to the origin of the superficial temporal and this artery may represent the transverse facial.

The major continuation of the main trunk of the external carotid is, as has been said, the common trunk for the lingual and external maxillary arteries. This latter divides in front of the digastric muscle into the rather narrow continuation of the named vessel and a much larger branch which bends cranially and medially and comes to lie medial to the pterygoid muscles. This large artery then gives rise to the inferior dental and a temporal muscular branch (presumably the deep temporal artery). It also often supplies a narrow vessel which runs backwards and may in some instances unite with the "transverse facial" described above, thus the true external carotid has been as it were replaced by an alternative pathway over the segment between the superficial and deep temporal vessels.

Anterior to the point of origin of the inferior dental artery the vessel enters the pterygoid canal and having given off the external ophthalmic (which supplies a branch to unite with the internal ophthalmic as well as the frontal and lachrymal artery) it continues into the face as the infra-orbital facial artery.

The artery which passes through the pterygoid canal also gives origin to the middle meningeal. It is clear that this artery of the pterygoid canal in fact represents the remains of the stapedial artery.

The Internal Carotid Artery

The internal carotid is absent or very small.

The Circle of Willis and the Vertebral Arteries

The Circle of Willis derives all, or almost all, of its blood from the well-developed spinal vertebral arteries.

Cynomys ludovicianus
Prairie Dog

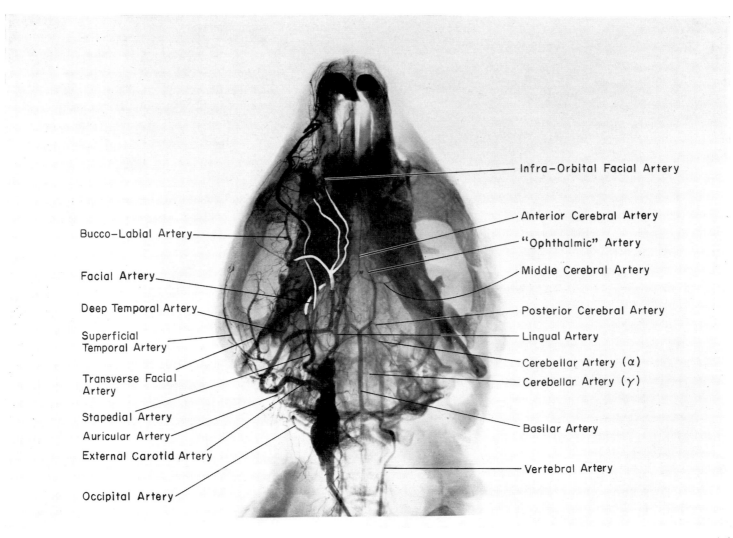

Infra-Orbital Facial Artery

Anterior Cerebral Artery

"Ophthalmic" Artery

Middle Cerebral Artery

Posterior Cerebral Artery

Lingual Artery

Cerebellar Artery (α)

Cerebellar Artery (γ)

Basilar Artery

Vertebral Artery

Bucco-Labial Artery

Facial Artery

Deep Temporal Artery

Superficial
Temporal Artery

Transverse Facial
Artery

Stapedial Artery

Auricular Artery

External Carotid Artery

Occipital Artery

$\times$ 1·6

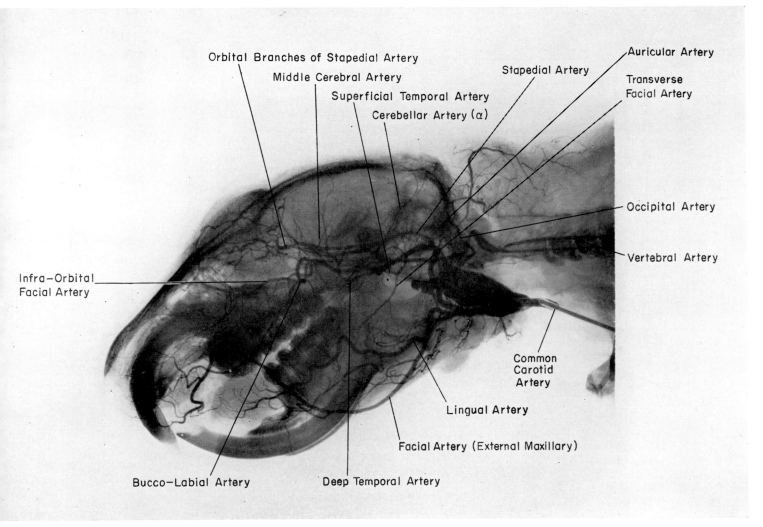

Orbital Branches of Stapedial Artery
Middle Cerebral Artery
Superficial Temporal Artery
Cerebellar Artery (α)
Stapedial Artery
Auricular Artery
Transverse Facial Artery
Occipital Artery
Vertebral Artery
Infra–Orbital Facial Artery
Common Carotid Artery
Lingual Artery
Facial Artery (External Maxillary)
Bucco–Labial Artery
Deep Temporal Artery

× 2·0

In these injection studies the origin of the external maxillary (facial) is superimposed upon the stapedial in the ventro-dorsal view. Extravasation obscures the region in two of the pictures.

Cynomys ludovicianus appears to be a typical Sciuromorph except that no major anastomotic connection has been shown between the internal maxillary and the end of the internal carotid. Instead there appears to be a large ophthalmic artery and it may be that this provides the useful anastomotic link between internal and external carotid circulations.

The inferior dental artery may arise directly from the deep temporal artery.

Classification of the intracranial branches cannot be given with certainty but it seems likely that the two posterior cerebral arteries arising from a common stem are γ and δ (Hofmann). The cerebellar arteries may be α or β and γ (Hofmann).

Cynomys ludovicianus

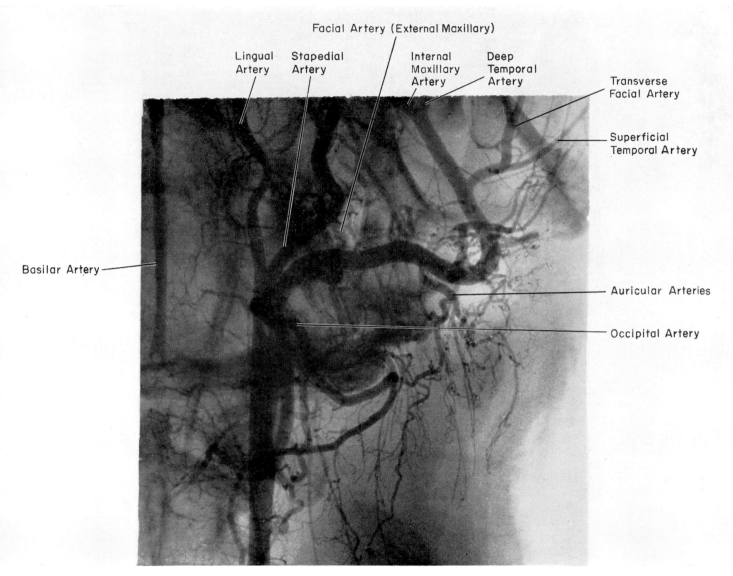

Facial Artery (External Maxillary)

Lingual Artery   Stapedial Artery   Internal Maxillary Artery   Deep Temporal Artery

Transverse Facial Artery

Superficial Temporal Artery

Basilar Artery

Auricular Arteries

Occipital Artery

× 4·0

Tamias striatus
Eastern Chipmunk

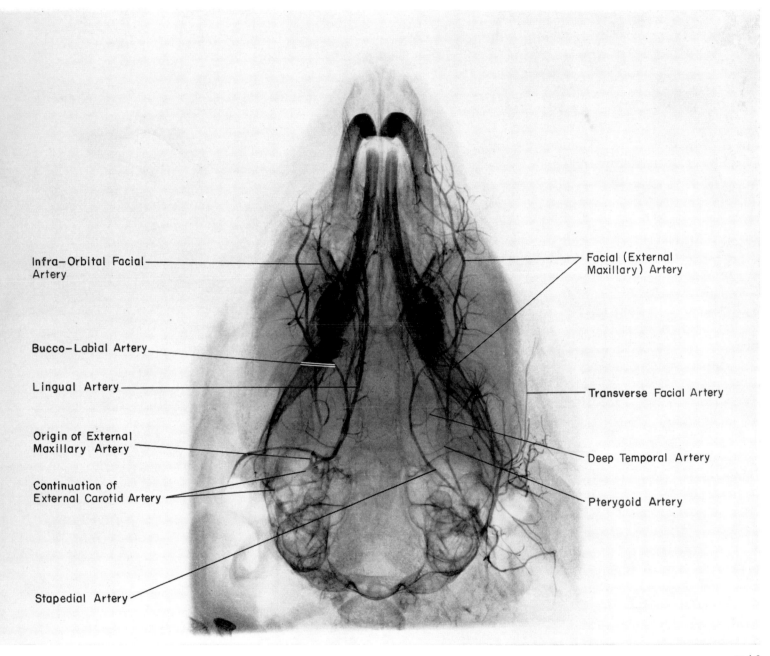

Infra–Orbital Facial Artery

Bucco–Labial Artery

Lingual Artery

Origin of External Maxillary Artery

Continuation of External Carotid Artery

Stapedial Artery

Facial (External Maxillary) Artery

Transverse Facial Artery

Deep Temporal Artery

Pterygoid Artery

× 4·0

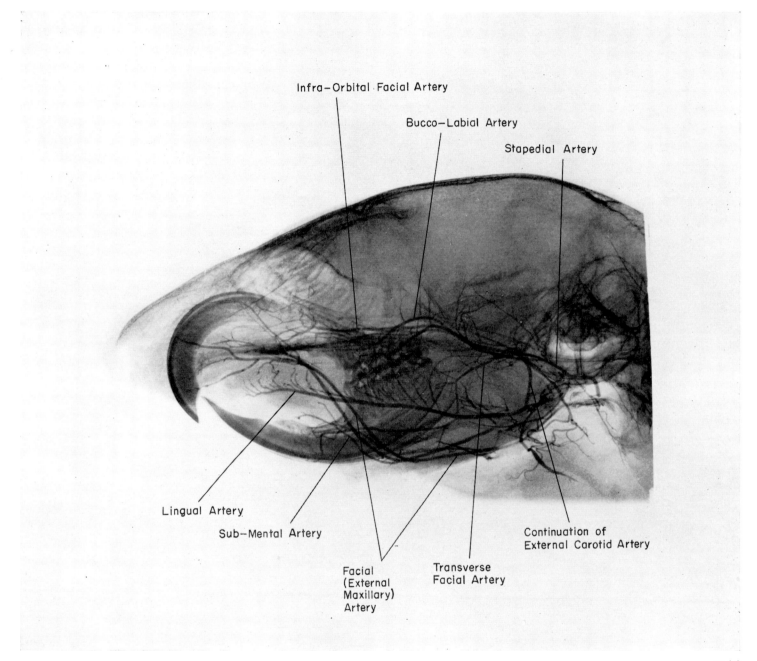

Infra-Orbital Facial Artery

Bucco-Labial Artery

Stapedial Artery

Lingual Artery

Sub-Mental Artery

Facial
(External
Maxillary)
Artery

Transverse
Facial Artery

Continuation of
External Carotid Artery

× 4·0

The external carotid circulation has been well-filled but no
barium has entered the cerebral vessels. This suggests that both
the arteria anastomotica and the ramus anastomoticus are
absent or very small. Tandler (1899) on the other hand describing what he called *Sciurus americanus* which has been identified
with *Tamias striatus* mentions a large anastomotic ramus.

Petaurista alborufus
Red and White Flying Squirrel

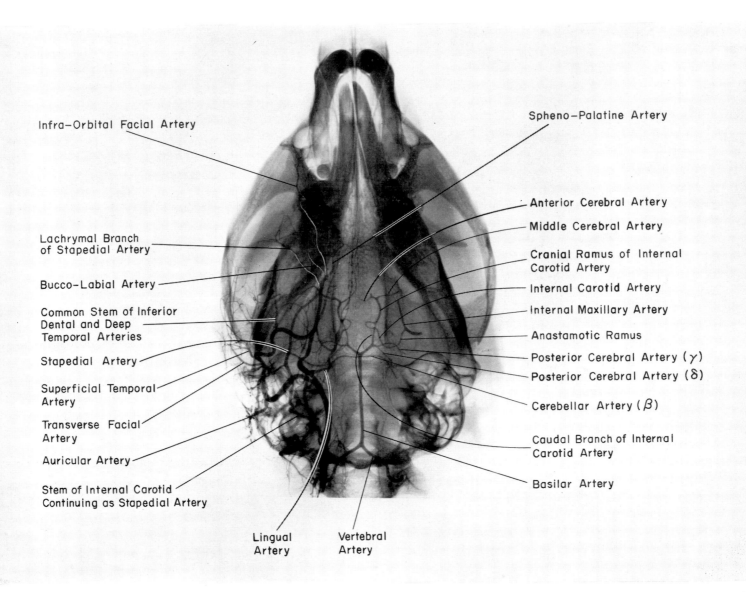

Infra–Orbital Facial Artery

Spheno–Palatine Artery

Lachrymal Branch of Stapedial Artery

Bucco-Labial Artery

Common Stem of Inferior Dental and Deep Temporal Arteries

Stapedial Artery

Superficial Temporal Artery

Transverse Facial Artery

Auricular Artery

Stem of Internal Carotid Continuing as Stapedial Artery

Anterior Cerebral Artery

Middle Cerebral Artery

Cranial Ramus of Internal Carotid Artery

Internal Carotid Artery

Internal Maxillary Artery

Anastamotic Ramus

Posterior Cerebral Artery (γ)

Posterior Cerebral Artery (δ)

Cerebellar Artery (β)

Caudal Branch of Internal Carotid Artery

Basilar Artery

Lingual Artery

Vertebral Artery

$\times$ 1·3

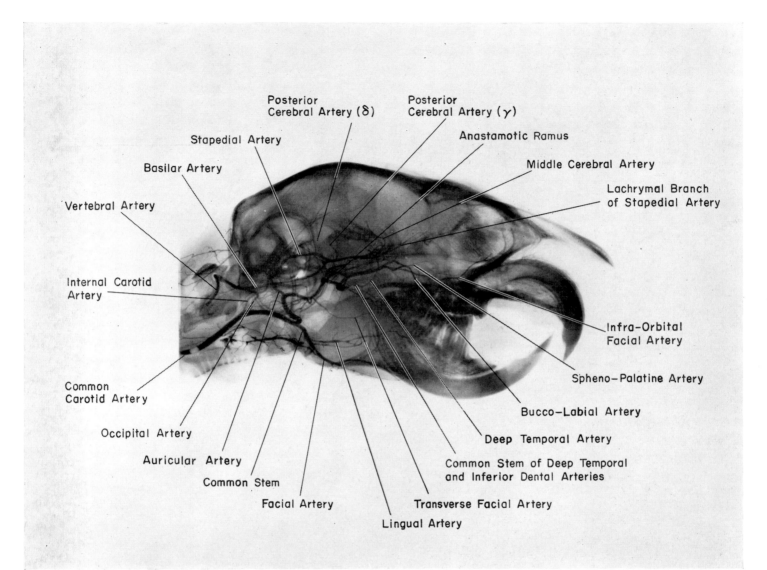

$\times 1.3$

The superficial temporal artery is obscured in the lateral view.
The cerebral part of the internal carotid appears to derive its
whole blood supply from the anastomotic ramus of the internal
maxillary.

Castor fiber
Beaver

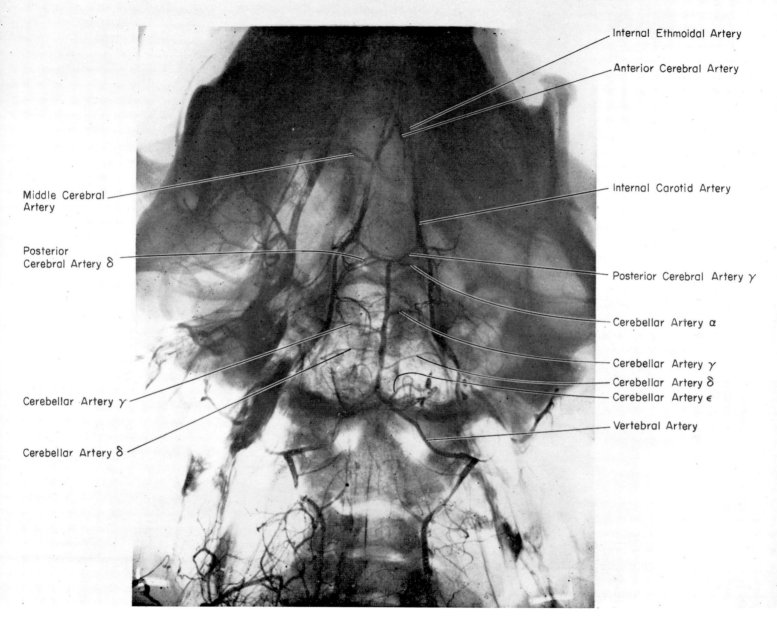

Internal Ethmoidal Artery

Anterior Cerebral Artery

Internal Carotid Artery

Middle Cerebral Artery

Posterior Cerebral Artery δ

Posterior Cerebral Artery γ

Cerebellar Artery α

Cerebellar Artery γ

Cerebellar Artery γ

Cerebellar Artery δ

Cerebellar Artery ε

Cerebellar Artery δ

Vertebral Artery

× 1·25

This view of the major vessels of the brain shows a most impressive row of cerebellar arteries.

Microtus agrestis
Short-tailed Vole

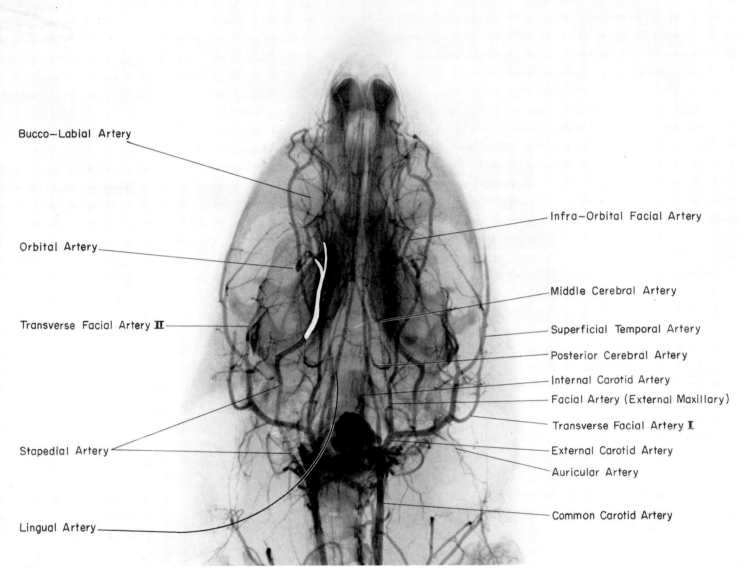

Bucco–Labial Artery

Orbital Artery

Transverse Facial Artery **II**

Stapedial Artery

Lingual Artery

Infra–Orbital Facial Artery

Middle Cerebral Artery

Superficial Temporal Artery

Posterior Cerebral Artery

Internal Carotid Artery

Facial Artery (External Maxillary)

Transverse Facial Artery **I**

External Carotid Artery

Auricular Artery

Common Carotid Artery

× 4·5

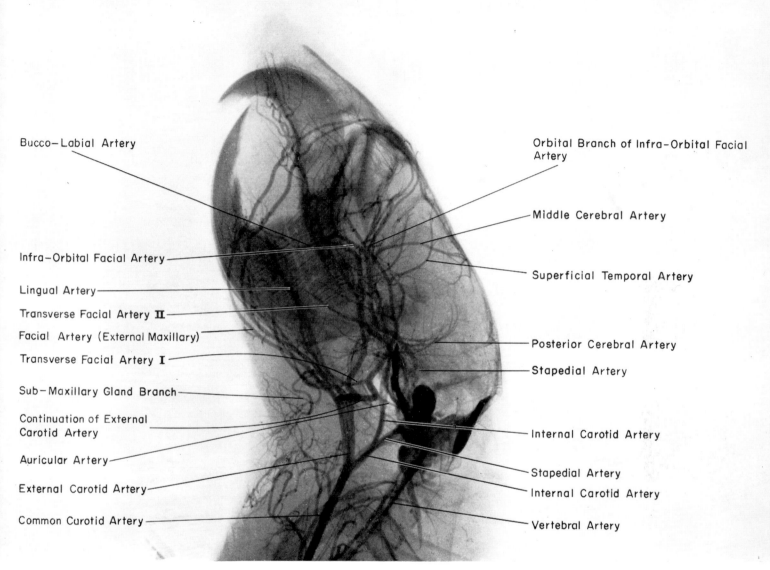

Bucco—Labial Artery

Orbital Branch of Infra—Orbital Facial Artery

Middle Cerebral Artery

Infra—Orbital Facial Artery

Superficial Temporal Artery

Lingual Artery

Transverse Facial Artery **II**

Facial Artery (External Maxillary)

Posterior Cerebral Artery

Transverse Facial Artery **I**

Stapedial Artery

Sub—Maxillary Gland Branch

Continuation of External Carotid Artery

Internal Carotid Artery

Auricular Artery

Stapedial Artery

External Carotid Artery

Internal Carotid Artery

Common Carotid Artery

Vertebral Artery

× 4·4

This animal apparently resembles *Arvicola terrestris* very closely in the arrangement of the extra-cranial vessels. The cerebral vessels, however, are difficult to see and it is not known for certain whether the similarity extends also to them.

In the main a typical myomorph but with one or two individual features. For instance, the superficial temporal is unusually large but the deep temporal has not been identified. There appear to be two arteries, both arising from the external carotid which might be named transverse facial. One of these, which is labelled as transverse facial I is a large branch coming off before the superficial temporal and running across the more ventral part of the face. Transverse facial II is more dorsally situated and is the direct continuation and termination of the external carotid artery after that has given off the superficial temporal.

Rattus norvegicus
The Brown Rat

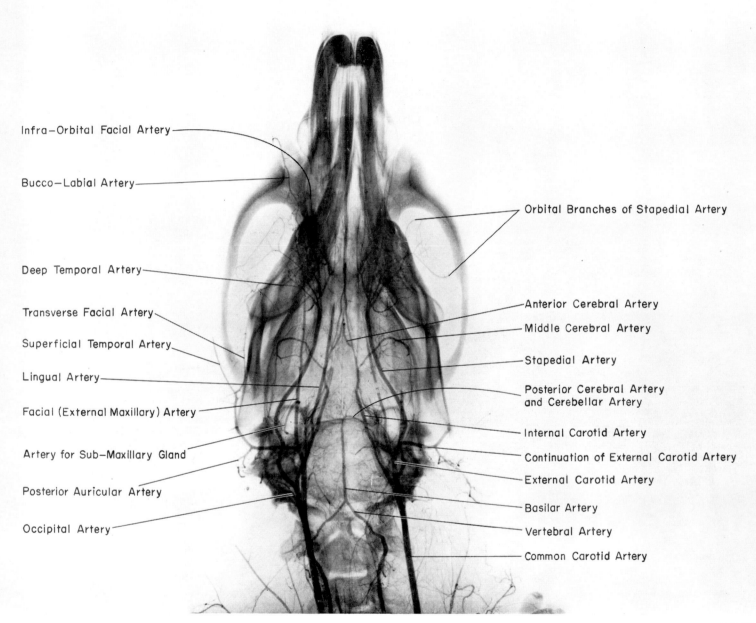

Infra–Orbital Facial Artery

Bucco–Labial Artery

Orbital Branches of Stapedial Artery

Deep Temporal Artery

Transverse Facial Artery

Superficial Temporal Artery

Lingual Artery

Facial (External Maxillary) Artery

Artery for Sub–Maxillary Gland

Posterior Auricular Artery

Occipital Artery

Anterior Cerebral Artery

Middle Cerebral Artery

Stapedial Artery

Posterior Cerebral Artery and Cerebellar Artery

Internal Carotid Artery

Continuation of External Carotid Artery

External Carotid Artery

Basilar Artery

Vertebral Artery

Common Carotid Artery

× 2·25

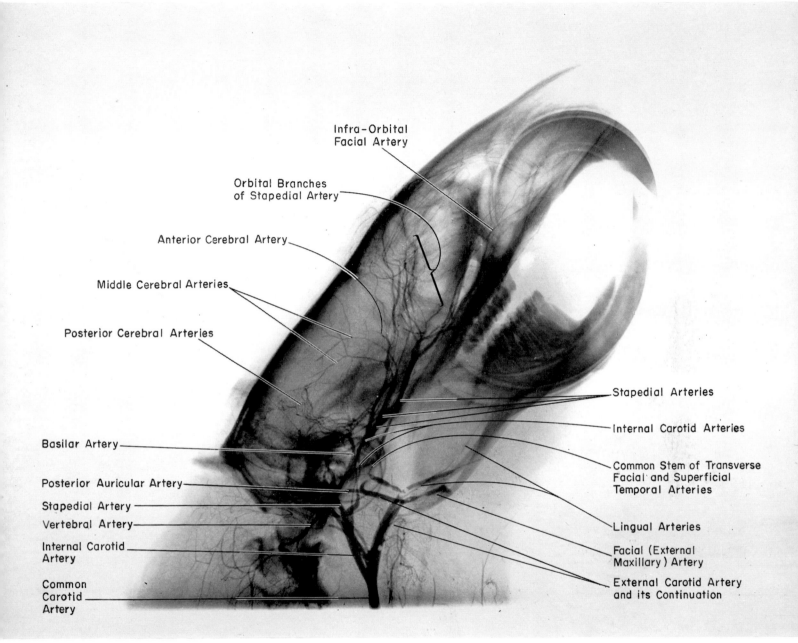

Infra-Orbital
Facial Artery

Orbital Branches
of Stapedial Artery

Anterior Cerebral Artery

Middle Cerebral Arteries

Posterior Cerebral Arteries

Stapedial Arteries

Internal Carotid Arteries

Basilar Artery

Common Stem of Transverse
Facial and Superficial
Temporal Arteries

Posterior Auricular Artery

Stapedial Artery

Vertebral Artery

Lingual Arteries

Internal Carotid
Artery

Facial (External
Maxillary) Artery

Common
Carotid
Artery

External Carotid Artery
and its Continuation

× 2·25

The standard myomorph pattern is illustrated. Internal carotid and vertebral arteries supply the Circle of Willis. There is a large stapedial artery.

The internal maxillary is rudimentary (and invisible in this specimen.

The large internal ethmoidal arteries are seen running forwards from the main stems of the anterior cerebral arteries.

Bucco-labial branches are too small to label.

There is less good filling of many branches, particularly the lingual, in the lateral view.

Hystrix leucura
Porcupine

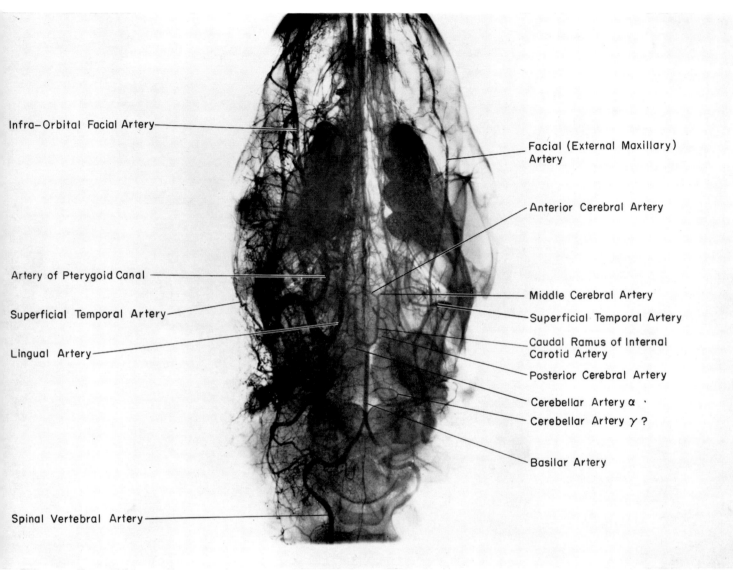

Infra–Orbital Facial Artery

Facial (External Maxillary) Artery

Anterior Cerebral Artery

Artery of Pterygoid Canal

Superficial Temporal Artery

Lingual Artery

Middle Cerebral Artery

Superficial Temporal Artery

Caudal Ramus of Internal Carotid Artery

Posterior Cerebral Artery

Cerebellar Artery α ·

Cerebellar Artery γ ?

Basilar Artery

Spinal Vertebral Artery

× 0·75

A typical hystricomorph.

Details of the blood vessels are hidden by the opacity of the quills and skull. Only the main vessels have been labelled.

The cerebral circulation is supplied solely by the vertebral arteries.

Cavia porcellus
Guinea Pig

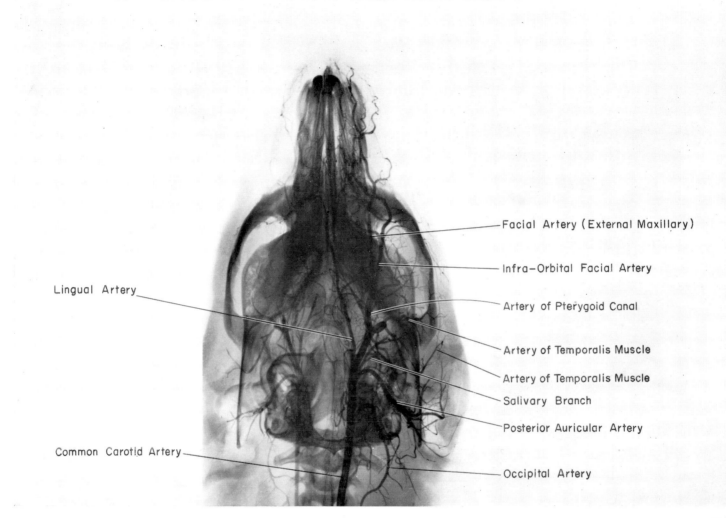

Facial Artery (External Maxillary)

Infra-Orbital Facial Artery

Lingual Artery

Artery of Pterygoid Canal

Artery of Temporalis Muscle

Artery of Temporalis Muscle

Salivary Branch

Posterior Auricular Artery

Common Carotid Artery

Occipital Artery

$\times$ 1·4

The typical hystricomorph pattern is illustrated. The posteriorly-running anastomotic vessel from the middle meningeal towards the external carotid is fairly well developed.

In the lateral view the auricular and superficial temporal branches of the external carotid are obscured by the density of the petrous bone.

The anterior cerebral is not filled in its pericallosal course so this too is unlabelled in the lateral view.

The identification of the posterior cerebral arteries as β and γ depends upon the rather anterior origin of the one and the curved course of the other.

The artery which Tandler called the artery for temporalis muscle looks remarkably like a normal superficial temporal artery in the distal part of its course.

The artery we have labelled buccinator is presumptive.

The extremely important pathway external opthalmic—internal ophthalmic—internal carotid is clearly illustrated.

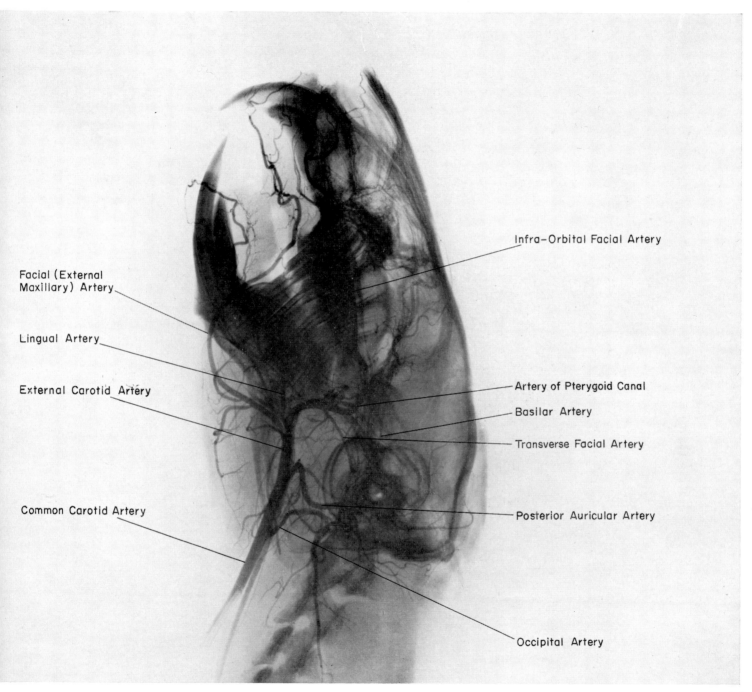

Infra-Orbital Facial Artery

Facial (External
Maxillary) Artery

Lingual Artery

External Carotid Artery

Artery of Pterygoid Canal

Basilar Artery

Transverse Facial Artery

Posterior Auricular Artery

Common Carotid Artery

Occipital Artery

× 2·6

Cavia porcellus

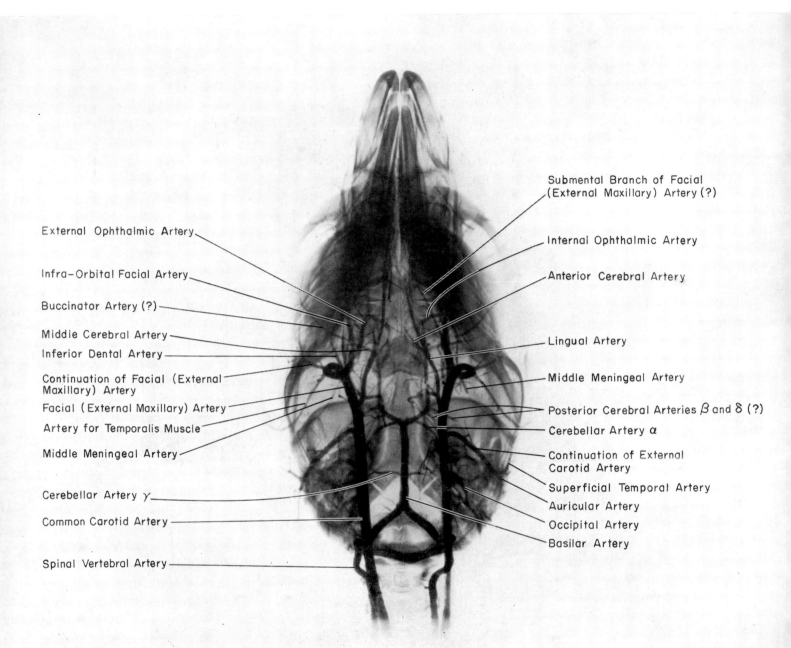

External Ophthalmic Artery

Infra–Orbital Facial Artery

Buccinator Artery (?)

Middle Cerebral Artery

Inferior Dental Artery

Continuation of Facial (External Maxillary) Artery

Facial (External Maxillary) Artery

Artery for Temporalis Muscle

Middle Meningeal Artery

Cerebellar Artery γ

Common Carotid Artery

Spinal Vertebral Artery

Submental Branch of Facial (External Maxillary) Artery (?)

Internal Ophthalmic Artery

Anterior Cerebral Artery

Lingual Artery

Middle Meningeal Artery

Posterior Cerebral Arteries β and δ (?)

Cerebellar Artery α

Continuation of External Carotid Artery

Superficial Temporal Artery

Auricular Artery

Occipital Artery

Basilar Artery

× 3·0

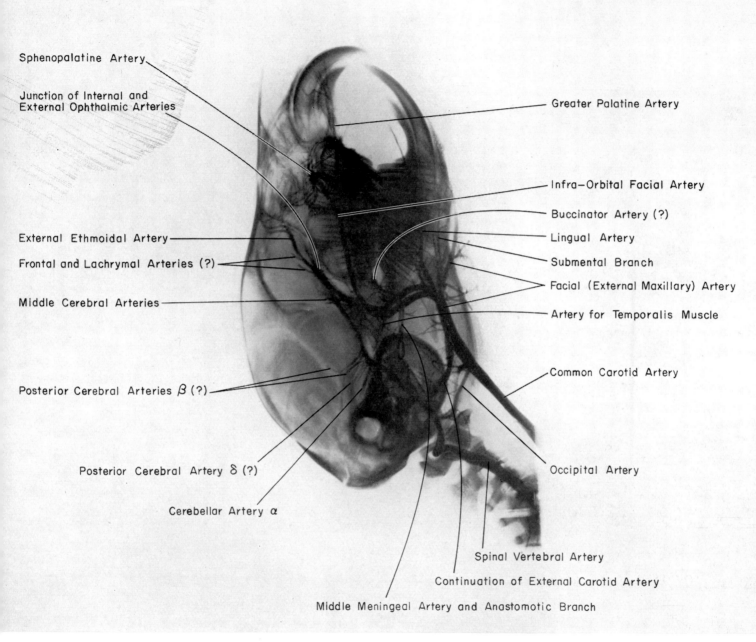

Sphenopalatine Artery

Junction of Internal and
External Ophthalmic Arteries

Greater Palatine Artery

Infra—Orbital Facial Artery

Buccinator Artery (?)

Lingual Artery

External Ethmoidal Artery

Frontal and Lachrymal Arteries (?)

Submental Branch

Facial (External Maxillary) Artery

Middle Cerebral Arteries

Artery for Temporalis Muscle

Common Carotid Artery

Posterior Cerebral Arteries β (?)

Posterior Cerebral Artery δ (?)

Occipital Artery

Cerebellar Artery α

Spinal Vertebral Artery

Continuation of External Carotid Artery

Middle Meningeal Artery and Anastomotic Branch

× 3·0

Galea musteloides
Cuis

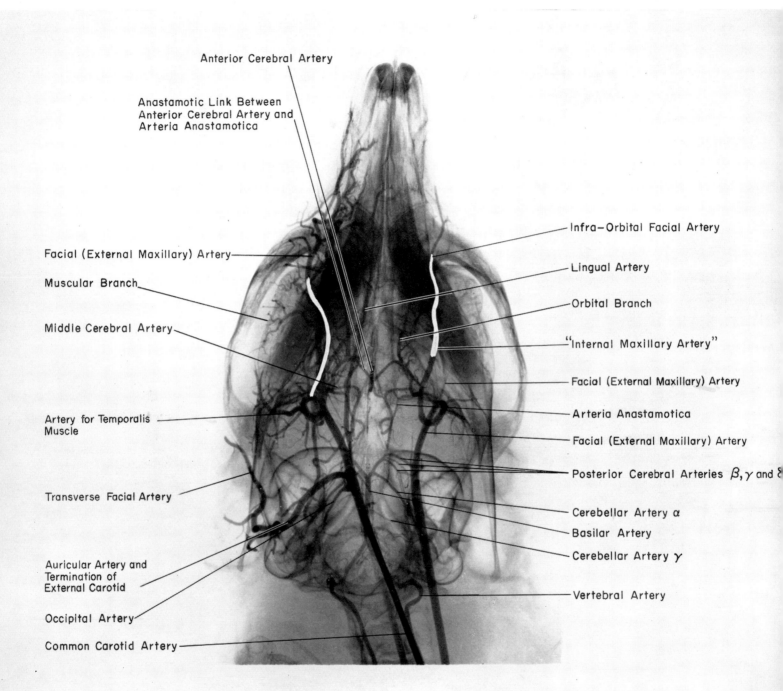

Anterior Cerebral Artery

Anastamotic Link Between
Anterior Cerebral Artery and
Arteria Anastamotica

Facial (External Maxillary) Artery

Muscular Branch

Middle Cerebral Artery

Artery for Temporalis
Muscle

Transverse Facial Artery

Auricular Artery and
Termination of
External Carotid

Occipital Artery

Common Carotid Artery

Infra-Orbital Facial Artery

Lingual Artery

Orbital Branch

"Internal Maxillary Artery"

Facial (External Maxillary) Artery

Arteria Anastamotica

Facial (External Maxillary) Artery

Posterior Cerebral Arteries β, γ and δ

Cerebellar Artery α

Basilar Artery

Cerebellar Artery γ

Vertebral Artery

× 2·5

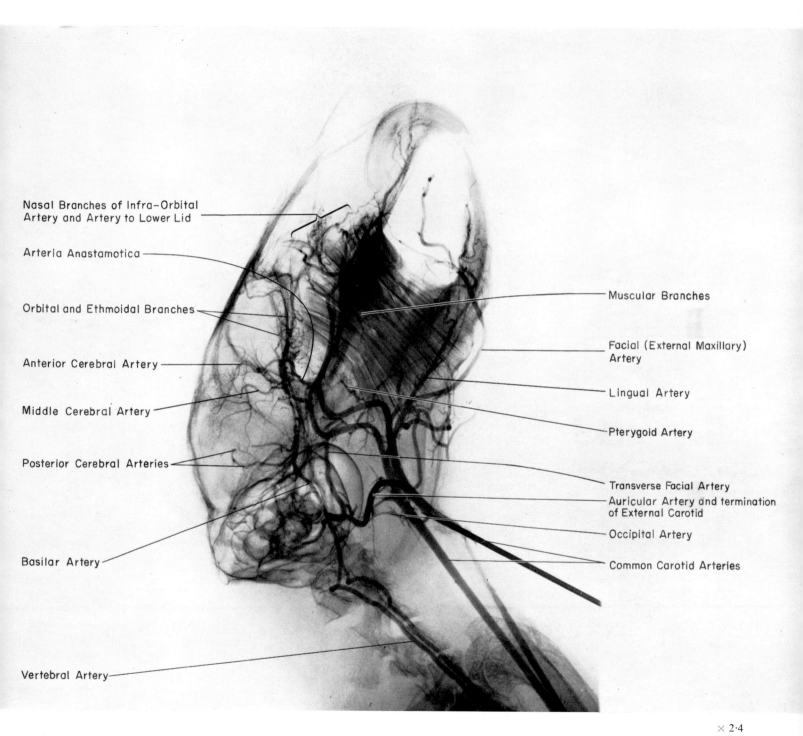

Nasal Branches of Infra-Orbital
Artery and Artery to Lower Lid

Arteria Anastamotica

Orbital and Ethmoidal Branches

Anterior Cerebral Artery

Middle Cerebral Artery

Posterior Cerebral Arteries

Basilar Artery

Vertebral Artery

Muscular Branches

Facial (External Maxillary)
Artery

Lingual Artery

Pterygoid Artery

Transverse Facial Artery

Auricular Artery and termination
of External Carotid

Occipital Artery

Common Carotid Arteries

× 2·4

A somewhat atypical hystricomorph.

The auricular artery is very large, from its anterior branch comes a forwardly directed superficial temporal. No deep temporal artery has been developed.

The arteria anastomotica, from the internal maxillary, supplies both the termination of the internal carotid and the main orbital branches, the largest of which is medially placed and seems to form a supra-orbital trunk with numerous ethmoidal and ciliary twigs. There may be a second connection to the Circle of Willis between the arteria anastomotica via the orbit and the anterior cerebral artery. The first part of one anterior cerebral artery in our specimen is hypoplastic; but two extra vessels run from the junction of the arteria anastomotica and the orbital artery to join the common anterior cerebral over the genu of the corpus callosum.

Dolichotis patagonum
Patagonian Cavey

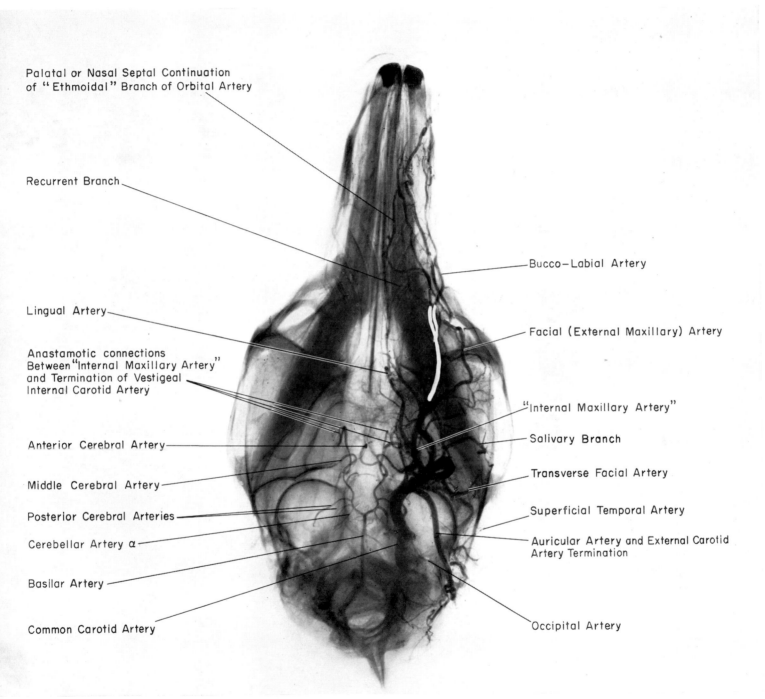

Palatal or Nasal Septal Continuation of "Ethmoidal" Branch of Orbital Artery

Recurrent Branch

Lingual Artery

Anastamotic connections Between "Internal Maxillary Artery" and Termination of Vestigeal Internal Carotid Artery

Anterior Cerebral Artery

Middle Cerebral Artery

Posterior Cerebral Arteries

Cerebellar Artery α

Basilar Artery

Common Carotid Artery

Bucco–Labial Artery

Facial (External Maxillary) Artery

"Internal Maxillary Artery"

Salivary Branch

Transverse Facial Artery

Superficial Temporal Artery

Auricular Artery and External Carotid Artery Termination

Occipital Artery

× 1·0

The Patagonian cavey does not resemble the standard hystricomorph pattern. Although the main stem of the internal carotid artery has disappeared, its distal end remains and, as in Sciuromorpha, derives its blood from an arteria anastomotica.

In this specimen it is noted that on one side (the right) there appear to be two such anastomotic arteries one of which supplies a large ophthalmic artery and thus acquires a secondary connection with the Circle of Willis. Thus something akin to a simple rete caroticum has developed.

The basilar artery is not particularly large.

The posterior cerebrals may be β and γ (Hofmann).

The very large auricular artery has more or less taken over from the occipital and also supplies a superficial temporal branch.

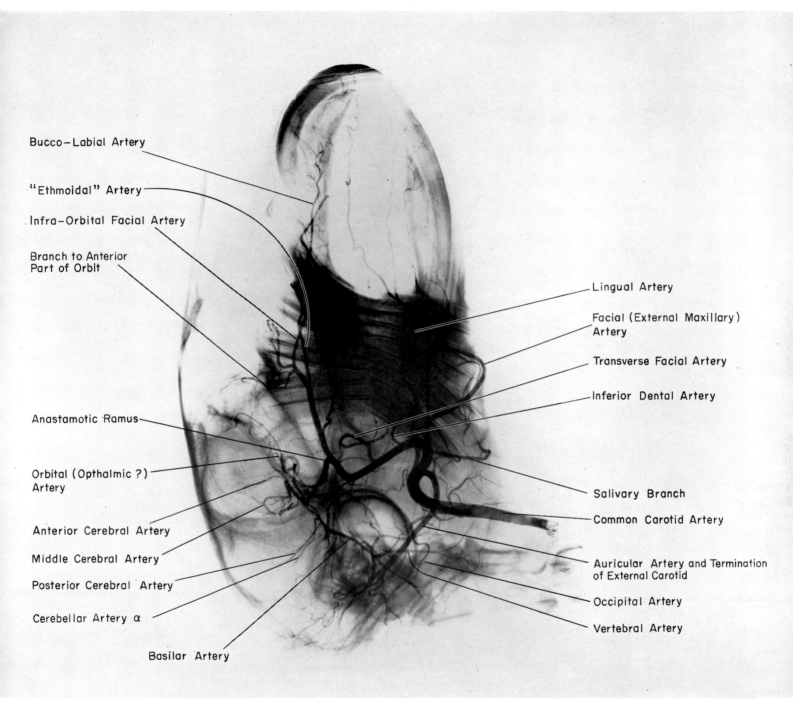

Bucco—Labial Artery

"Ethmoidal" Artery

Infra—Orbital Facial Artery

Branch to Anterior
Part of Orbit

Anastamotic Ramus

Orbital (Opthalmic ?)
Artery

Anterior Cerebral Artery

Middle Cerebral Artery

Posterior Cerebral Artery

Cerebellar Artery α

Basilar Artery

Lingual Artery

Facial (External Maxillary)
Artery

Transverse Facial Artery

Inferior Dental Artery

Salivary Branch

Common Carotid Artery

Auricular Artery and Termination
of External Carotid

Occipital Artery

Vertebral Artery

× 1·0

Myoprocta pratti
Green Acouchy

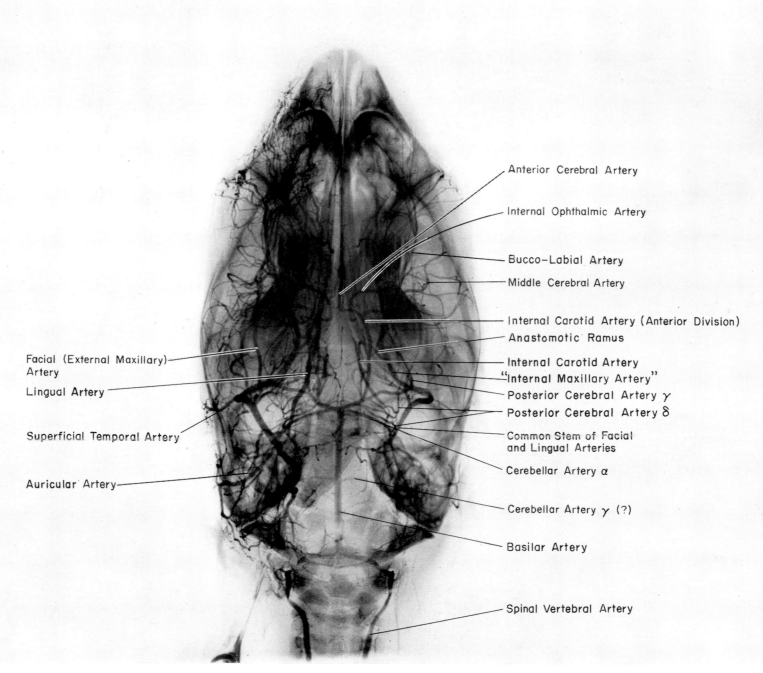

Anterior Cerebral Artery

Internal Ophthalmic Artery

Bucco-Labial Artery

Middle Cerebral Artery

Internal Carotid Artery (Anterior Division)

Anastomotic Ramus

Internal Carotid Artery

"Internal Maxillary Artery"

Posterior Cerebral Artery γ

Posterior Cerebral Artery δ

Common Stem of Facial
and Lingual Arteries

Cerebellar Artery α

Cerebellar Artery γ (?)

Basilar Artery

Spinal Vertebral Artery

Facial (External Maxillary)
Artery

Lingual Artery

Superficial Temporal Artery

Auricular Artery

$\times 3 \cdot 4$

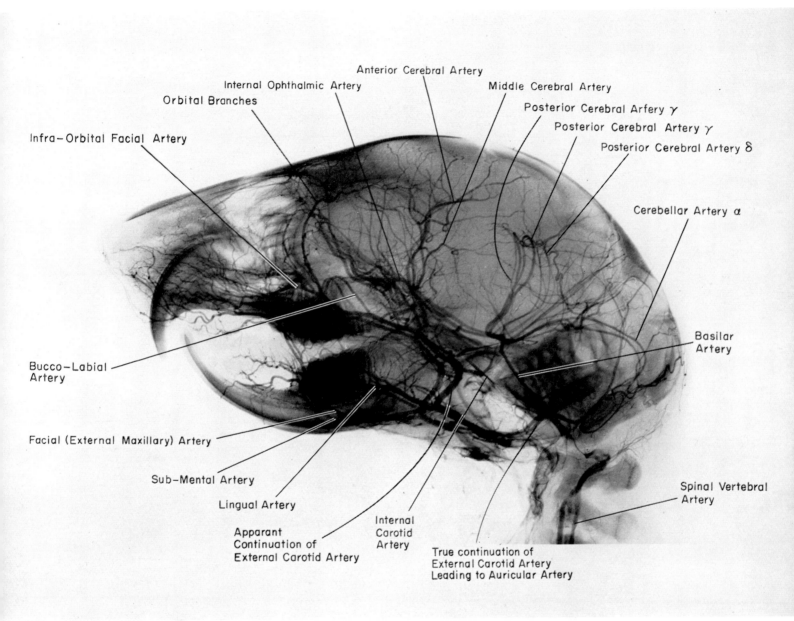

Anterior Cerebral Artery

Internal Ophthalmic Artery

Middle Cerebral Artery

Orbital Branches

Posterior Cerebral Artery γ

Infra-Orbital Facial Artery

Posterior Cerebral Artery γ

Posterior Cerebral Artery δ

Cerebellar Artery α

Basilar Artery

Bucco-Labial Artery

Facial (External Maxillary) Artery

Spinal Vertebral Artery

Sub-Mental Artery

Lingual Artery

Internal Carotid Artery

Apparant Continuation of External Carotid Artery

True continuation of External Carotid Artery Leading to Auricular Artery

× 3·5

A fairly typical hystricomorph.

Injection has filled the intracranial and orbital vessels better than the occipital and auricular supply. The eye and brain seem large in comparison with the size of the head.

The common carotid divides unequally into a small internal and a large external carotid.

The internal ophthalmic arteries are very large. The infra-orbital facial continuation of the "internal maxillary" artery also supplies what appear to be large branches to the lower lid and large supra-orbital branches which course around the anterior orbital margin and also supply twigs to the ethmoid air-cells.

The Circle of Willis in this specimen is barely complete since the right anterior cerebral is hypoplastic.

There appears to be β, γ and δ posterior cerebral arteries.

The very long course of the cerebellar artery γ (or β) is well shown.

In the ventro-dorsal view the name "internal maxillary" has been used for brevity, though it is realised that this section of artery is not strictly speaking the internal maxillary.

Lagostomus maximus
Plains Viscacha

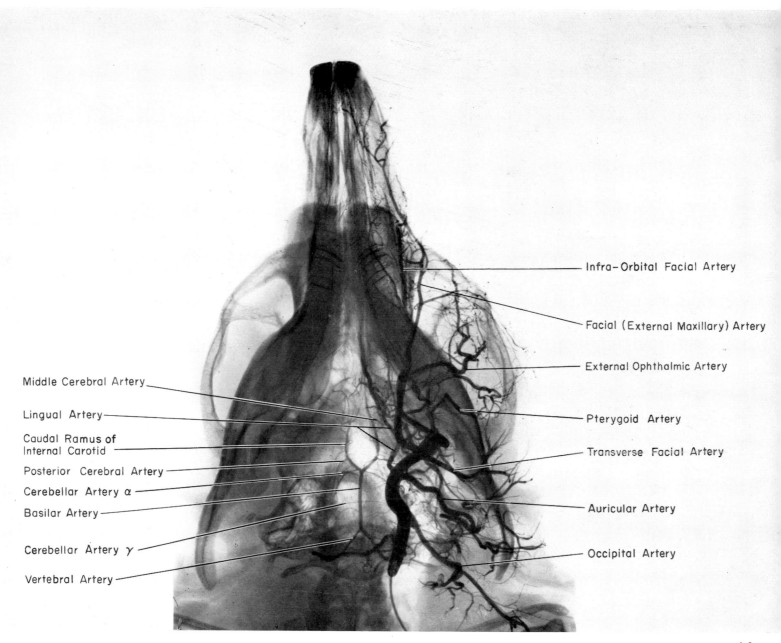

Infra-Orbital Facial Artery

Facial (External Maxillary) Artery

External Ophthalmic Artery

Pterygoid Artery

Transverse Facial Artery

Auricular Artery

Occipital Artery

Middle Cerebral Artery

Lingual Artery

Caudal Ramus of Internal Carotid

Posterior Cerebral Artery

Cerebellar Artery α

Basilar Artery

Cerebellar Artery γ

Vertebral Artery

× 1·0

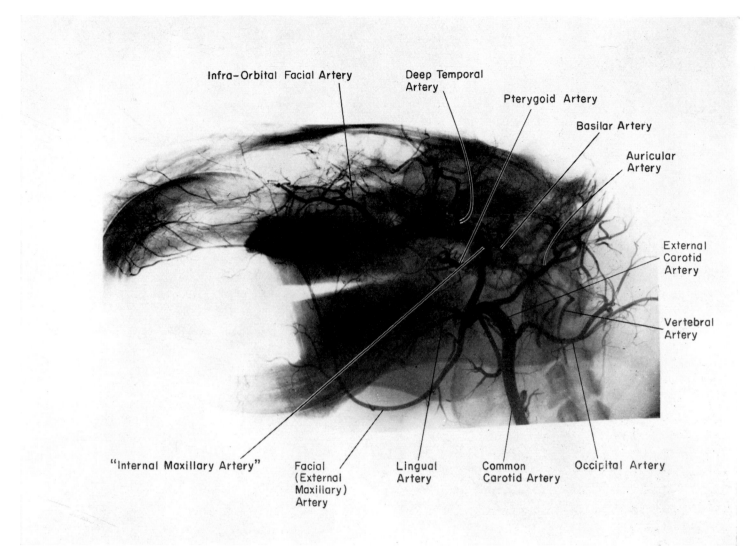

Infra-Orbital Facial Artery

Deep Temporal Artery

Pterygoid Artery

Basilar Artery

Auricular Artery

External Carotid Artery

Vertebral Artery

"Internal Maxillary Artery"

Facial (External Maxillary) Artery

Lingual Artery

Common Carotid Artery

Occipital Artery

× 1·0

A typical hystricomorph.

Posterior cerebral arteries may be β, γ and δ (Hofmann).

Cerebellar arteries may be α, γ and δ.

In the illustration the connection between the common trunk of the facial (external maxillary) and lingual and the artery of the pterygoid canal has been called "internal maxillary artery".

Lagidium pervanum
Mountain Viscacha

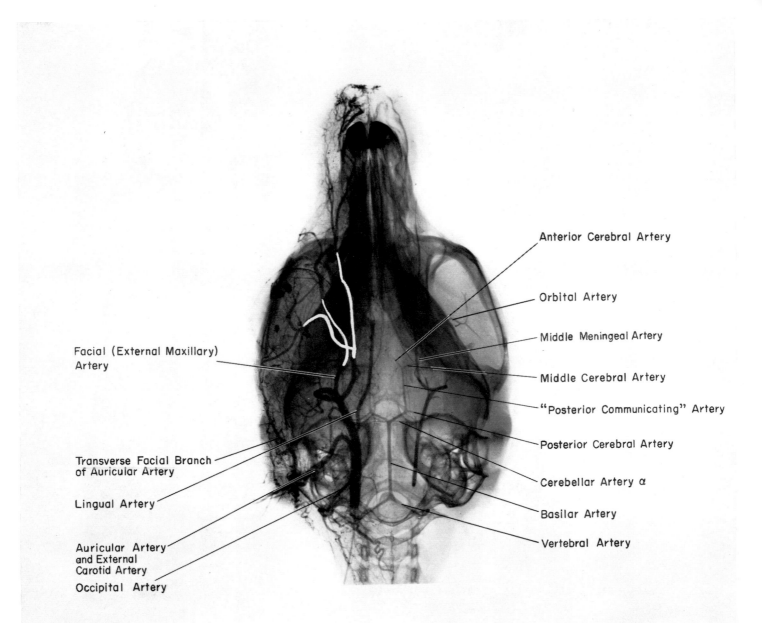

Anterior Cerebral Artery

Orbital Artery

Middle Meningeal Artery

Middle Cerebral Artery

"Posterior Communicating" Artery

Posterior Cerebral Artery

Cerebellar Artery α

Basilar Artery

Vertebral Artery

Facial (External Maxillary) Artery

Transverse Facial Branch of Auricular Artery

Lingual Artery

Auricular Artery and External Carotid Artery

Occipital Artery

× 1·8

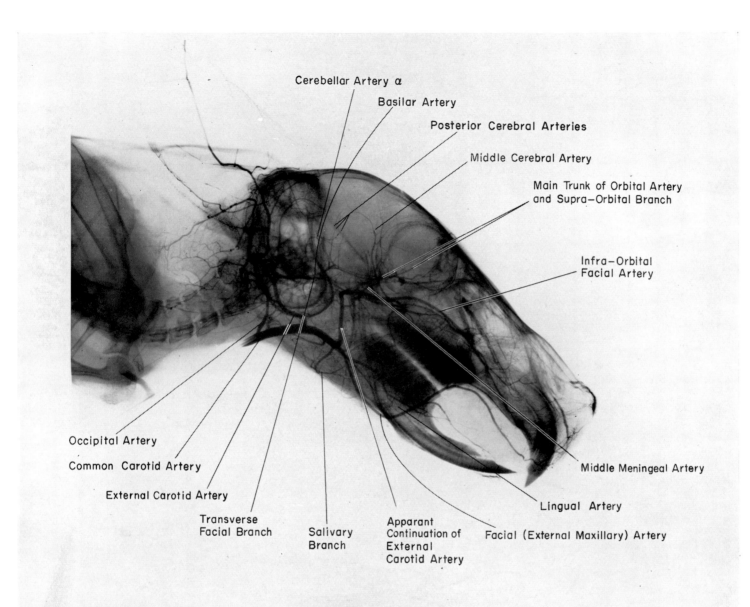

Cerebellar Artery α

Basilar Artery

Posterior Cerebral Arteries

Middle Cerebral Artery

Main Trunk of Orbital Artery
and Supra—Orbital Branch

Infra—Orbital
Facial Artery

Occipital Artery

Common Carotid Artery

External Carotid Artery

Transverse
Facial Branch

Salivary
Branch

Apparant
Continuation of
External
Carotid Artery

Middle Meningeal Artery

Lingual Artery

Facial (External Maxillary) Artery

× 1·6

In the main pattern a typical hystricomorph.

The whole cerebral supply comes from the vertebral arteries which have been shown to have free communication with the occipital arteries.

In order to provide a comparison with man the caudal limb of the internal carotid has been labelled "the posterior communicating artery".

The posterior cerebral arteries are probably γ and δ (Hofmann).

The anterior cerebral is very poorly outlined.

Myocastor coypus
Coypu Rat

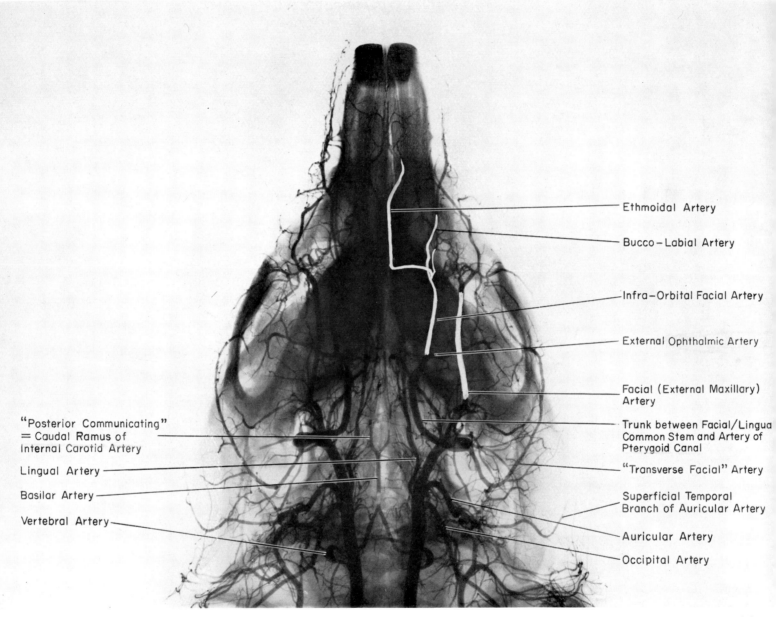

Ethmoidal Artery

Bucco-Labial Artery

Infra-Orbital Facial Artery

External Ophthalmic Artery

Facial (External Maxillary) Artery

Trunk between Facial/Lingua Common Stem and Artery of Pterygoid Canal

"Transverse Facial" Artery

Superficial Temporal Branch of Auricular Artery

Auricular Artery

Occipital Artery

"Posterior Communicating" = Caudal Ramus of Internal Carotid Artery

Lingual Artery

Basilar Artery

Vertebral Artery

× 1·0

A typical hystricomorph, resembling *Cavia porcellus*.

The internal carotid is entirely absent. The cerebral circulation is derived from the vertebral arteries. In the basal view their large spinal parts are obscured by the common carotids.

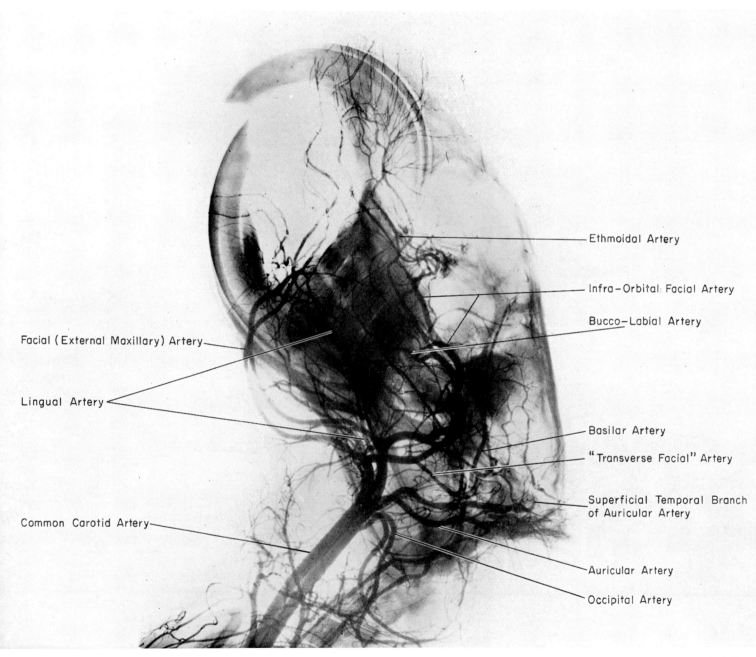

Ethmoidal Artery

Infra-Orbital Facial Artery

Bucco-Labial Artery

Facial (External Maxillary) Artery

Lingual Artery

Basilar Artery

"Transverse Facial" Artery

Superficial Temporal Branch of Auricular Artery

Common Carotid Artery

Auricular Artery

Occipital Artery

× 1·0

Octodon degus
Degu

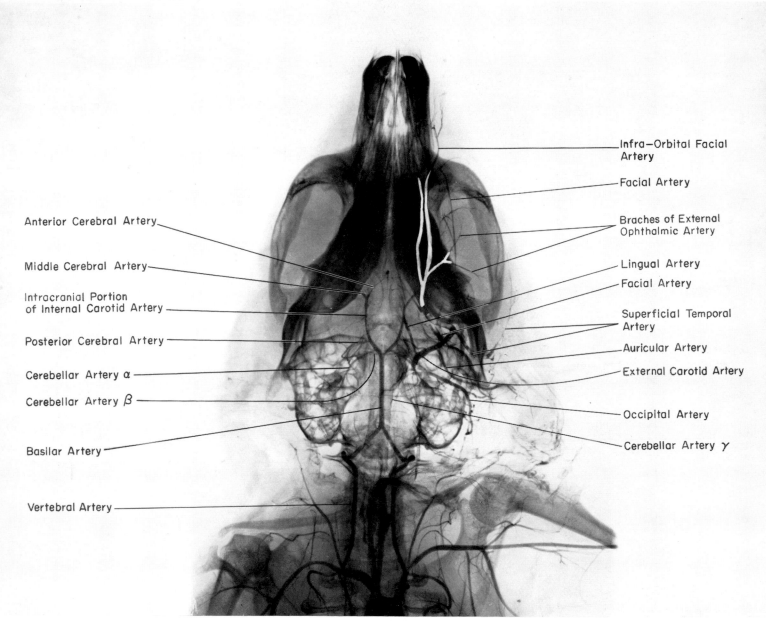

Infra–Orbital Facial Artery

Facial Artery

Braches of External Ophthalmic Artery

Lingual Artery

Facial Artery

Superficial Temporal Artery

Auricular Artery

External Carotid Artery

Occipital Artery

Cerebellar Artery γ

Anterior Cerebral Artery

Middle Cerebral Artery

Intracranial Portion of Internal Carotid Artery

Posterior Cerebral Artery

Cerebellar Artery α

Cerebellar Artery β

Basilar Artery

Vertebral Artery

× 2·6

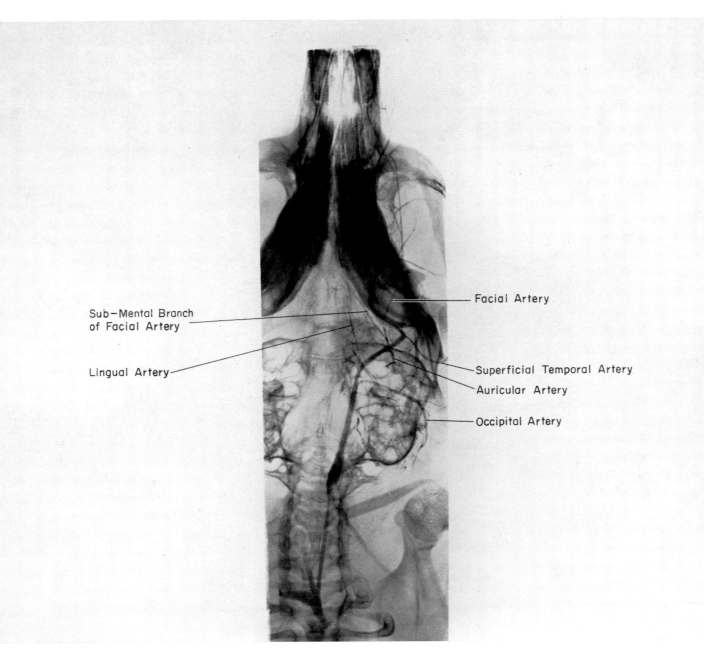

Sub–Mental Branch
of Facial Artery

Lingual Artery

Facial Artery

Superficial Temporal Artery

Auricular Artery

Occipital Artery

× 3·0

The external carotid is unlike that of *Cavia porcellus* but resembles the usual mammalian pattern.

One of the main branches of the external carotid in the neck, probably displaced during dissection, has not been identified.

The whole cerebral blood supply appears to derive from the spinal vertebral arteries.

The forward continuations from the basilar towards the anterior parts of the Circle of Willis, which must represent the caudal branches of the embryonic internal carotids have been labelled "posterior communicating arteries" in the lateral view.

Octogon degus

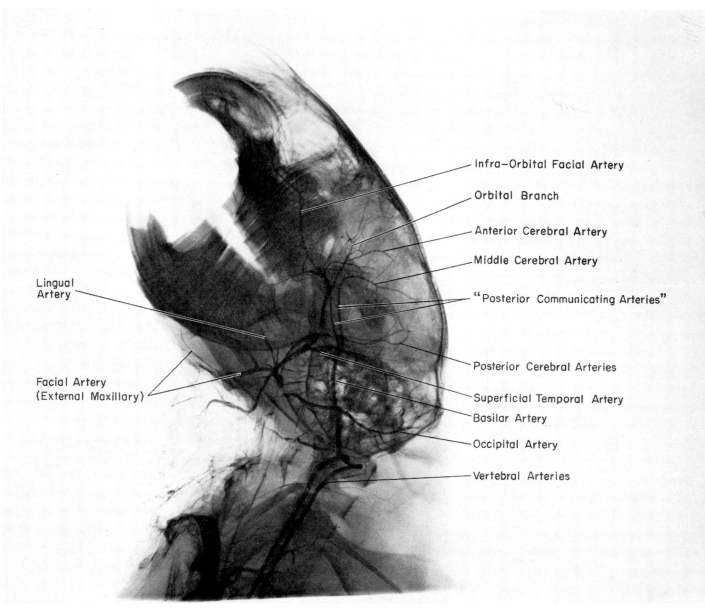

Infra–Orbital Facial Artery

Orbital Branch

Anterior Cerebral Artery

Middle Cerebral Artery

"Posterior Communicating Arteries"

Posterior Cerebral Arteries

Superficial Temporal Artery

Basilar Artery

Occipital Artery

Vertebral Arteries

Lingual Artery

Facial Artery (External Maxillary)

× 2·7

Ctenomys talarum mendocina
Tuco Tuco

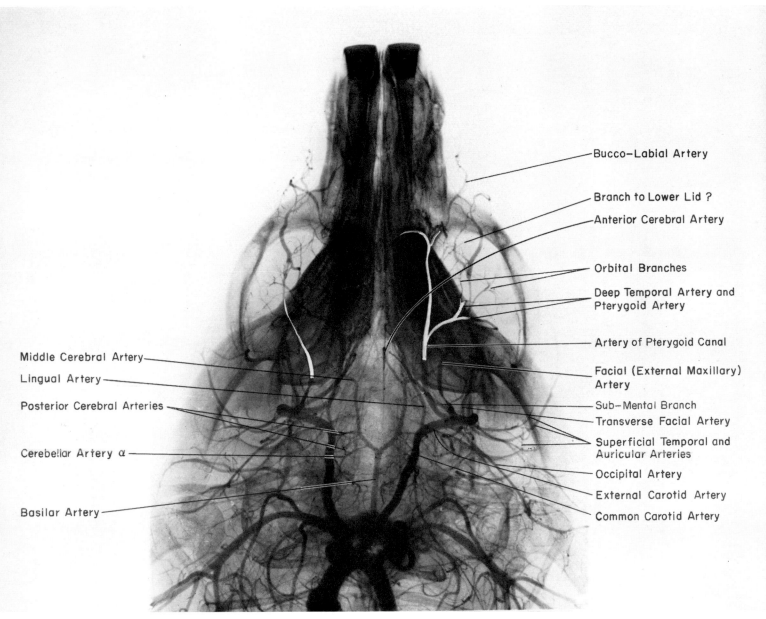

Bucco–Labial Artery

Branch to Lower Lid ?

Anterior Cerebral Artery

Orbital Branches

Deep Temporal Artery and
Pterygoid Artery

Artery of Pterygoid Canal

Facial (External Maxillary)
Artery

Sub–Mental Branch

Transverse Facial Artery

Superficial Temporal and
Auricular Arteries

Occipital Artery

External Carotid Artery

Common Carotid Artery

Middle Cerebral Artery

Lingual Artery

Posterior Cerebral Arteries

Cerebellar Artery α

Basilar Artery

× 3·0

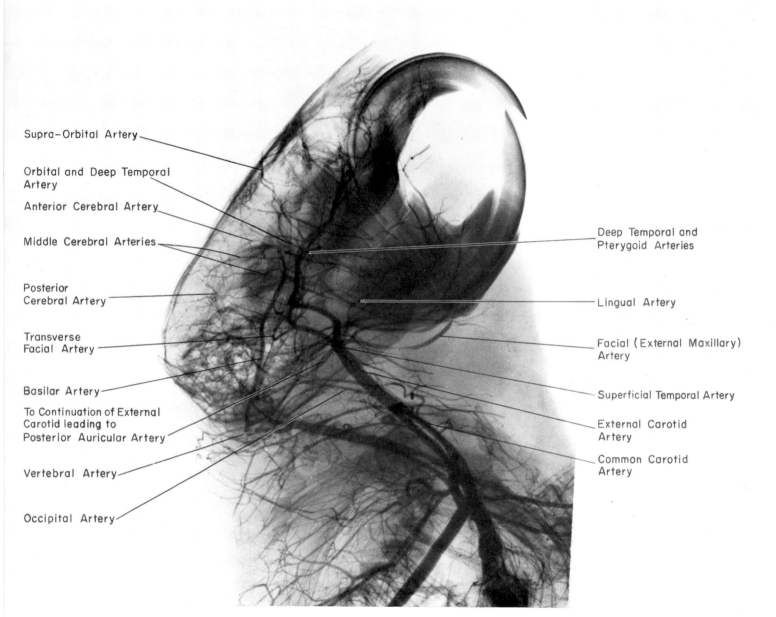

Supra–Orbital Artery

Orbital and Deep Temporal Artery

Anterior Cerebral Artery

Middle Cerebral Arteries

Posterior Cerebral Artery

Transverse Facial Artery

Basilar Artery

To Continuation of External Carotid leading to Posterior Auricular Artery

Vertebral Artery

Occipital Artery

Deep Temporal and Pterygoid Arteries

Lingual Artery

Facial (External Maxillary) Artery

Superficial Temporal Artery

External Carotid Artery

Common Carotid Artery

× 2·7

This is a typical hystricomorph with the usual reservations about the superficial temporal artery.

The internal carotid and the main stem and divisions of the stapedial artery have disappeared.

There is neither an arteria anastomotica nor a ramus anastomoticus and the whole of the brain's blood supply appears to come from the vertebral arteries.

The posterior cerebral arteries are probably β, γ and δ, the β being the largest.

The γ cerebellar artery may be seen in the original radiograph.

It appears probable that a deep temporal branch arises from the same area as the orbital branches of the internal maxillary artery.

Tursiops truncatus
Bottlenosed Dolphin

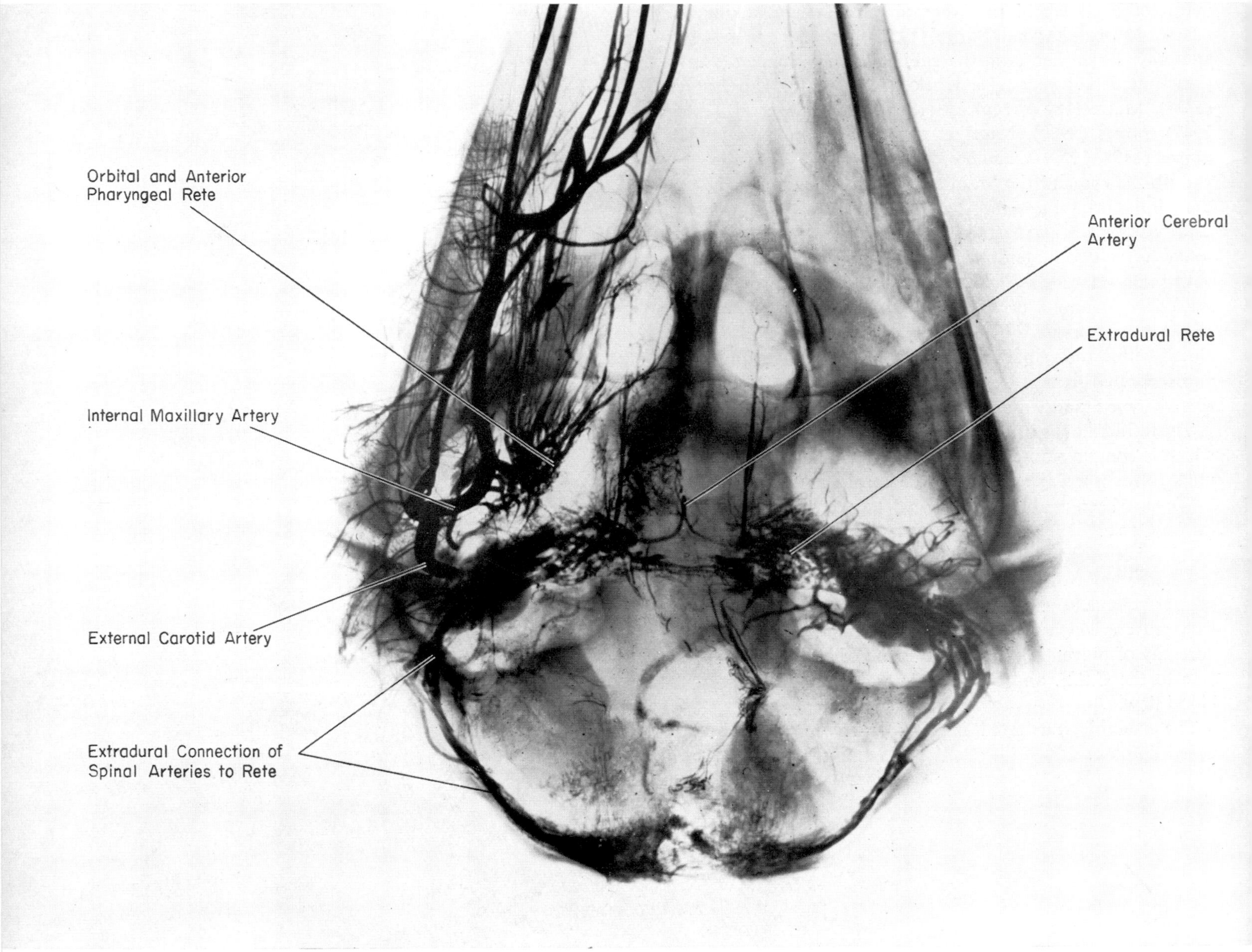

Orbital and Anterior
Pharyngeal Rete

Anterior Cerebral
Artery

Extradural Rete

Internal Maxillary Artery

External Carotid Artery

Extradural Connection of
Spinal Arteries to Rete

× 0·6

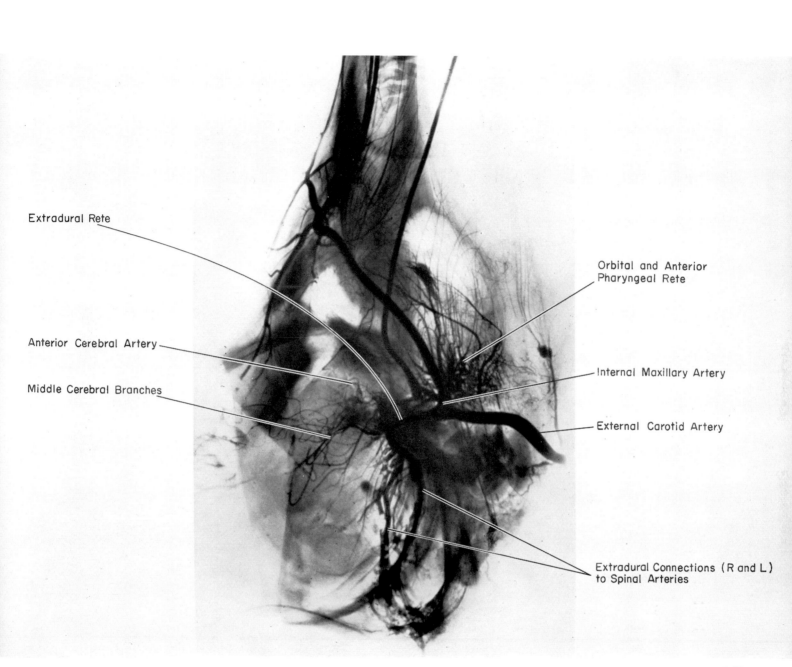

Extradural Rete

Orbital and Anterior
Pharyngeal Rete

Anterior Cerebral Artery

Internal Maxillary Artery

Middle Cerebral Branches

External Carotid Artery

Extradural Connections (R and L)
to Spinal Arteries

× 0·55

Carnivora

The variety of form exhibited by the normal arterial tree is so great that generalisations are apt to be more misleading than helpful.

The most arresting of peculiarities, a rete is possessed by all the *Felidae* but does not occur in any well developed form among other families in the order except the *Hyaenidae*. Nevertheless, free communications between the external and internal carotid systems are the rule rather than the exception among Carnivora and it would not be surprising to find that these anastomotic channels serve part of the function of the rete in controlling cerebral blood flow in a way rather different from that of primates. Apart from the major peculiarity of the cerebral blood supply in *Felidae*, less obvious family characteristics distinguish the Carnivora as will appear.

There are also a few general tendencies which seem to unite the Carnivora, though they are not quite universal throughout the order. These are firstly that the occipital artery is often relatively small and much of the blood supply to the posterior part of the scalp is taken over by the auricular (posterior auricular) and secondly that both the facial (external maxillary) and the transverse facial arteries are usually small and unimportant vessels.

Reasons for the diminuation of size of the occipital artery may be found in the relatively posterior placement of the external ears dictated presumably by the very extensive origin of the muscles of mastication. Furthermore, in many species the occipital arteries provide only a little reinforcement to the vertebral/anterior spinal/basilar anterial complex whose main connections with the cervical extra-spinal arteries lie at C.3 rather than C.1.

The reason for the small size of the facial arteries may also be connected with the carnivorous habit and consequent adaptations of the mouth which is nearly always wide and capable of a large gape. This interferes with the course taken by the facial artery towards the medial side of the orbit. In these circumstances those branches of the facial (external maxillary artery) which supply structures in the floor of the mouth tend to be larger than the small artery which crosses the mandible and ascends over the cheek.

Davies and Story (1943) who made the most comprehensive account of the cranial arterial anatomy of the cat so far published have summed up the relationships between *Felidae* and the rest of the Carnivora in the following terms. "All the important adaptations found in the domestic cat are present in some form in all except the bears and giant panda; the latter appear to exhibit an entirely different trend.

(a) The three anastomoses (arteria anastomotica, ramus anastomoticus, ascending pharyngeal) are present in *Bassariscus* in the form of thread like vessels. These vessels presumably come from nutrient twigs to surrounding structures and are known to occur in non-carnivora.

(b) In *Viverridae* the caliber of the internal carotid is much reduced and the calibers of the anastomotic vessels are increased proportionately. There are also incipient retia mirabilia. Thus the condition in the *Viverridae* is almost exactly intermediate between the primitive pattern of *Bassariscus* and the highly specialised pattern of the *Felis domestica*.

(c) The large cats (*Panthera*) resemble *Felis* closely, but are slightly less extensive: the minute internal carotid is often (usually?) perforate and the distal end of the ascending pharyngeal resembles that of non-felid carnivora.

(d) The pattern of the *Hyaenidae* is known only from Tandler's incomplete description, but as far as is known agrees with that of the *Felidae*.

(e) Thus the Carnivora may be arranged in a closely graded series leading from the least aberrant pattern (*Bassariscus*) which differs little from that of other mammals to the extremely specialised pattern of *Felis domestica*. The transition thus exhibited agrees closely with the changes that take place in the pattern during ontogenesis in *Felis*.

(f) Therefore the cause for the carotid specialisation in *Felis* is probably to be sought in such a form as *Bassariscus*, rather than in the highly specialised *Felis* itself."

The pattern in the *Hyaenidae* referred to above is newly illustrated in this chapter.

Canidae

The anatomy of the cranial arteries of the dog is well-known and has been described on many previous occasions. Tandler (1899) and Hofmann (1900) were among the first to write detailed accounts of the extra- and intracranial vessels. Jewell (1952) and de la Torre *et al.* (1959) have added to our knowledge.

Very little variation from their basic description has been found in the injection radiographs of other species of *Canidae* published here.

Because of its frequent use for experimental purposes and because veterinary surgery is sometimes concerned with the diagnosis of intracranial tumours in dogs by means of angiography, a moderately detailed description of the cranial arteries of the dog is given.

It might be wise to consider the physiological implications of the free communication of internal maxillary artery and internal carotid and not to take for granted that the dog provides an adequate model for experiments designed to throw light upon human physiology.

After giving off the thyroid artery, the common carotid divides into external and internal carotids.

The external carotid—This represents the continuation of the main stem of the common carotid. It usually gives immediate origin to the occipital artery, though this may also arise in the angle between the external and internal carotids. Cervical branches of the occipital artery anastomose with cervical branches of the vertebral. Continuing towards the head, the external carotid gives off the lingual artery, a small sub-lingual and then the facial (external maxillary). It bends behind the mandible, gives off a large posterior auricular artery and the superficial temporal and then continues medial to the lower jaw as the internal maxillary artery.

The first branches of the internal maxillary (the inferior dental and the deep temporal) leave it almost at once. It then crosses the third division of the 5th nerve to continue on its medial side giving off the ramus anastomoticus which enters the head through foramen ovale and after giving rise to a middle meningeal artery of variable size, anastomoses with the arteria anastomotica within the cavernous sinus, thus supplying the internal carotid. Either the arteria anastomotica or the ramus anastomoticus may be small in any individual.

The internal maxillary then passes through the short pterygoid canal and joins the second division of the 5th nerve. Immediately after leaving the pterygoid canal, the internal maxillary artery gives rise to a large orbital ramus which runs from below into the orbit. Either from the main stem of this or from one of its branches comes the arteria anastomotica which turns backwards into the head through the orbital fissure to join the internal carotid. There is also an anastomosis between the arteria anastomotica and the external ophthalmic after that artery has entered the orbit via the optic foramen. The orbital ramus of the internal maxillary artery also gives off the ethmoidal, frontal, lachrymal and ciliary arteries. Finally the internal maxillary artery, after giving off the bucco-labial branch comes to lie in the infra-orbital canal.

The internal carotid artery divides immediately after perforating the dura into a large cranial branch and a weak caudal one.

The first branch of the cranial ramus is a moderately large internal ophthalmic which enters the orbit through the optic canal. The cranial ramus then divides into a large middle cerebral artery and a small anterior cerebral. This latter joins with the opposite anterior cerebral to complete the Circle of Willis; but often again separates so that there may either be one or two pericallosal arteries for part or all of the distance to the splenium where their terminal branches unite with those of the posterior cerebral γ.

The middle cerebral is said to give off one, or occasionally two weak anterior choroidal arteries; it turns around the front of the uncus and sends an anterior olfactory artery forwards and one or more posterior olfactory branches.

In the Sylvian fissure the main stem of the middle cerebral divides into three branches, anterior, middle and posterior which supply between them the lateral side of the cerebral cortex, the anterior branch providing pial anastomosis with the anterior cerebral artery over the frontal lobe.

The anterior cerebral first supplies a narrow lateral artery to the olfactory bulb. Close to the midline it supplies an ethmoidal artery, a twig from which anastomoses in the region of the cribriform plate with the ethmoidal branch of the internal maxillary.

Close to the midline, while still on the brain's base, the anterior cerebral gives rise to a marginal artery which follows the edge of the cortex to the medial side of the occipital pole. Soon after its origin this artery often gives rise to a medial artery of the olfactory bulb. The terminal branch of the anterior cerebral artery is the artery of the corpus callosum (pericallosal artery) which supplies twigs to the medial surface of the hemisphere, some turning over the top onto the lateral cortex where they join the pial branches of the middle cerebral.

The caudal rami of the internal carotid turn backwards and after giving off numerous small arteries to the hypothalamus, the posterior perforated substance and the cerebral peduncles unite with one another at the top of the basilar artery.

Laterally the caudal rami supply—
1. A weak anterior choroidal unless that has sprung from the middle cerebral.
2. Small vessels on the lateral side of the brainstem.
3. A small vessel which anastomoses with the posterior cerebral γ in front of the medial geniculate body.
4. A posterior cerebral artery γ (Hofmann) which, as well as numerous other branches, gives rise near its origin to a medial posterior choroidal artery.
5. The cerebellar artery α (Hofmann) which is large and in addition to numerous branches has anastomoses to the cerebellar artery δ.

The basilar artery is formed by the union of the two vertebrals which in turn receive their blood supply partly from the ventral rami of the two first spinal nerve arteries which in turn take it partly from the occipital vessels. These ventral rami have caudal and cranial branches and it is the cranial rami which unite to make the basilar. The caudal rami unite as the ventral spinal tract.

The basilar artery gives off—
1. Three or four pontine arteries.
2. A large superior trigeminal to the nerve root.
3. A narrow cerebellar artery β which stops short on the medulla.
4. One or two branches to the trapezoid body.
5. A narrow cerebellar artery γ often sharing a common stem with the internal auditory artery.
6. A row of branches to the medulla.
7. A cerebellar artery δ.
8. A whole row of central perforating arteries to the brain-stem.

The first spinal nerve root arteries also have dorsal rami, the larger caudal rami of which unite to form the upper part of the dorsal spinal arterial tract.

The ventral spinal tract is not a single vessel but forms a series of large meshes, the largest of which has been called the spinal arterial circle.

The 3rd spinal nerve artery is different from the others because of its great enlargement and represents the essential end of the spinal vertebral artery uniting by means of its ventral rami the ventral spinal arterial tract and the spinal vertebral arteries.

Canis lupus occidentalis
Timber Wolf

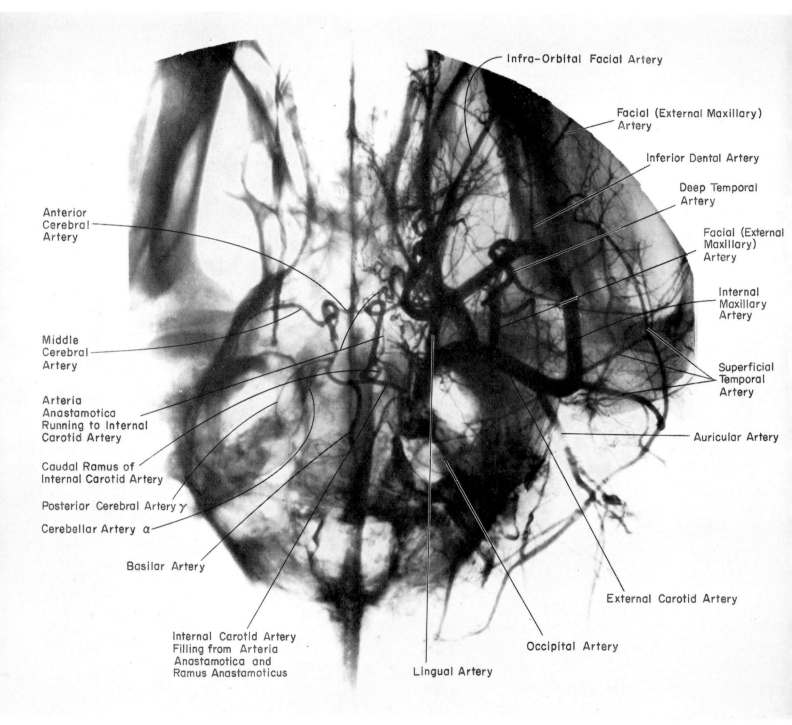

Infra-Orbital Facial Artery

Facial (External Maxillary) Artery

Inferior Dental Artery

Deep Temporal Artery

Facial (External Maxillary) Artery

Internal Maxillary Artery

Superficial Temporal Artery

Anterior Cerebral Artery

Middle Cerebral Artery

Arteria Anastamotica Running to Internal Carotid Artery

Caudal Ramus of Internal Carotid Artery

Posterior Cerebral Artery γ

Cerebellar Artery α

Basilar Artery

Auricular Artery

External Carotid Artery

Occipital Artery

Lingual Artery

Internal Carotid Artery Filling from Arteria Anastamotica and Ramus Anastamoticus

× 1·0

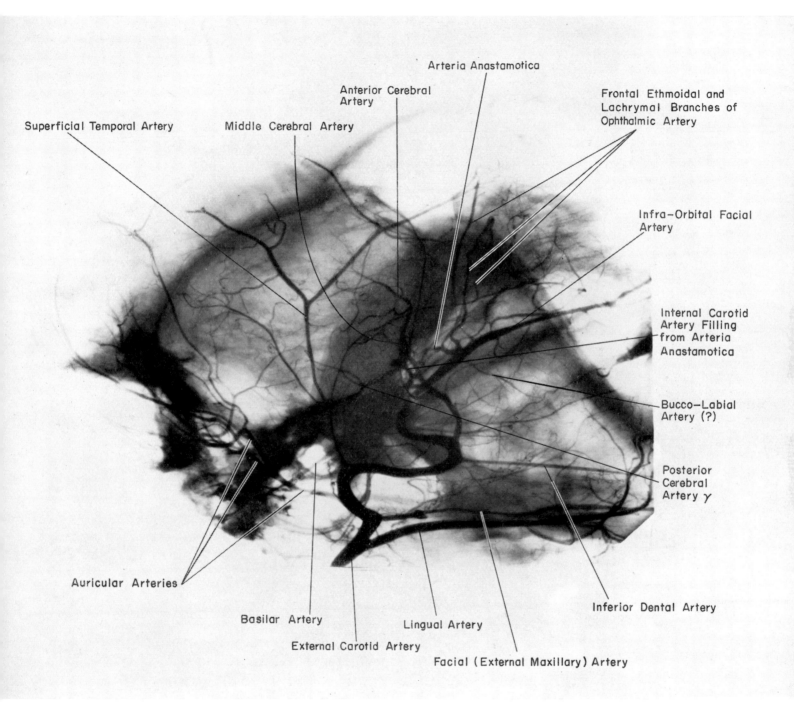

Arteria Anastamotica

Anterior Cerebral
Artery

Frontal Ethmoidal and
Lachrymal Branches of
Ophthalmic Artery

Superficial Temporal Artery

Middle Cerebral Artery

Infra—Orbital Facial
Artery

Internal Carotid
Artery Filling
from Arteria
Anastamotica

Bucco—Labial
Artery (?)

Posterior
Cerebral
Artery γ

Auricular Arteries

Inferior Dental Artery

Basilar Artery

Lingual Artery

External Carotid Artery

Facial (External Maxillary) Artery

× 1·0

The arrangement of the cranial arteries is characteristic of the *Canidae*. In this specimen the cervical portion of the internal carotid has not filled from below because of prior damage to the common carotid; but the intracranial portion of the internal carotid and the Circle of Willis are well outlined. The free communication which exists between the internal maxillary artery and the intracranial arterial system via the arteria anastomotica and the ramus anastomoticus in *Canidae* is thus very clearly shown.

The elaborate branching of the lingual artery is separately illustrated.

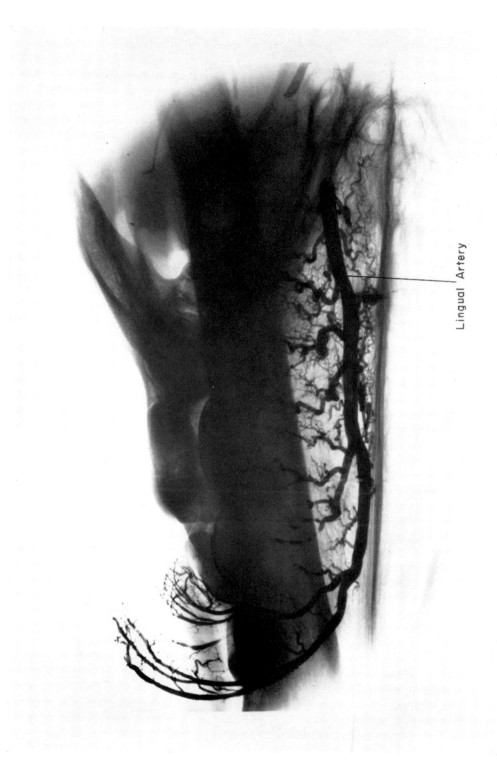

Lingual Artery

× 1·25

Canis latrans
Coyote

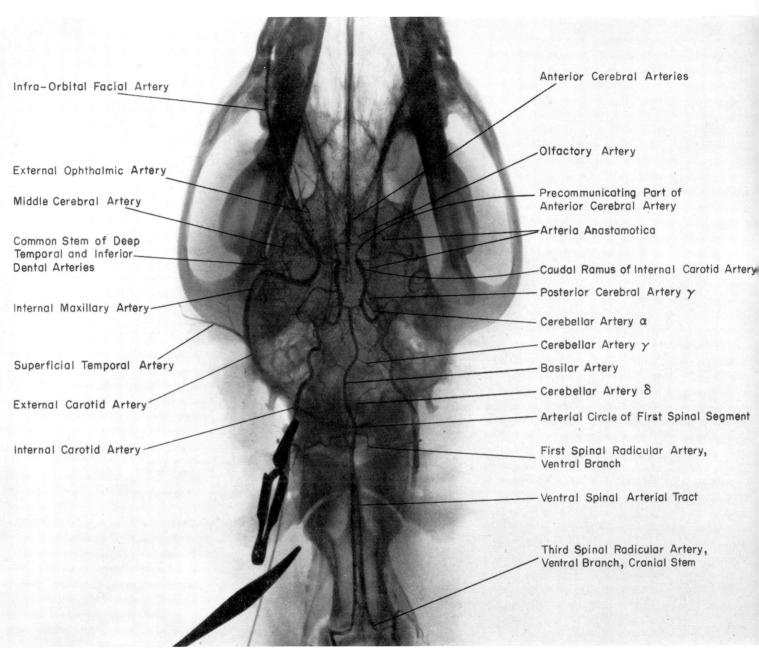

Infra-Orbital Facial Artery

External Ophthalmic Artery

Middle Cerebral Artery

Common Stem of Deep
Temporal and Inferior
Dental Arteries

Internal Maxillary Artery

Superficial Temporal Artery

External Carotid Artery

Internal Carotid Artery

Anterior Cerebral Arteries

Olfactory Artery

Precommunicating Part of
Anterior Cerebral Artery

Arteria Anastamotica

Caudal Ramus of Internal Carotid Artery

Posterior Cerebral Artery γ

Cerebellar Artery α

Cerebellar Artery γ

Basilar Artery

Cerebellar Artery δ

Arterial Circle of First Spinal Segment

First Spinal Radicular Artery,
Ventral Branch

Ventral Spinal Arterial Tract

Third Spinal Radicular Artery,
Ventral Branch, Cranial Stem

× 1·0

The external carotid branches are not well outlined, but the
intracranial circulation, which is typical, is well shown.

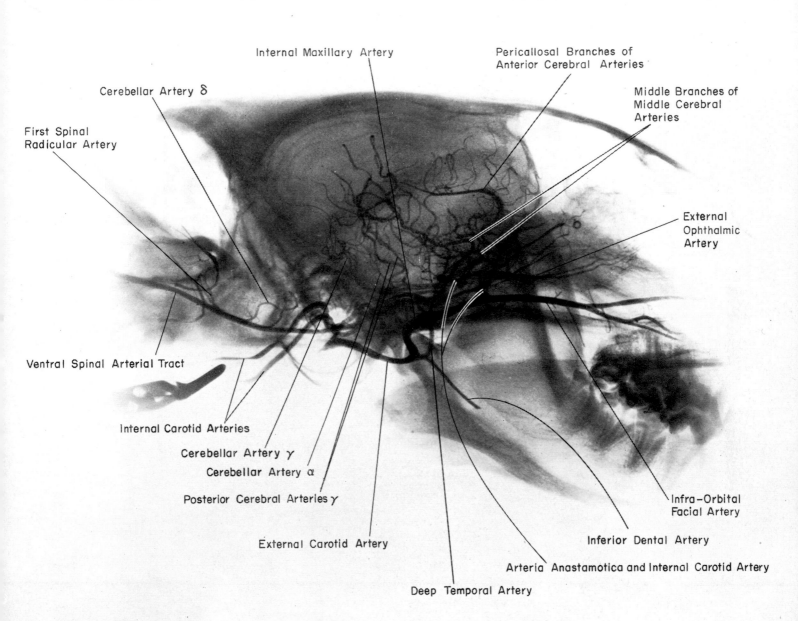

Internal Maxillary Artery

Pericallosal Branches of
Anterior Cerebral Arteries

Cerebellar Artery δ

Middle Branches of
Middle Cerebral
Arteries

First Spinal
Radicular Artery

External
Ophthalmic
Artery

Ventral Spinal Arterial Tract

Internal Carotid Arteries

Cerebellar Artery γ

Cerebellar Artery α

Infra–Orbital
Facial Artery

Posterior Cerebral Arteries γ

Inferior Dental Artery

External Carotid Artery

Arteria Anastamotica and Internal Carotid Artery

Deep Temporal Artery

× 1·0

Canis familiaris
Greyhound

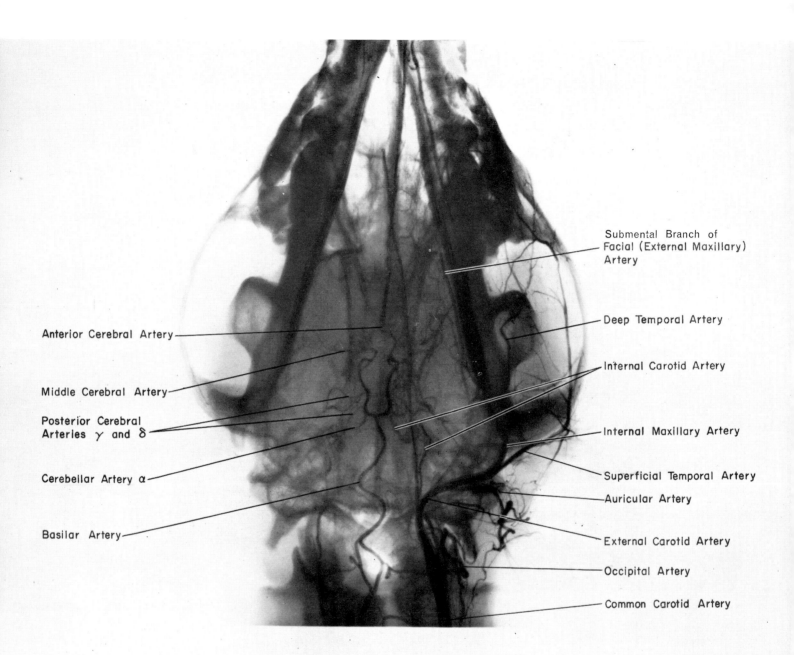

Submental Branch of Facial (External Maxillary) Artery

Deep Temporal Artery

Internal Carotid Artery

Internal Maxillary Artery

Superficial Temporal Artery

Auricular Artery

External Carotid Artery

Occipital Artery

Common Carotid Artery

Anterior Cerebral Artery

Middle Cerebral Artery

Posterior Cerebral Arteries γ and δ

Cerebellar Artery α

Basilar Artery

× 0·9

The arrangement of the vessels is similar to other *Canidae*. On the authority of Hofmann the largest posterior cerebral artery has been named γ.

In this specimen the anastomosis between the internal maxillary and the internal carotid is difficult to see.

The main trunk of the facial (external maxillary) continuing after the branch which Tandler called "sublingual" has left it, though filled with barium, is very faintly shown in the print. It is, as usual, a small vessel. The "sublingual" artery would be better called "submental".

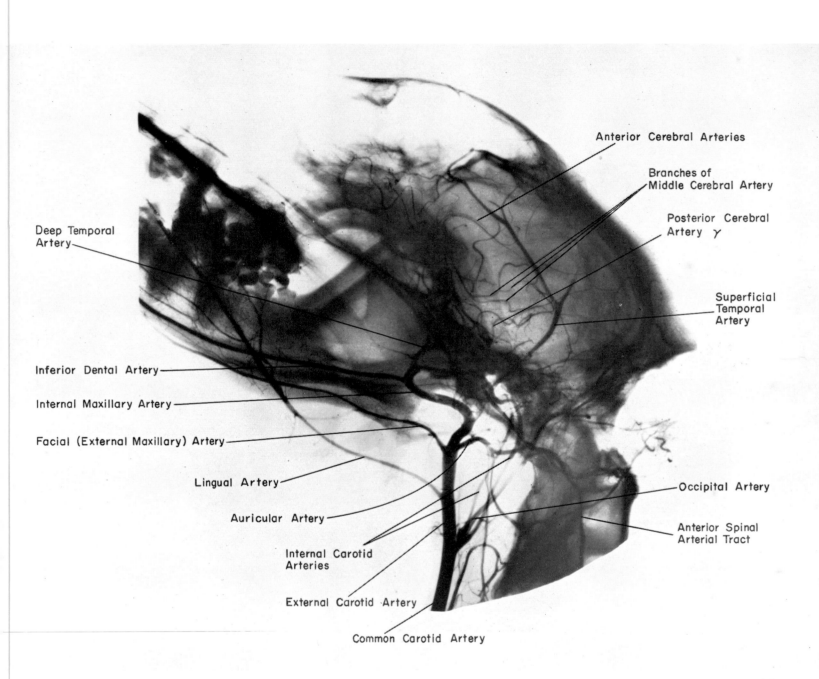

Deep Temporal Artery

Inferior Dental Artery

Internal Maxillary Artery

Facial (External Maxillary) Artery

Lingual Artery

Auricular Artery

Internal Carotid Arteries

External Carotid Artery

Common Carotid Artery

Anterior Cerebral Arteries

Branches of Middle Cerebral Artery

Posterior Cerebral Artery γ

Superficial Temporal Artery

Occipital Artery

Anterior Spinal Arterial Tract

× 0·8

Procyon lotor
North American Raccoon

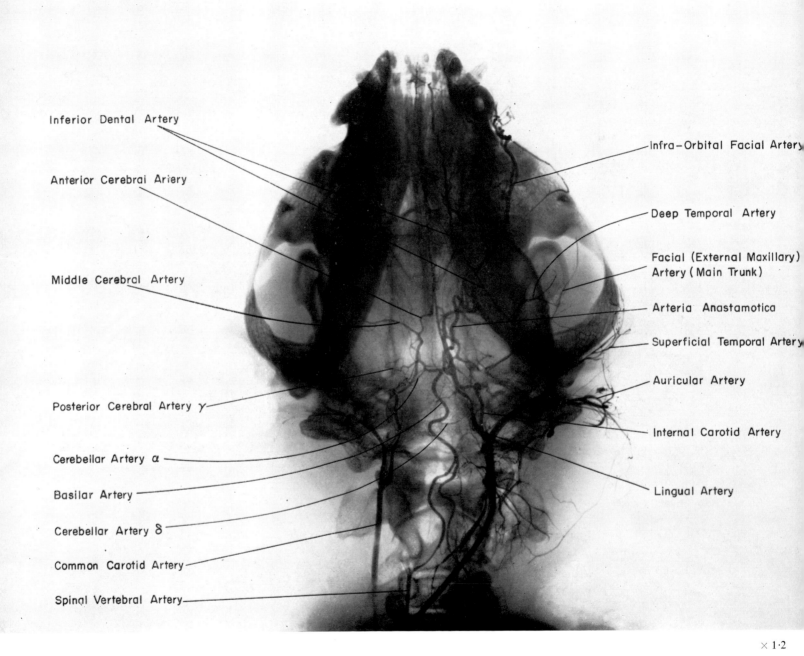

Inferior Dental Artery

Anterior Cerebral Artery

Middle Cerebral Artery

Posterior Cerebral Artery γ

Cerebellar Artery α

Basilar Artery

Cerebellar Artery δ

Common Carotid Artery

Spinal Vertebral Artery

Infra-Orbital Facial Artery

Deep Temporal Artery

Facial (External Maxillary) Artery (Main Trunk)

Arteria Anastamotica

Superficial Temporal Artery

Auricular Artery

Internal Carotid Artery

Lingual Artery

× 1·2

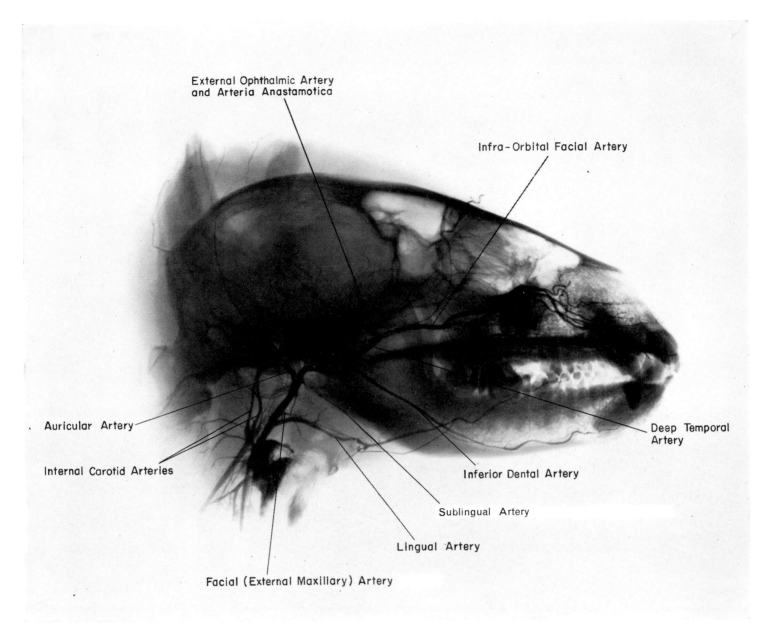

External Ophthalmic Artery
and Arteria Anastamotica

Infra-Orbital Facial Artery

Auricular Artery

Internal Carotid Arteries

Deep Temporal
Artery

Inferior Dental Artery

Sublingual Artery

Lingual Artery

Facial (External Maxillary) Artery

× 1·0

The vertebral and carotid arterial supply to the Circle of Willis
are of equal importance. There are some further comments
upon the arterial patterns of Procyonidae in the account of the
giant panda on the following page.

Ailuropoda melanoleuca
Giant Panda

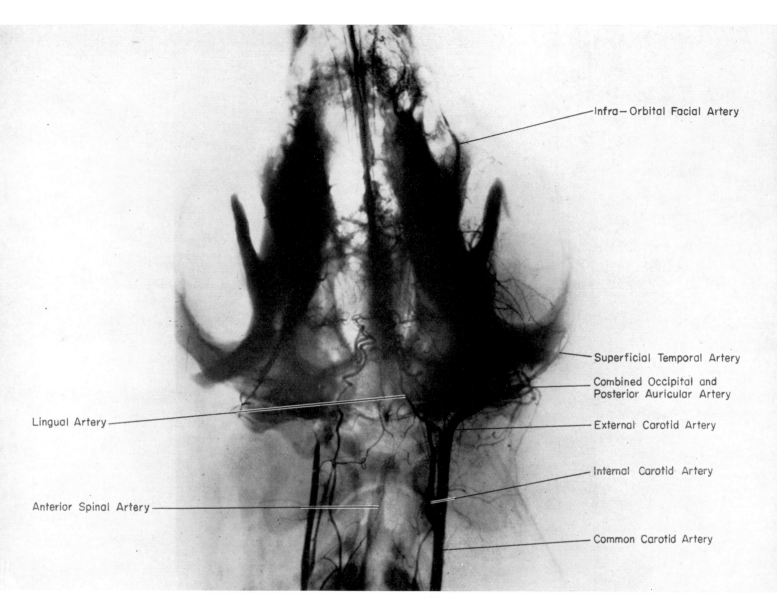

Infra—Orbital Facial Artery

Superficial Temporal Artery

Combined Occipital and Posterior Auricular Artery

External Carotid Artery

Internal Carotid Artery

Common Carotid Artery

Lingual Artery

Anterior Spinal Artery

× 0·5

The reason why studies of the cranial arteries of mammals are so rare is that the skull is so precious.

The Giant Panda provides an outstanding example of the rivalry between osteology and vascular anatomy.

Of all the Giant Pandas which have been shot or captured, there are records of only four in which the brain has definitely been examined. Even in them the neural anatomy has been studied more closely than the blood vessels. Only Davis (1964) and Davis and Storey (1943) give a clear and detailed description of the cranial arteries and this seems to be based upon the finding in one single Panda (Su lin ♂).

Indeed, fully to document the arterial system by dissection demands considerable destruction of the skull base.

Radiology offers a way in which the pattern of the arteries may be photographed after a simple non-destructive dissection of the neck.

The injection of radio-opaque material may even be followed with great advantage, after radiographs have been made, by perfusion with a formalin solution to preserve the brain.

There is, of course, no radiology in the wilderness, but, for those interested in the intracranial vascular (and neurological) anatomy of wild-shot animals, we would suggest intracarotid perfusion with formalin in the field followed (months later if necessary) by injection of radio-opaque material and radiography prior to opening the skull.

Because of past discussions about the relationships between

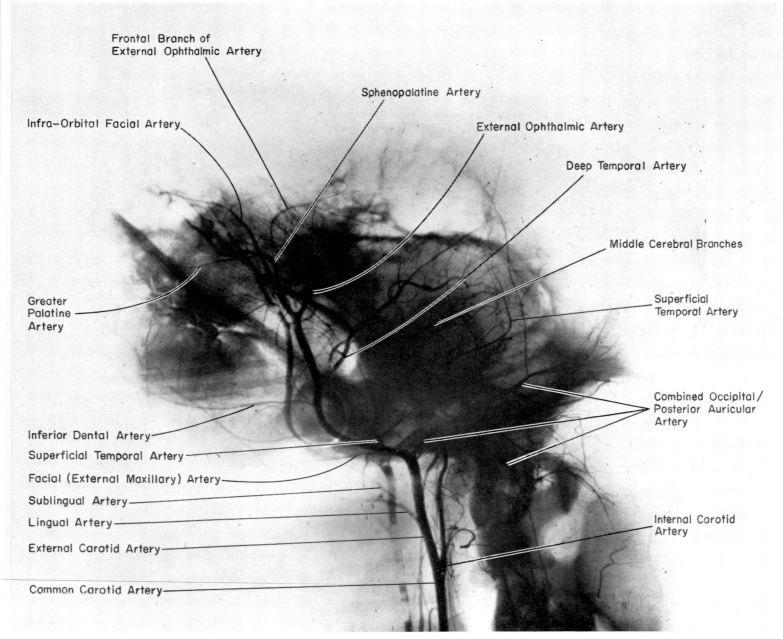

Frontal Branch of
External Ophthalmic Artery

Sphenopalatine Artery

Infra-Orbital Facial Artery

External Ophthalmic Artery

Deep Temporal Artery

Middle Cerebral Branches

Superficial
Temporal Artery

Greater
Palatine
Artery

Combined Occipital/
Posterior Auricular
Artery

Inferior Dental Artery

Superficial Temporal Artery

Facial (External Maxillary) Artery

Sublingual Artery

Lingual Artery

Internal Carotid
Artery

External Carotid Artery

Common Carotid Artery

× 0·55

Melogale moschata
Chinese Ferret-badger

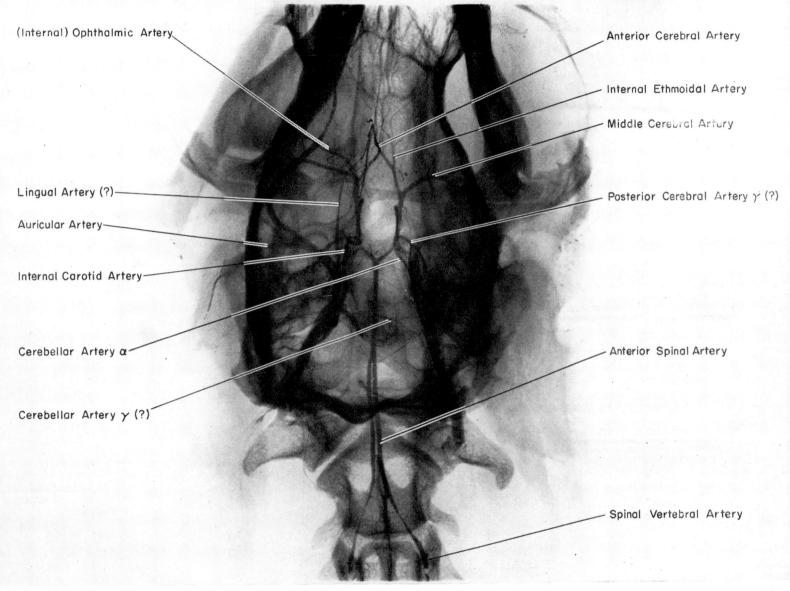

(Internal) Ophthalmic Artery

Lingual Artery (?)

Auricular Artery

Internal Carotid Artery

Cerebellar Artery α

Cerebellar Artery γ (?)

Anterior Cerebral Artery

Internal Ethmoidal Artery

Middle Cerebral Artery

Posterior Cerebral Artery γ (?)

Anterior Spinal Artery

Spinal Vertebral Artery

× 2·5

Only the Circle of Willis is usefully outlined. There does not seem to be any great contribution from the occipital artery to the vertebral and anterior spinal arterial system. The occipital artery arises from the internal carotid.

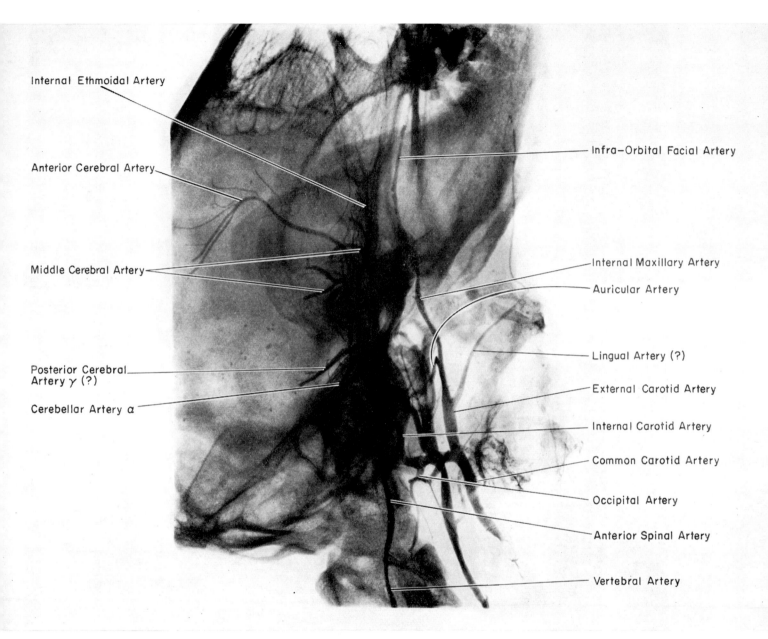

Internal Ethmoidal Artery

Anterior Cerebral Artery

Middle Cerebral Artery

Posterior Cerebral
Artery γ (?)

Cerebellar Artery α

Infra–Orbital Facial Artery

Internal Maxillary Artery

Auricular Artery

Lingual Artery (?)

External Carotid Artery

Internal Carotid Artery

Common Carotid Artery

Occipital Artery

Anterior Spinal Artery

Vertebral Artery

× 2·0

Lutra lutra
Otter

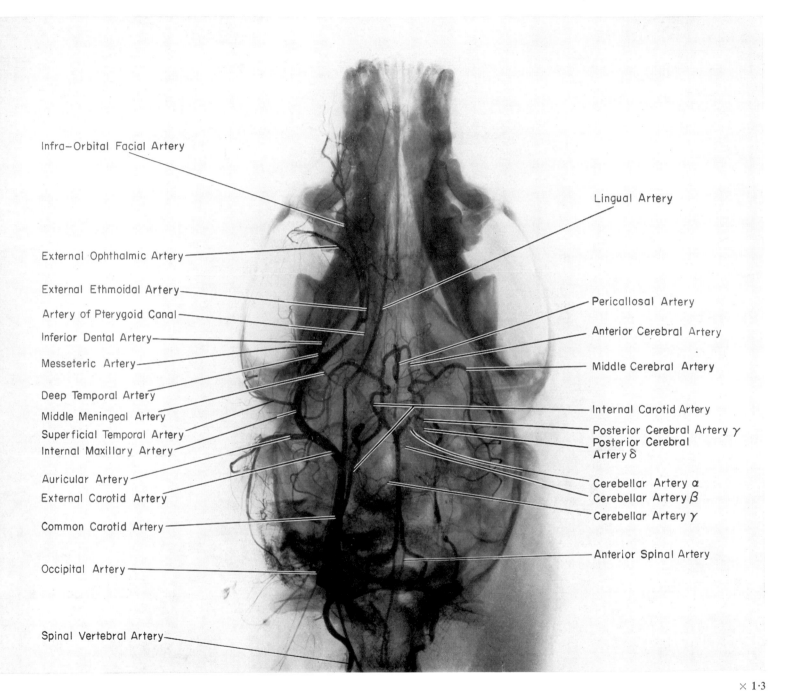

Infra–Orbital Facial Artery

External Ophthalmic Artery

External Ethmoidal Artery

Artery of Pterygoid Canal

Inferior Dental Artery

Messeteric Artery

Deep Temporal Artery

Middle Meningeal Artery

Superficial Temporal Artery

Internal Maxillary Artery

Auricular Artery

External Carotid Artery

Common Carotid Artery

Occipital Artery

Spinal Vertebral Artery

Lingual Artery

Pericallosal Artery

Anterior Cerebral Artery

Middle Cerebral Artery

Internal Carotid Artery

Posterior Cerebral Artery γ

Posterior Cerebral Artery δ

Cerebellar Artery α

Cerebellar Artery β

Cerebellar Artery γ

Anterior Spinal Artery

× 1·3

The common carotid divides into two unequal stems, the external carotid being the larger and the common stem for the internal carotid and occipital arteries the smaller. The branching of the external carotid resembles that of the *Mustelidae*. The terminal branches of the internal maxillary artery appear to be: an external ethmoidal which takes over part of the usual territory of the spheno-palatine artery and gives rise to a narrow recurrent branch through the pterygoid canal (this latter artery can be traced back on the original radiograph along the usual course of the stapedial artery to the temporal bone).

A large external ophthalmic artery, cerebellar arteries α, β, γ, δ and ε are all identifiable, but the last two are extremely small.

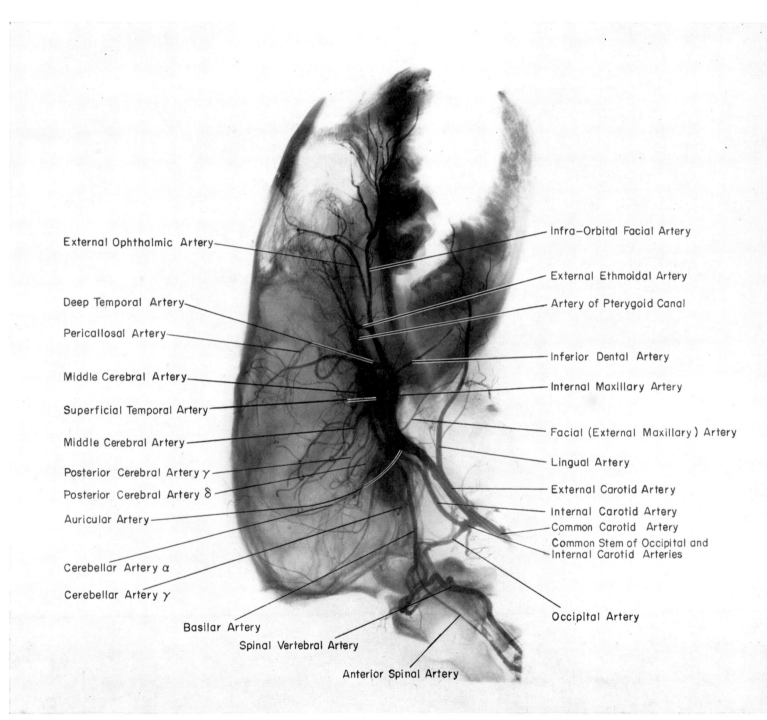

External Ophthalmic Artery

Deep Temporal Artery

Pericallosal Artery

Middle Cerebral Artery

Superficial Temporal Artery

Middle Cerebral Artery

Posterior Cerebral Artery γ

Posterior Cerebral Artery δ

Auricular Artery

Cerebellar Artery α

Cerebellar Artery γ

Basilar Artery

Spinal Vertebral Artery

Anterior Spinal Artery

Infra–Orbital Facial Artery

External Ethmoidal Artery

Artery of Pterygoid Canal

Inferior Dental Artery

Internal Maxillary Artery

Facial (External Maxillary) Artery

Lingual Artery

External Carotid Artery

Internal Carotid Artery

Common Carotid Artery

Common Stem of Occipital and Internal Carotid Arteries

Occipital Artery

× 1·3

Paguma larvata
Masked Palm Civet

External Ophthalmic Artery

Inferior Dental Artery

Infra-Orbital Facial Artery

Middle Cerebral Artery

Deep Temporal Artery

Superficial Temporal Artery

Internal Maxillary Artery

Auricular Artery

External Carotid Artery

Occipital Artery

Common Carotid Artery

Spinal Vertebral Artery

Anterior Cerebral Artery

Arteria Anastamotica

Posterior Cerebral Artery γ

Internal Maxillary Artery

Ramus Anastamoticus

Cerebellar Artery α

Internal Carotid Artery

Posterior Cerebral Artery δ

Cerebellar Artery γ (?)

Basilar Artery

Anterior Spinal Artery

× 1·7

The lingual artery has not been outlined.

The configuration of the cranial arterial tree is very like that seen in the Canidae.

It is of interest to see a well developed arteria anastomotica on one side, but not on the other. The arteria anastomotica is larger than the cervical internal carotid.

On the original radiographs it is possible to see a well developed anastomosis between the superior and anterior-inferior cerebellar arteries (cerebellar arteries α and γ (?)).

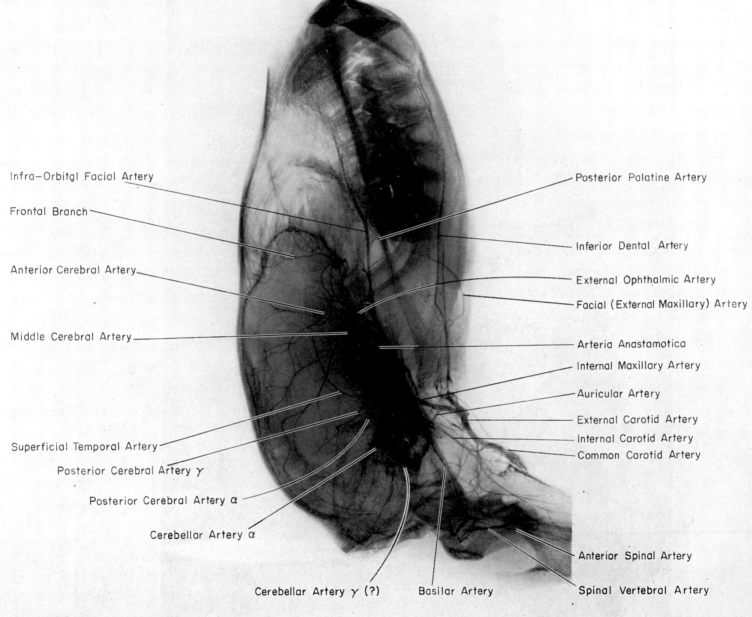

Infra–Orbital Facial Artery

Frontal Branch

Anterior Cerebral Artery

Middle Cerebral Artery

Superficial Temporal Artery

Posterior Cerebral Artery γ

Posterior Cerebral Artery α

Cerebellar Artery α

Cerebellar Artery γ (?)

Basilar Artery

Posterior Palatine Artery

Inferior Dental Artery

External Ophthalmic Artery

Facial (External Maxillary) Artery

Arteria Anastamotica

Internal Maxillary Artery

Auricular Artery

External Carotid Artery

Internal Carotid Artery

Common Carotid Artery

Anterior Spinal Artery

Spinal Vertebral Artery

× 1·7

Cynictis penicillata
Yellow Mongoose

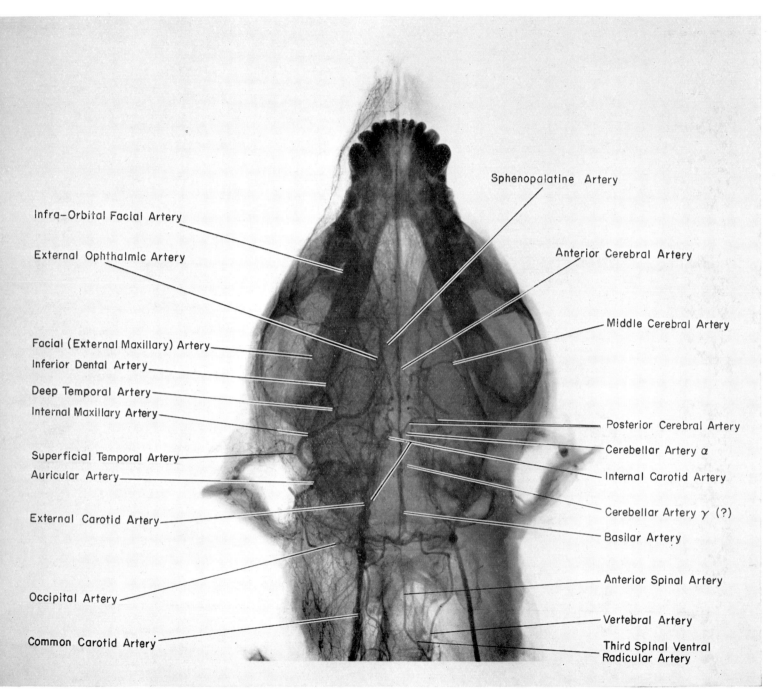

Infra-Orbital Facial Artery

External Ophthalmic Artery

Facial (External Maxillary) Artery

Inferior Dental Artery

Deep Temporal Artery

Internal Maxillary Artery

Superficial Temporal Artery

Auricular Artery

External Carotid Artery

Occipital Artery

Common Carotid Artery

Sphenopalatine Artery

Anterior Cerebral Artery

Middle Cerebral Artery

Posterior Cerebral Artery

Cerebellar Artery α

Internal Carotid Artery

Cerebellar Artery γ (?)

Basilar Artery

Anterior Spinal Artery

Vertebral Artery

Third Spinal Ventral Radicular Artery

× 1·6

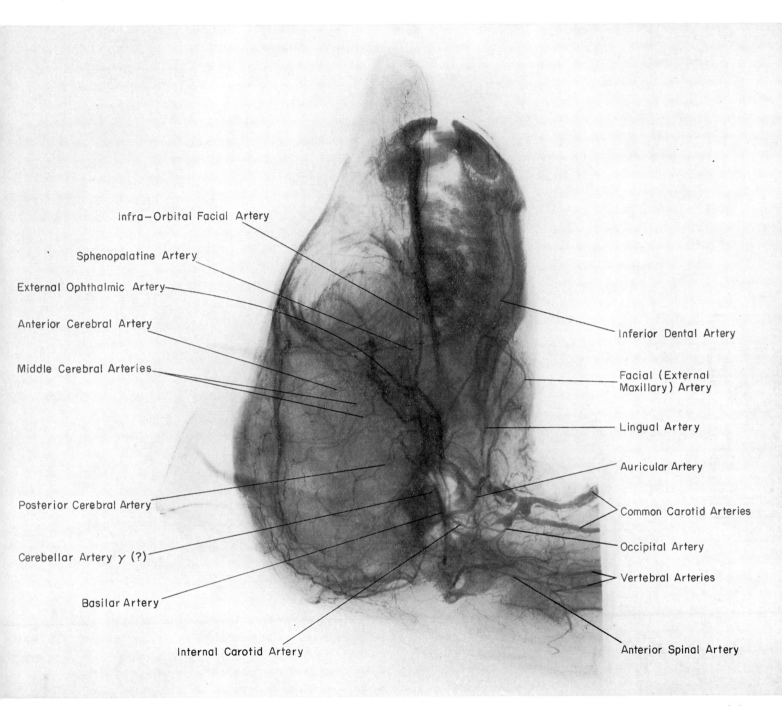

Infra–Orbital Facial Artery

Sphenopalatine Artery

External Ophthalmic Artery

Anterior Cerebral Artery

Middle Cerebral Arteries

Posterior Cerebral Artery

Cerebellar Artery γ (?)

Basilar Artery

Internal Carotid Artery

Inferior Dental Artery

Facial (External Maxillary) Artery

Lingual Artery

Auricular Artery

Common Carotid Arteries

Occipital Artery

Vertebral Arteries

Anterior Spinal Artery

× 1·6

The pictures show the small peripheral ramifications of the arteries; but it is difficult to see the main trunks of some of them. In the lateral view the superficial and deep temporal arteries have not been labelled, and in both views it is very difficult to see the lingual artery.

Nomenclature (by Hofmann's classification) of the posterior cerebral and cerebellar arteries is conjectural, but by human analogy, as so often the cerebellar arteries are "superior" and "anterior inferior".

Suricata suricatta
Grey Meerkat

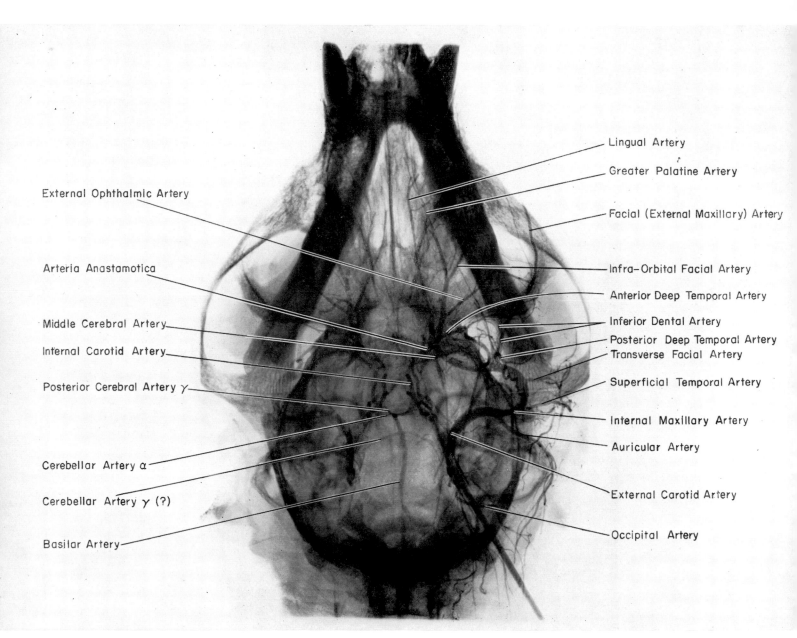

External Ophthalmic Artery

Arteria Anastamotica

Middle Cerebral Artery

Internal Carotid Artery

Posterior Cerebral Artery γ

Cerebellar Artery α

Cerebellar Artery γ (?)

Basilar Artery

Lingual Artery

Greater Palatine Artery

Facial (External Maxillary) Artery

Infra-Orbital Facial Artery

Anterior Deep Temporal Artery

Inferior Dental Artery

Posterior Deep Temporal Artery

Transverse Facial Artery

Superficial Temporal Artery

Internal Maxillary Artery

Auricular Artery

External Carotid Artery

Occipital Artery

× 2·0

The arterial anatomy is rather different from the mongoose, particularly in the region of the orbit. A large artery, which we have named the anterior deep temporal from its distribution, arises from the internal maxillary almost simultaneously with an arteria anastomotica. The orbital branch named here the external ophthalmic artery arises quite separately and does not appear to have a direct connection with the arteria anastomotica.

There is probably also an internal ophthalmic artery.

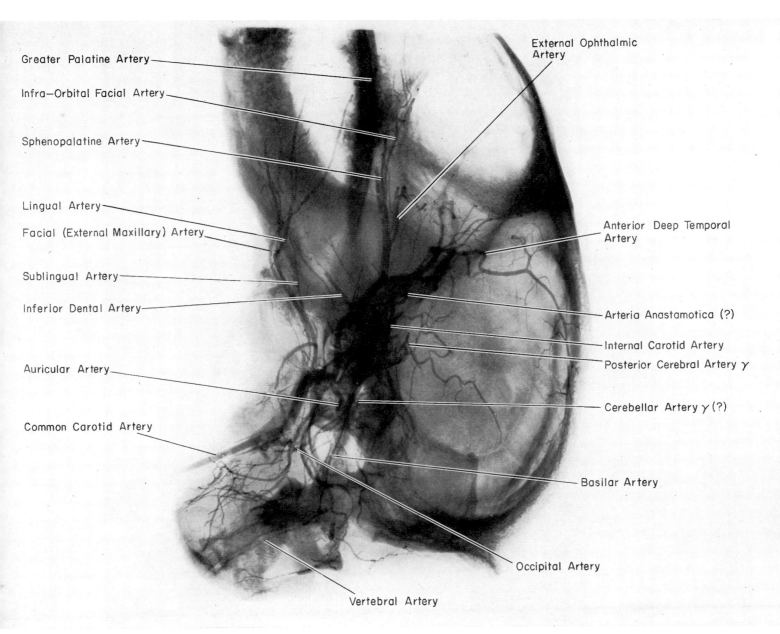

Greater Palatine Artery

Infra—Orbital Facial Artery

Sphenopalatine Artery

Lingual Artery

Facial (External Maxillary) Artery

Sublingual Artery

Inferior Dental Artery

Auricular Artery

Common Carotid Artery

External Ophthalmic Artery

Anterior Deep Temporal Artery

Arteria Anastamotica (?)

Internal Carotid Artery

Posterior Cerebral Artery γ

Cerebellar Artery γ (?)

Basilar Artery

Occipital Artery

Vertebral Artery

× 2·0

Crocuta crocuta
Hyaena

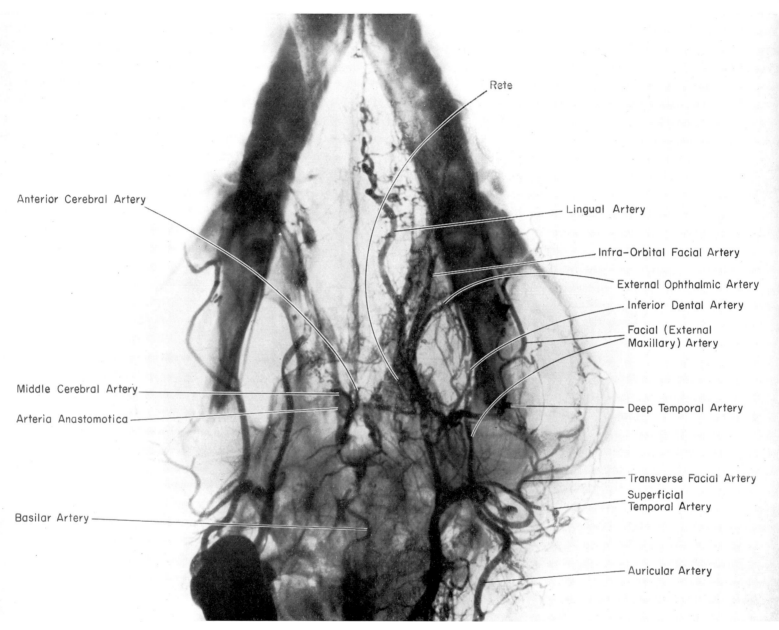

Rete

Anterior Cerebral Artery

Lingual Artery

Infra-Orbital Facial Artery

External Ophthalmic Artery

Inferior Dental Artery

Facial (External
Maxillary) Artery

Middle Cerebral Artery

Arteria Anastomotica

Deep Temporal Artery

Transverse Facial Artery

Superficial
Temporal Artery

Basilar Artery

Auricular Artery

× 0·5

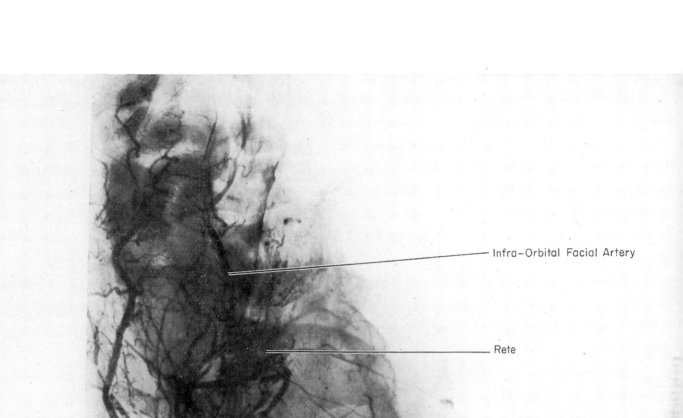

Infra-Orbital Facial Artery

Rete

Lingual Artery

Facial (External Maxillary) Artery

External Carotid Artery

Internal Carotid Artery

Common Carotid Artery

Auricular Artery

Occipital Artery

× 0·5

The internal maxillary artery is incompletely filled even on the left; making identification of several of the branches very difficult in the lateral view.

Note the similarity of the wide carotid sinus to that of the dog. Note, also, the existence of an extensive rete in the orbital and retro-orbital regions. This fills from the external ophthalmic artery or its parent vessel and communicates with the extradural portion of the internal carotid by way of one large arteria anastomotica.

Felis catus
Domestic Cat

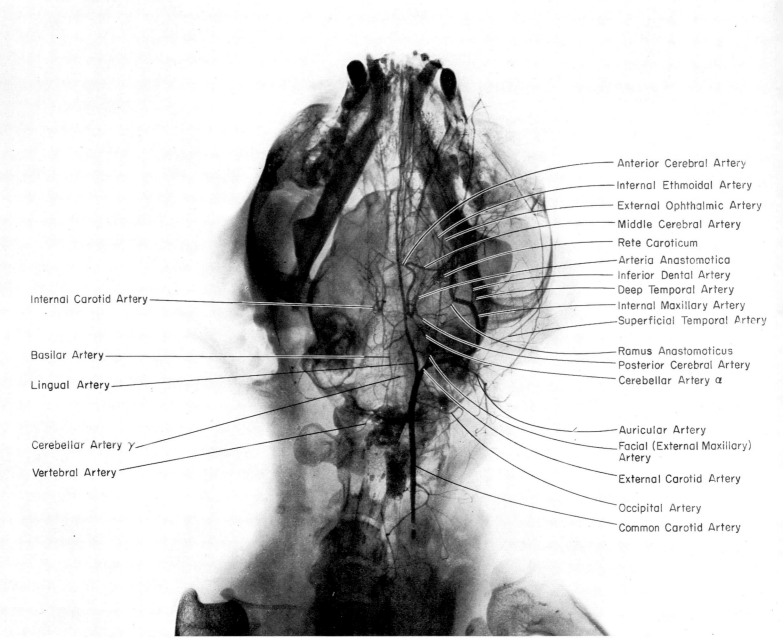

Anterior Cerebral Artery
Internal Ethmoidal Artery
External Ophthalmic Artery
Middle Cerebral Artery
Rete Caroticum
Arteria Anastomotica
Inferior Dental Artery
Deep Temporal Artery
Internal Maxillary Artery
Superficial Temporal Artery

Ramus Anastomoticus
Posterior Cerebral Artery
Cerebellar Artery α

Auricular Artery
Facial (External Maxillary) Artery
External Carotid Artery

Occipital Artery
Common Carotid Artery

Internal Carotid Artery

Basilar Artery

Lingual Artery

Cerebellar Artery γ

Vertebral Artery

× 1·1

This animal has had a myelogram and there is some contrast-medium (Myodil) within the spinal canal.

The rete and its branches are difficult to see in the lateral view so that no names have been attached to the arteria anastomotica (which consists of a leash of small vessels), the internal ethmoidal and the orbital branches.

The deep temporal is a very small artery.

In this specimen no vestige of a ramus anastomoticus can be seen although the middle menigeal has been filled. The ascending pharyngeal taking origin from the occipital artery does not appear to reach the rete. The internal carotid is still preserved

in the neck as an exceedingly fine vessel which may be traced from its origin up to the mastoid bulla.

Davis and Story (1943) and Daniel, Dawes and Prichard (1953) do not differ materially in their description of the anatomy of the cranial arteries of the cat from Tandler (1899), though they add a good deal.

Davis and Story give the following branches. The common carotid supplies near its termination a few small muscular twigs and then the internal carotid, which in the adult is usually represented in the neck by an imperforate cord. The ascending pharyngeal arising from the occipital artery a little further

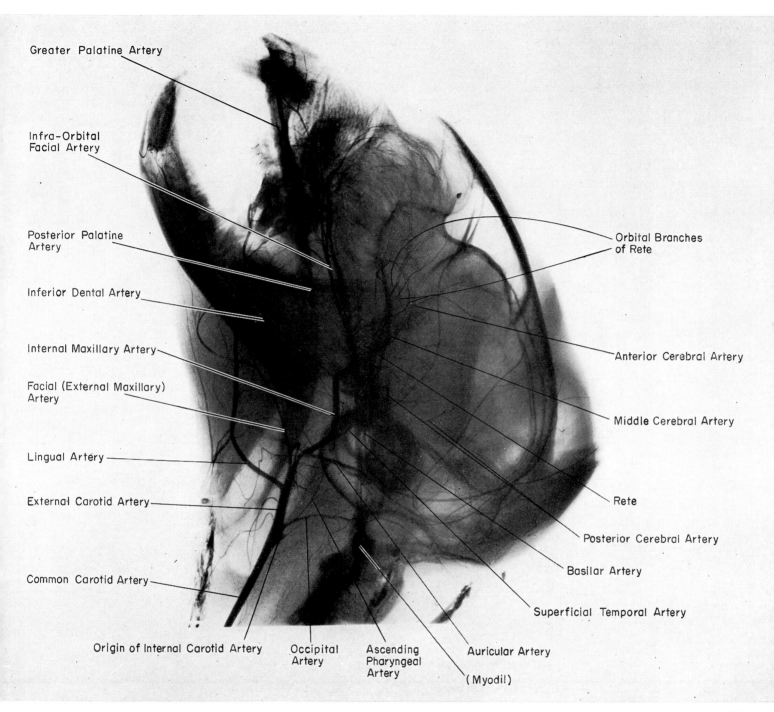

Greater Palatine Artery

Infra-Orbital Facial Artery

Posterior Palatine Artery

Inferior Dental Artery

Internal Maxillary Artery

Facial (External Maxillary) Artery

Lingual Artery

External Carotid Artery

Common Carotid Artery

Origin of Internal Carotid Artery

Occipital Artery

Ascending Pharyngeal Artery

(Myodil)

Auricular Artery

Superficial Temporal Artery

Basilar Artery

Posterior Cerebral Artery

Rete

Middle Cerebral Artery

Anterior Cerebral Artery

Orbital Branches of Rete

× 2·0

along takes over the function of the internal carotid, by forming a connection with its carvernous position via foramen lacerum medium.

Nevertheless, the volume of blood passing through the narrow vessel must be small. Some of it is directed along a twig to the promontory of the middle ear, this twig representing the osseous portion of the internal carotid, in which blood flow has been reversed.

The ascending pharyngeal also supplies pharyngeal muscular branches, a palatine branch and eustachian branches.

The occipital artery, also a rather small vessel has a large number of small branches arising close to its origin, viz. a glandular ramus to the large cervical lymph node, a twig

(inconstant) accompanying the internal carotid nerve onto the promontory and minute twigs to the nodose and superior cervical ganglia and the cranial nerves emerging from foramen lacerum posterior.

Further cranially the occipital artery gives rise to a muscular twig accompanying the spinal accessory nerve to the cleido-mastoid muscle, a vertebral muscular branch and a branch which divides into the posterior meningeal artery, entering the head via the hypoglossal foramen, and the inferior tymparic (the further course and connection of which Davis and Stony give in detail). The occipital artery then runs on across the mastoid process to which and to surrounding muscles it gives off twigs. Finally it divides into a superficial and deep branch.

Felis manul
Pallas's Cat

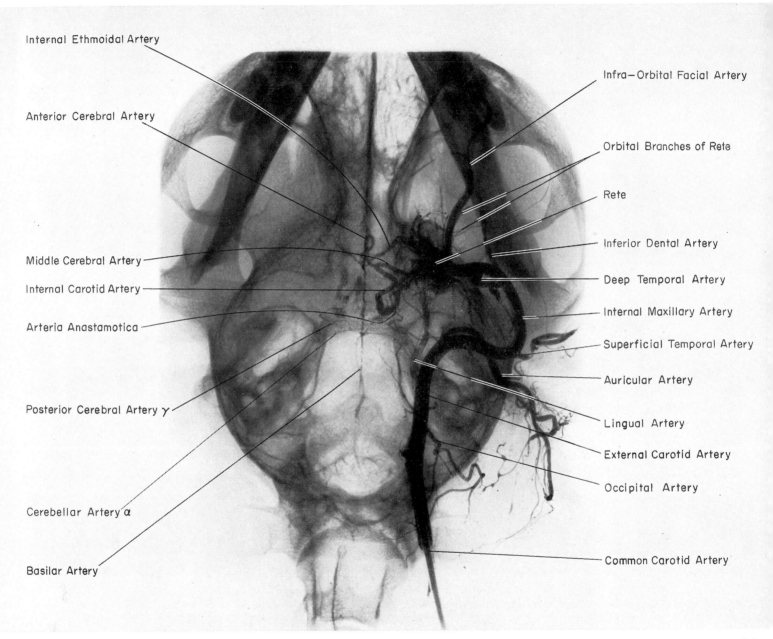

Internal Ethmoidal Artery

Anterior Cerebral Artery

Middle Cerebral Artery

Internal Carotid Artery

Arteria Anastamotica

Posterior Cerebral Artery γ

Cerebellar Artery α

Basilar Artery

Infra–Orbital Facial Artery

Orbital Branches of Rete

Rete

Inferior Dental Artery

Deep Temporal Artery

Internal Maxillary Artery

Superficial Temporal Artery

Auricular Artery

Lingual Artery

External Carotid Artery

Occipital Artery

Common Carotid Artery

× 1·1

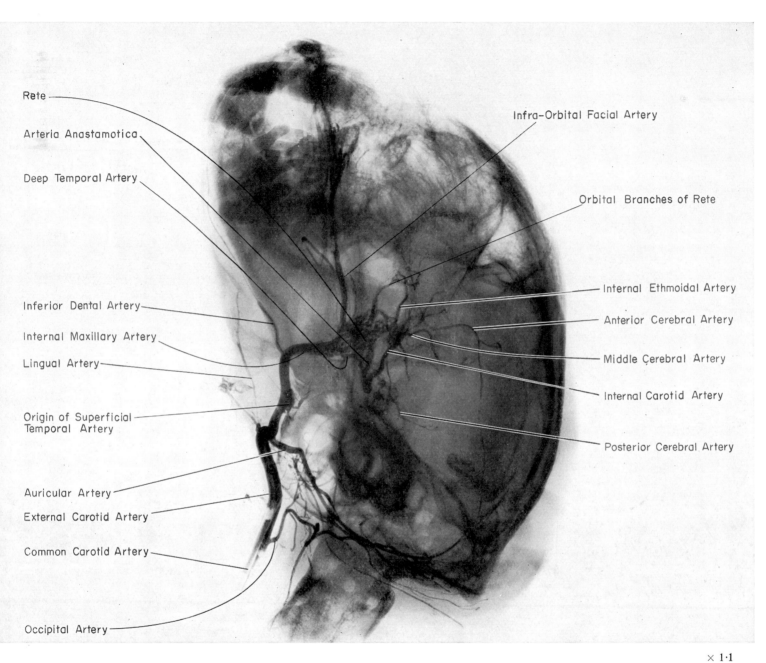

Rete

Arteria Anastamotica

Deep Temporal Artery

Inferior Dental Artery

Internal Maxillary Artery

Lingual Artery

Origin of Superficial
Temporal Artery

Auricular Artery

External Carotid Artery

Common Carotid Artery

Occipital Artery

Infra-Orbital Facial Artery

Orbital Branches of Rete

Internal Ethmoidal Artery

Anterior Cerebral Artery

Middle Cerebral Artery

Internal Carotid Artery

Posterior Cerebral Artery

× 1·1

A typical example of the *Felidae*.

Felis concolor
Puma (cub)

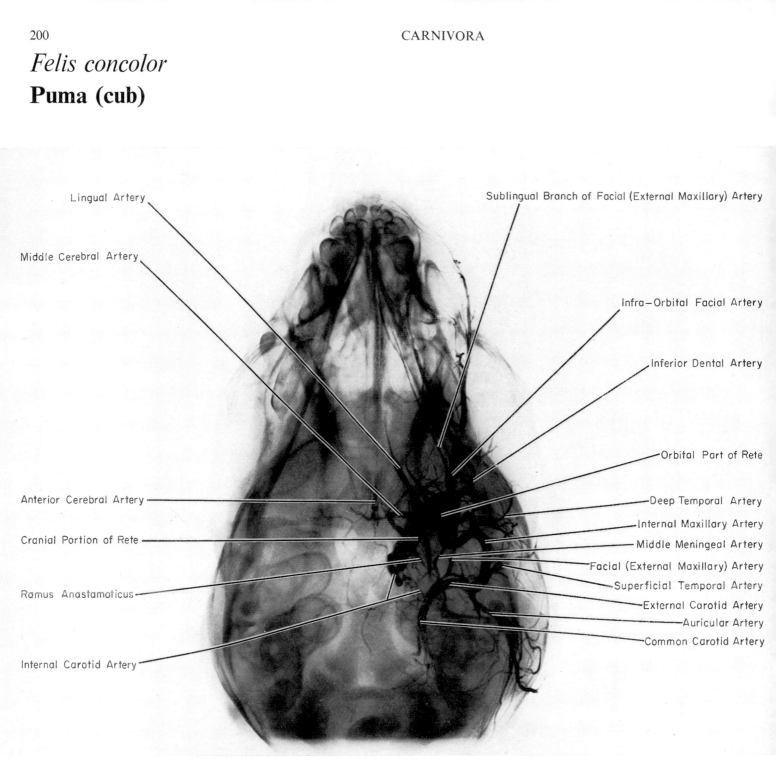

Lingual Artery

Middle Cerebral Artery

Anterior Cerebral Artery

Cranial Portion of Rete

Ramus Anastamoticus

Internal Carotid Artery

Sublingual Branch of Facial (External Maxillary) Artery

Infra–Orbital Facial Artery

Inferior Dental Artery

Orbital Part of Rete

Deep Temporal Artery

Internal Maxillary Artery

Middle Meningeal Artery

Facial (External Maxillary) Artery

Superficial Temporal Artery

External Carotid Artery

Auricular Artery

Common Carotid Artery

× 2·0

The posterior part of the Circle of Willis is very poorly shown.

This specimen of a cub only a few days old shows the internal carotid artery in the neck already very narrow. It also shows the ramus anastomoticus and the cranial position of the rete corresponding to the arteria anastomotica.

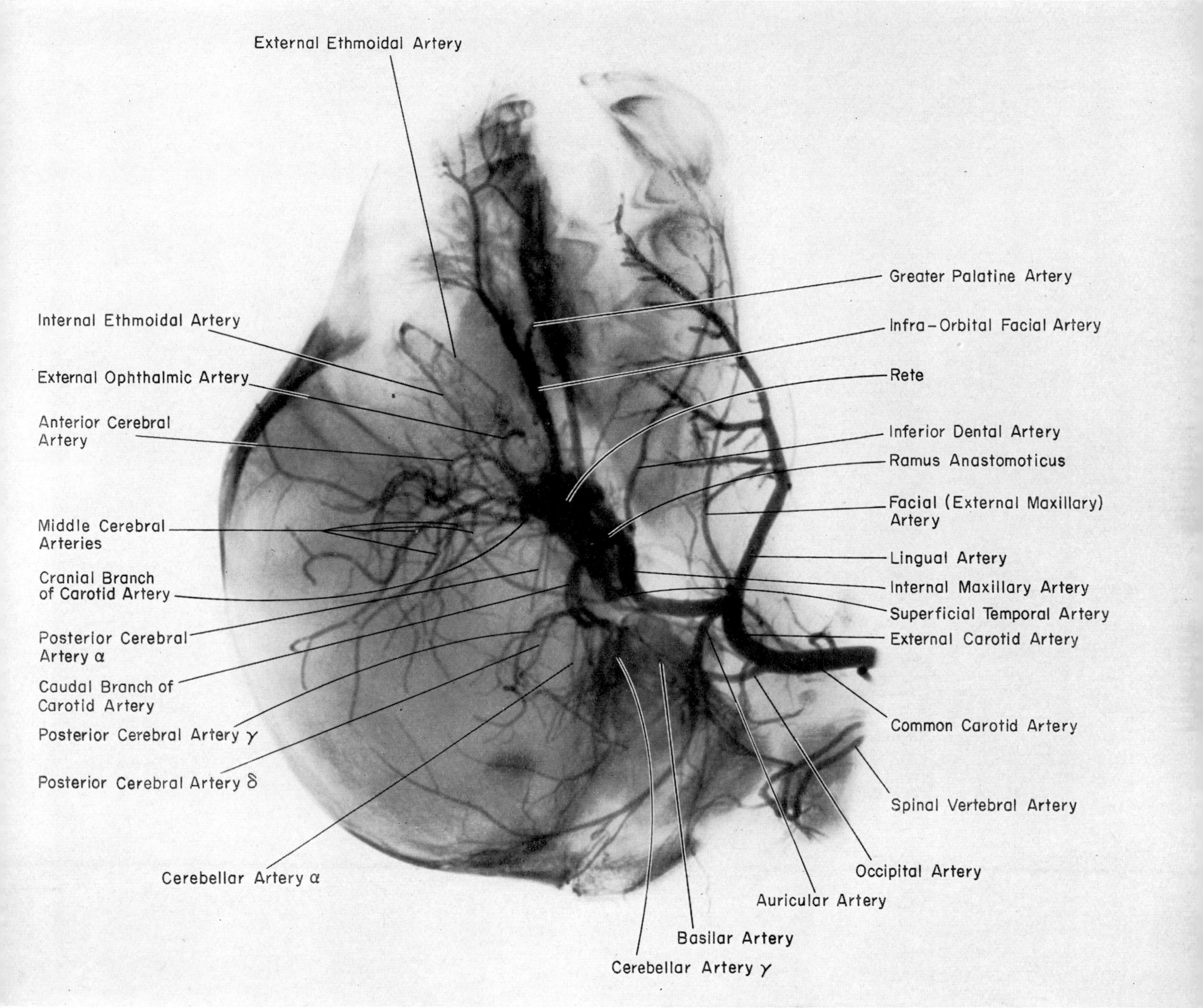

External Ethmoidal Artery

Internal Ethmoidal Artery

External Ophthalmic Artery

Anterior Cerebral
Artery

Middle Cerebral
Arteries

Cranial Branch
of Carotid Artery

Posterior Cerebral
Artery α

Caudal Branch of
Carotid Artery

Posterior Cerebral Artery γ

Posterior Cerebral Artery δ

Cerebellar Artery α

Greater Palatine Artery

Infra-Orbital Facial Artery

Rete

Inferior Dental Artery

Ramus Anastomoticus

Facial (External Maxillary)
Artery

Lingual Artery

Internal Maxillary Artery

Superficial Temporal Artery

External Carotid Artery

Common Carotid Artery

Spinal Vertebral Artery

Occipital Artery

Auricular Artery

Basilar Artery

Cerebellar Artery γ

× 2·0

Felis concolor
Puma (cub)

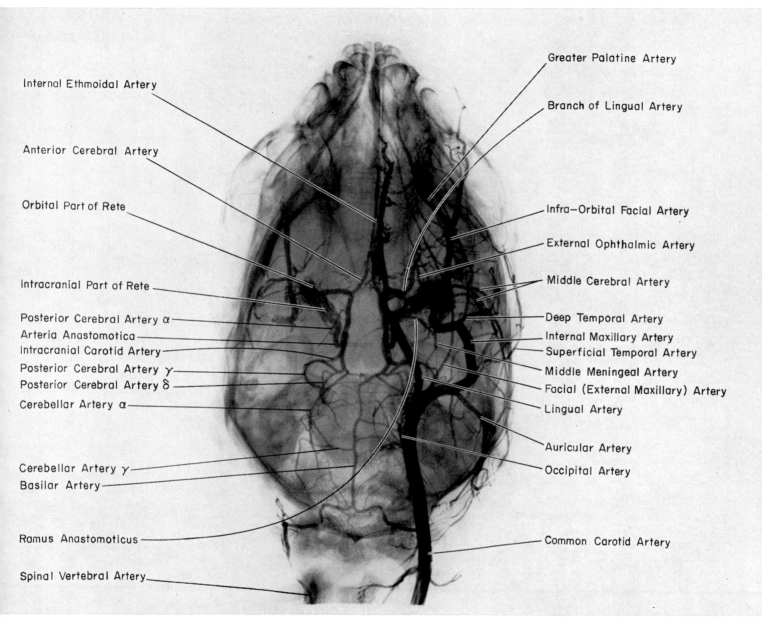

Internal Ethmoidal Artery

Anterior Cerebral Artery

Orbital Part of Rete

Intracranial Part of Rete

Posterior Cerebral Artery α
Arteria Anastomotica
Intracranial Carotid Artery
Posterior Cerebral Artery γ
Posterior Cerebral Artery δ
Cerebellar Artery α

Cerebellar Artery γ
Basilar Artery

Ramus Anastomoticus

Spinal Vertebral Artery

Greater Palatine Artery

Branch of Lingual Artery

Infra–Orbital Facial Artery

External Ophthalmic Artery

Middle Cerebral Artery

Deep Temporal Artery
Internal Maxillary Artery
Superficial Temporal Artery
Middle Meningeal Artery
Facial (External Maxillary) Artery
Lingual Artery

Auricular Artery
Occipital Artery

Common Carotid Artery

× 2·0

This puma cub differs from the other illustrated in having completely lost the cervical connection to the intracranial carotid.

In most respects the arterial tree is typical of the cat family, but the usual internal ethmoidal stem from the rete seems to be lacking. Instead there is a well-developed internal ethmoidal arising directly from the anterior cerebral artery.

The posterior cerebral α consists of little more than an anterior choroidal artery. On the original radiograph it is possible to see the internal auditory artery arising from the cerebellar artery γ on one side.

Panthera leo
Lion (cub)

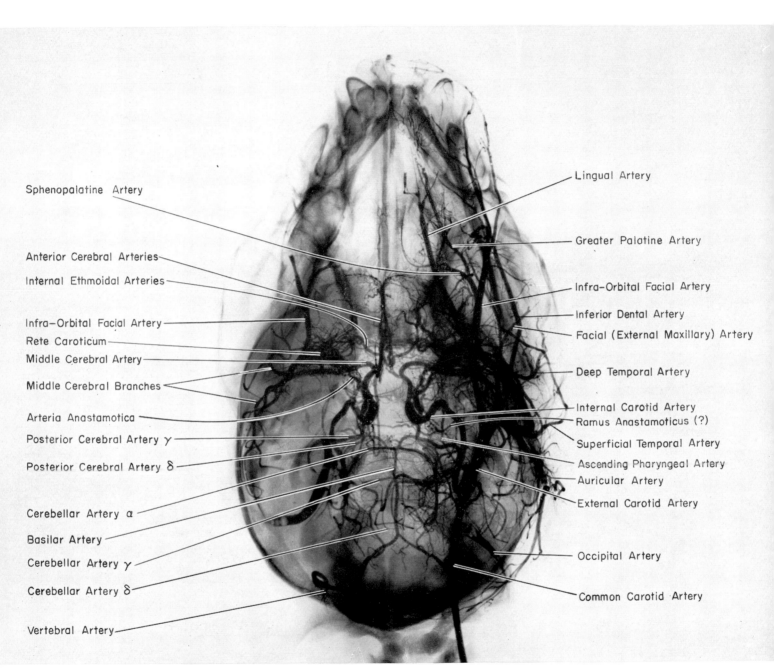

Sphenopalatine Artery

Anterior Cerebral Arteries

Internal Ethmoidal Arteries

Infra-Orbital Facial Artery
Rete Caroticum
Middle Cerebral Artery

Middle Cerebral Branches

Arteria Anastamotica

Posterior Cerebral Artery γ

Posterior Cerebral Artery δ

Cerebellar Artery α

Basilar Artery

Cerebellar Artery γ

Cerebellar Artery δ

Vertebral Artery

Lingual Artery

Greater Palatine Artery

Infra-Orbital Facial Artery

Inferior Dental Artery
Facial (External Maxillary) Artery

Deep Temporal Artery

Internal Carotid Artery
Ramus Anastamoticus (?)

Superficial Temporal Artery

Ascending Pharyngeal Artery
Auricular Artery

External Carotid Artery

Occipital Artery

Common Carotid Artery

× 1·8

This cub, at most a few days old, shows clearly the dual supply of the Circle of Willis from internal and external carotid arteries. At this stage the internal carotid was very large; but it was destined to atrophy as the lion grew.

Note how the rete, which lies largely at the back of the orbit, receives blood from the internal maxillary artery and from the ascending pharyngeal artery. Principally it supplies a leash of vessels running to the extradural intracranial part of the internal carotid, this leash representing the arteria anastomotica. Into the leash or the carotid close to its junction with the leash, empties a small ramus anastomoticus.

The internal ethmoidal arteries, which are very large, also originate from the orbital carotid rete, but as in the cat, have a connection with the Circle of Willis (via the anterior cerebral arteries).

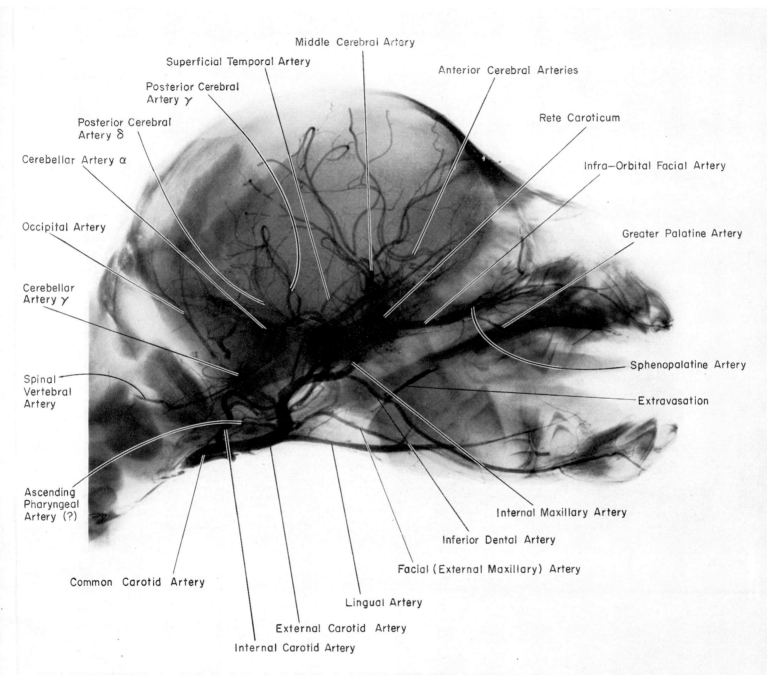

Middle Cerebral Artery

Superficial Temporal Artery

Posterior Cerebral
Artery γ

Anterior Cerebral Arteries

Posterior Cerebral
Artery δ

Rete Caroticum

Cerebellar Artery α

Infra—Orbital Facial Artery

Occipital Artery

Greater Palatine Artery

Cerebellar
Artery γ

Spinal
Vertebral
Artery

Sphenopalatine Artery

Extravasation

Ascending
Pharyngeal
Artery (?)

Internal Maxillary Artery

Inferior Dental Artery

Common Carotid Artery

Facial (External Maxillary) Artery

Lingual Artery

External Carotid Artery

Internal Carotid Artery

× 1·8

Note how the injection material has flowed through the
rete on one side from internal carotid to infra-orbital facial
artery, a reversal of the physiological direction of flow.

Panthera tigris
Tiger

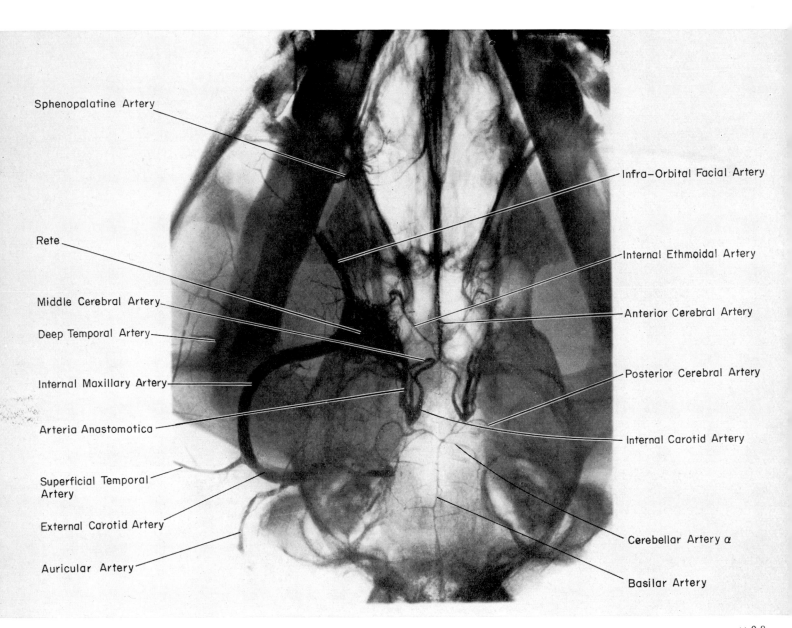

Sphenopalatine Artery

Rete

Middle Cerebral Artery

Deep Temporal Artery

Internal Maxillary Artery

Arteria Anastomotica

Superficial Temporal Artery

External Carotid Artery

Auricular Artery

Infra-Orbital Facial Artery

Internal Ethmoidal Artery

Anterior Cerebral Artery

Posterior Cerebral Artery

Internal Carotid Artery

Cerebellar Artery α

Basilar Artery

× 0·8

In general we have followed Davis and Story (1943) in naming the arteries in the vicinity of the orbit; but some are poorly filled and others not visible. Consequently it has been necessary to indicate the tentative nature of some of the identifications.

We have made no attempt to name:

The anterior meningeal artery.
The artery of the olfactory bulb.
The external ethmoidal artery.
The ophthalmic artery.
The muscular branches in the orbit.
The ciliary artery.
The supraorbital artery.
The frontal artery.

The trochlear branch.
Palpebral branches.
The angular artery.
Masseteric arteries.
The posterior deep temporal artery.

Some of these vessels are probably filled and visible, but so superimposed upon the orbital part of the rete as to defy certain recognition. Others, notably the angular artery and the posterior deep temporal do not seem to be filled.

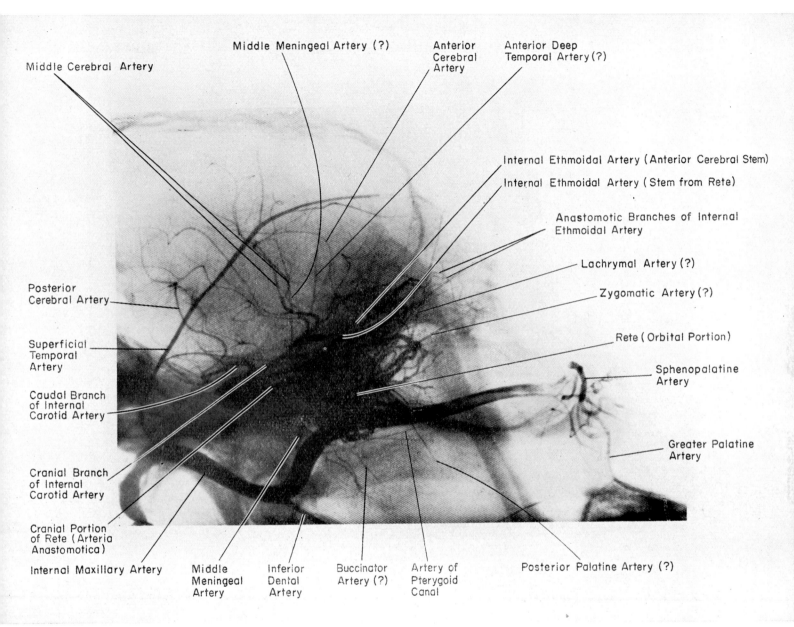

Middle Cerebral Artery

Middle Meningeal Artery (?)

Anterior Cerebral Artery

Anterior Deep Temporal Artery (?)

Internal Ethmoidal Artery (Anterior Cerebral Stem)

Internal Ethmoidal Artery (Stem from Rete)

Anastomotic Branches of Internal Ethmoidal Artery

Lachrymal Artery (?)

Zygomatic Artery (?)

Rete (Orbital Portion)

Sphenopalatine Artery

Greater Palatine Artery

Posterior Cerebral Artery

Superficial Temporal Artery

Caudal Branch of Internal Carotid Artery

Cranial Branch of Internal Carotid Artery

Cranial Portion of Rete (Arteria Anastomotica)

Internal Maxillary Artery

Middle Meningeal Artery

Inferior Dental Artery

Buccinator Artery (?)

Artery of Pterygoid Canal

Posterior Palatine Artery (?)

× 1·2

Panthera pardus
Leopard, Black Panther

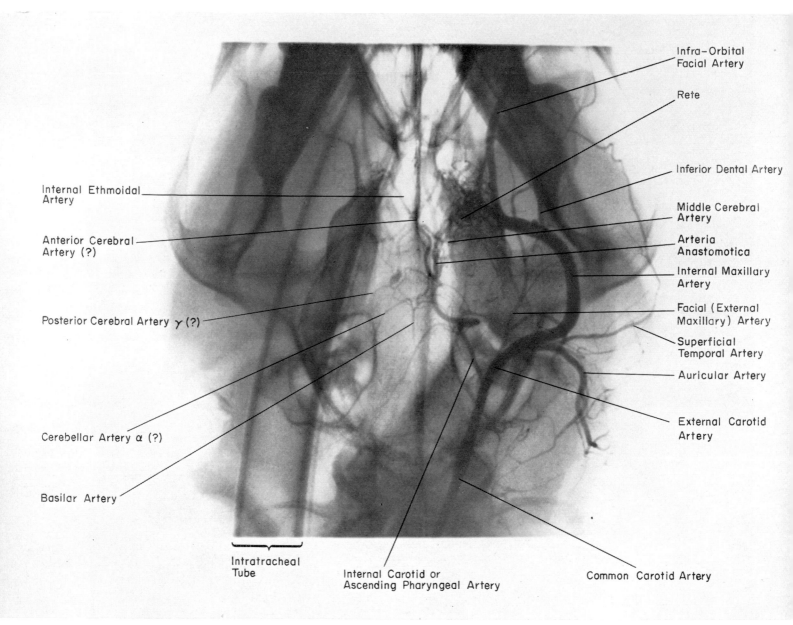

Infra-Orbital Facial Artery

Rete

Inferior Dental Artery

Middle Cerebral Artery

Arteria Anastomotica

Internal Maxillary Artery

Facial (External Maxillary) Artery

Superficial Temporal Artery

Auricular Artery

External Carotid Artery

Internal Ethmoidal Artery

Anterior Cerebral Artery (?)

Posterior Cerebral Artery γ (?)

Cerebellar Artery α (?)

Basilar Artery

Intratracheal Tube

Internal Carotid or Ascending Pharyngeal Artery

Common Carotid Artery

× 0·75

This ventro-dorsal view is taken from a percutaneous common carotid angiogram done in life for diagnostic purposes.

Only a proportion of the known branches are visible; the deep temporal arteries, for instance, have not been outlined.

A very small cervical internal carotid persists but neither the ramus anastomoticus nor the ascending pharyngeal artery are seen.

It was notable that the external carotid branches filled well before contrast medium had passed through the rete into the Circle of Willis.

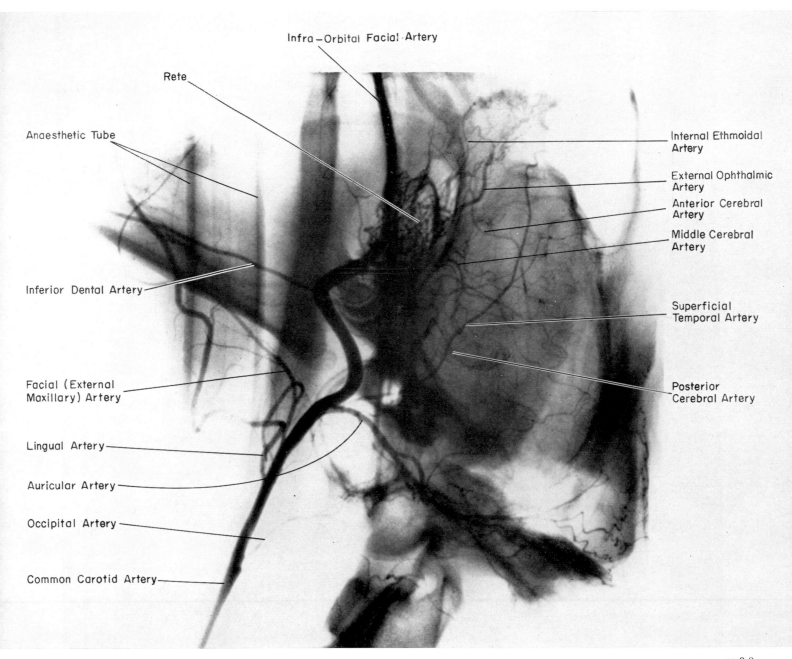

Infra—Orbital Facial Artery

Rete

Anaesthetic Tube

Inferior Dental Artery

Facial (External Maxillary) Artery

Lingual Artery

Auricular Artery

Occipital Artery

Common Carotid Artery

Internal Ethmoidal Artery

External Ophthalmic Artery

Anterior Cerebral Artery

Middle Cerebral Artery

Superficial Temporal Artery

Posterior Cerebral Artery

× 0·8

Pinnipedia

Examples of each of the three families which have been examined, together with Tandler's descriptions of two of them exhibit certain common features. The most obvious of these is the very large size of the brain with its double blood supply from internal carotids and vertebral arteries.

The origin of the middle meningeal artery in the orbit is another common feature.

Seals of the family *Phocidae* have particularly large and well developed orbital retia; but none of the Pinnipedia has a cerebral rete.

Murie (1874) wrote about the sea-lion as well as other diving mammals.

Zalophus californianus
Californian Sea-lion

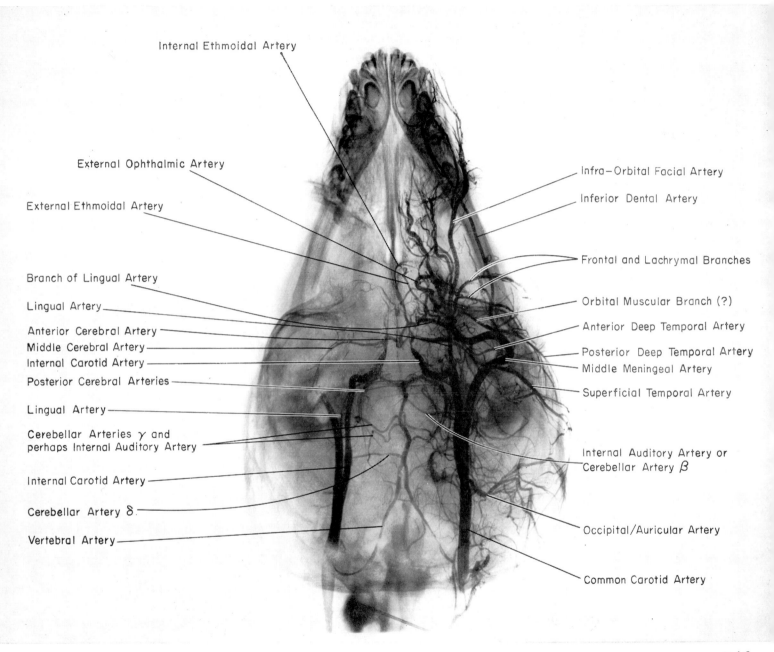

Internal Ethmoidal Artery

External Ophthalmic Artery

External Ethmoidal Artery

Branch of Lingual Artery

Lingual Artery

Anterior Cerebral Artery

Middle Cerebral Artery

Internal Carotid Artery

Posterior Cerebral Arteries

Lingual Artery

Cerebellar Arteries γ and perhaps Internal Auditory Artery

Internal Carotid Artery

Cerebellar Artery δ

Vertebral Artery

Infra–Orbital Facial Artery

Inferior Dental Artery

Frontal and Lachrymal Branches

Orbital Muscular Branch (?)

Anterior Deep Temporal Artery

Posterior Deep Temporal Artery

Middle Meningeal Artery

Superficial Temporal Artery

Internal Auditory Artery or Cerebellar Artery β

Occipital/Auricular Artery

Common Carotid Artery

× 1·0

Tandler's description of *Otaria jubata*, the Southern Sea-lion might be expected to resemble this injection of a related species. There are, however, some points of difference and some difficulties.

The external carotid gives rise to a combined auricular and occipital artery. No facial (external maxillary) artery has been identified. There appear to be both anterior and posterior deep temporals though neither is easy to see in the lateral view. No middle meningeal has been found but the other arteries in the orbit are well filled.

The large vessel tentatively identified as the lachrymal branch is superimposed on the infra-orbital facial for some distance in the lateral view.

Cerebellar arteries are asymmetrical. The internal auditory arteries are less obviously hypertrophied than in the Baikal seal.

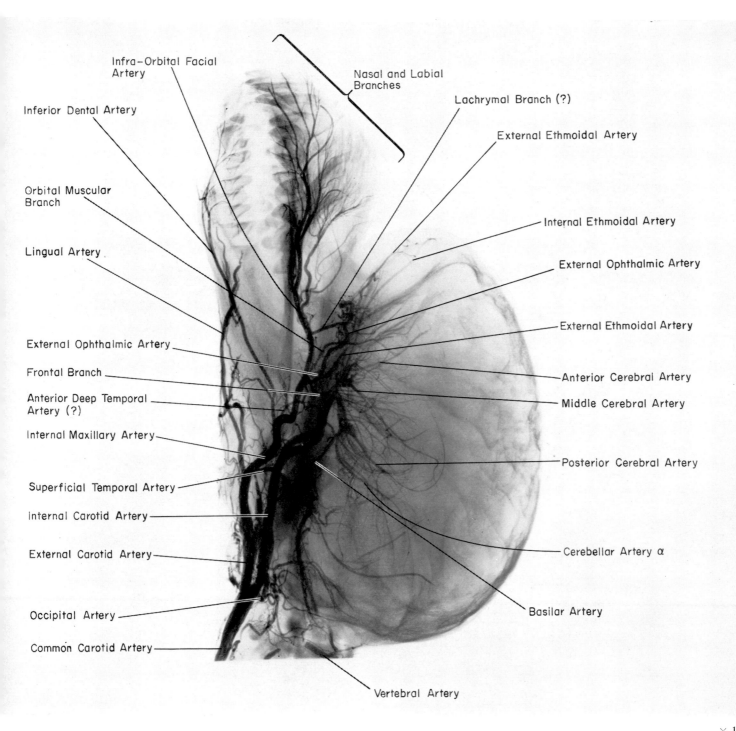

Infra-Orbital Facial
Artery

Inferior Dental Artery

Orbital Muscular
Branch

Lingual Artery

External Ophthalmic Artery

Frontal Branch

Anterior Deep Temporal
Artery (?)

Internal Maxillary Artery

Superficial Temporal Artery

Internal Carotid Artery

External Carotid Artery

Occipital Artery

Common Carotid Artery

Nasal and Labial
Branches

Lachrymal Branch (?)

External Ethmoidal Artery

Internal Ethmoidal Artery

External Ophthalmic Artery

External Ethmoidal Artery

Anterior Cerebral Artery

Middle Cerebral Artery

Posterior Cerebral Artery

Cerebellar Artery α

Basilar Artery

Vertebral Artery

× 1·0

Odobenus rosmarus
Walrus

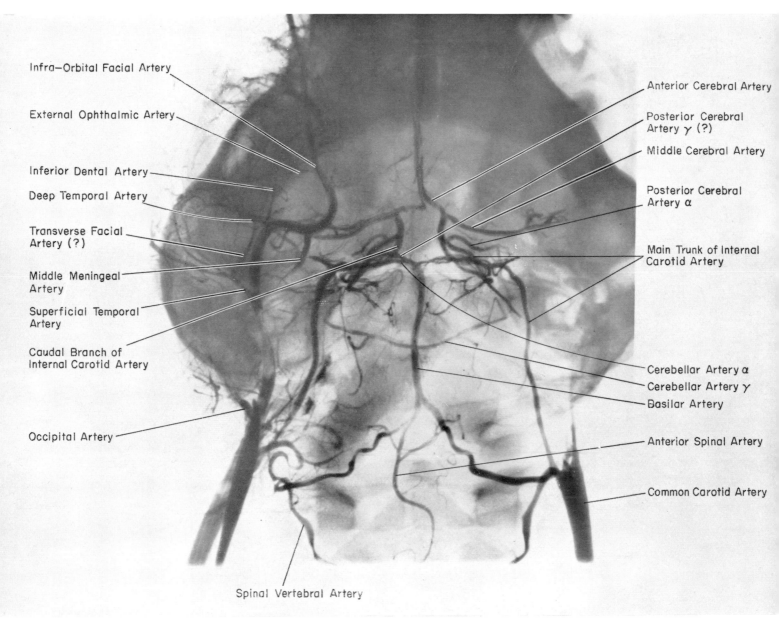

Infra—Orbital Facial Artery

External Ophthalmic Artery

Inferior Dental Artery

Deep Temporal Artery

Transverse Facial Artery (?)

Middle Meningeal Artery

Superficial Temporal Artery

Caudal Branch of Internal Carotid Artery

Occipital Artery

Spinal Vertebral Artery

Anterior Cerebral Artery

Posterior Cerebral Artery γ (?)

Middle Cerebral Artery

Posterior Cerebral Artery α

Main Trunk of Internal Carotid Artery

Cerebellar Artery α

Cerebellar Artery γ

Basilar Artery

Anterior Spinal Artery

Common Carotid Artery

$\times$ 0·58

For a reason not understood the lingual arteries have completely failed to fill in this specimen. The size and importance of the facial (external maxillary) artery is therefore also unknown.

Note the absence of the auricular artery. No doubt a small twig exists to supply the region of the external auditory meatus.

In most ways the arterial tree resembles that of seal and sea-lion. Note the very large middle meningeal trunk passing backwards from the orbital region.

Note, also, the anterior choroidal artery (posterior cerebral artery α) arising from the main trunk of the internal carotid.

There may also be a posterior cerebral artery δ (unlabelled) in addition to the large posterior cerebral γ.

The cerebellar artery γ is very large and may be the source of the internal auditory artery.

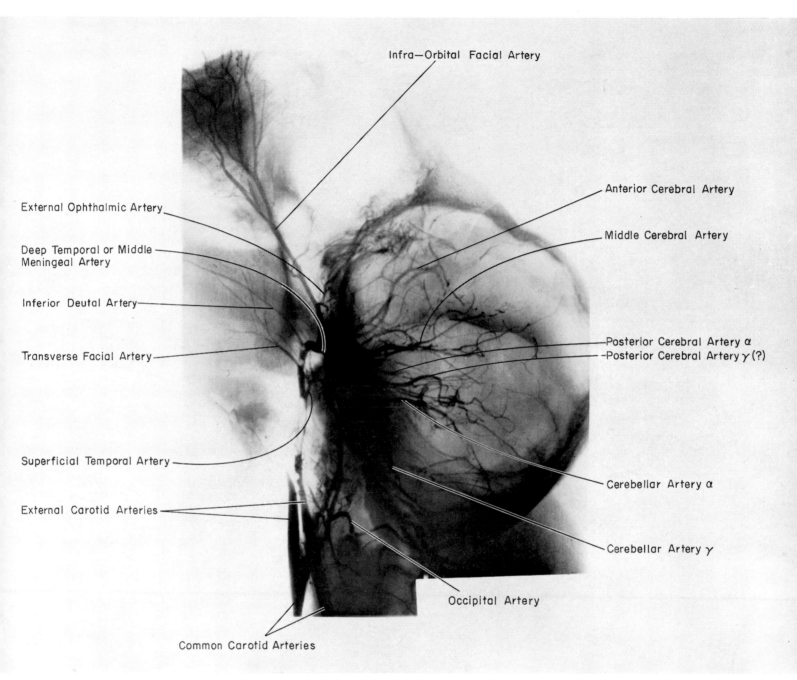

Infra—Orbital Facial Artery

Anterior Cerebral Artery

Middle Cerebral Artery

External Ophthalmic Artery

Deep Temporal or Middle Meningeal Artery

Inferior Deutal Artery

Posterior Cerebral Artery α

Posterior Cerebral Artery γ (?)

Transverse Facial Artery

Superficial Temporal Artery

Cerebellar Artery α

External Carotid Arteries

Cerebellar Artery γ

Occipital Artery

Common Carotid Arteries

× 0·5

Pusa sibirica
Baikal Seal

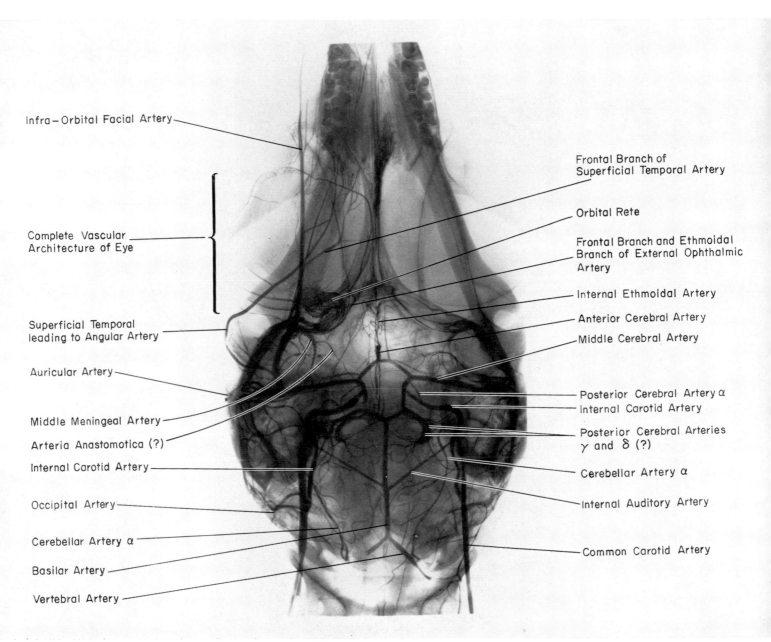

Infra—Orbital Facial Artery

Complete Vascular Architecture of Eye

Superficial Temporal leading to Angular Artery

Auricular Artery

Middle Meningeal Artery

Arteria Anastomotica (?)

Internal Carotid Artery

Occipital Artery

Cerebellar Artery α

Basilar Artery

Vertebral Artery

Frontal Branch of Superficial Temporal Artery

Orbital Rete

Frontal Branch and Ethmoidal Branch of External Ophthalmic Artery

Internal Ethmoidal Artery

Anterior Cerebral Artery

Middle Cerebral Artery

Posterior Cerebral Artery α

Internal Carotid Artery

Posterior Cerebral Arteries γ and δ (?)

Cerebellar Artery α

Internal Auditory Artery

Common Carotid Artery

× 0·85

The segment of external carotid artery which crosses the mastoid bulla is compressed and poorly filled. This in turn has led to very poor filling of the lingual artery and may also be partly responsible for what seems to be an excessively narrowed auricular artery.

The extremely good filling of the arteries of the (enormous) eye, bear witness to the vascular system needed to maintain perfusion under high submersion pressure. No doubt the orbital rete developed from the same stimulus. The huge internal auditory arteries are also presumably connected with the adaptations to diving, for the seal's inner ear is protected by a system sf surrounding veins. Tandler (1899) in one of his

illustrations to a description of *Phoca vitulina* shows the origins of these large branches from the basilar artery; but without comment.

This specimen of the Baikal seal differs from Tandler's description of the common seal in several respects.

1. The auricular (posterior auricular) artery is apparently much larger in Phoca vitulina.

2. We have not been able to identify a facial (external maxillary) artery.

3. The external ophthalmic artery of this Baikal Seal is reduplicated. It seems that the rete with its retinal, choroidal and ciliary branches is supplied by the anterior branch while

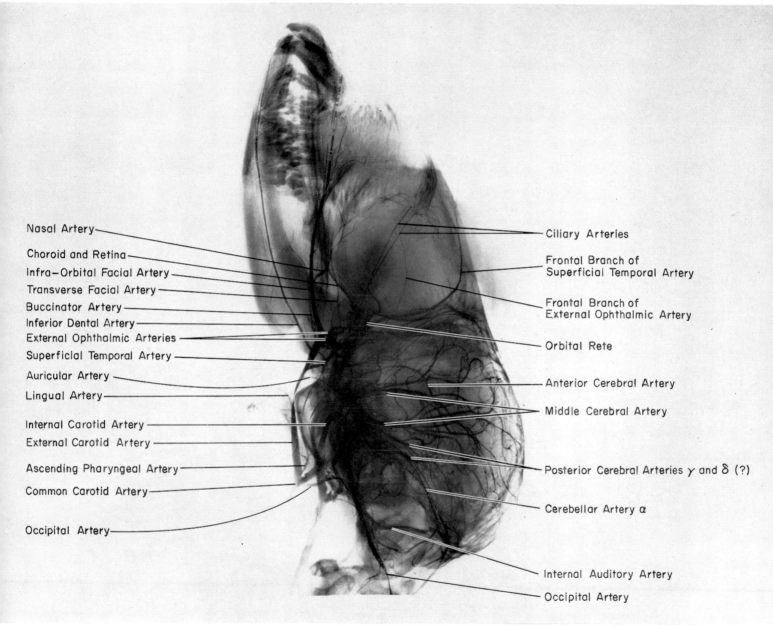

Nasal Artery

Choroid and Retina

Infra-Orbital Facial Artery

Transverse Facial Artery

Buccinator Artery

Inferior Dental Artery

External Ophthalmic Arteries

Superficial Temporal Artery

Auricular Artery

Lingual Artery

Internal Carotid Artery

External Carotid Artery

Ascending Pharyngeal Artery

Common Carotid Artery

Occipital Artery

Ciliary Arteries

Frontal Branch of
Superficial Temporal Artery

Frontal Branch of
External Ophthalmic Artery

Orbital Rete

Anterior Cerebral Artery

Middle Cerebral Artery

Posterior Cerebral Arteries γ and δ (?)

Cerebellar Artery α

Internal Auditory Artery

Occipital Artery

× 0·85

the posterior of the two branches supplies the large recurrent middle meningeal artery and the frontal and external ethmoidal branches. In *Phoca vitulina* all come from a single stem.

One of the small branches which arises from the middle meningeal artery may well be the arteria anastomotica (which in the common seal, Tandler says, is a small branch of an intra-orbital muscular twig).

4. The internal ophthalmic artery must be absent or extremely small.

Two posterior cerebral arteries arise close together and are presumably γ and δ. Posterior cerebral arteries α are only anterior choroidal vessels.

Apart from the internal auditory artery the major posterior fossa arteries are cerebellar α and have a very long course.

220

Halichoerus grypus
Grey Seal

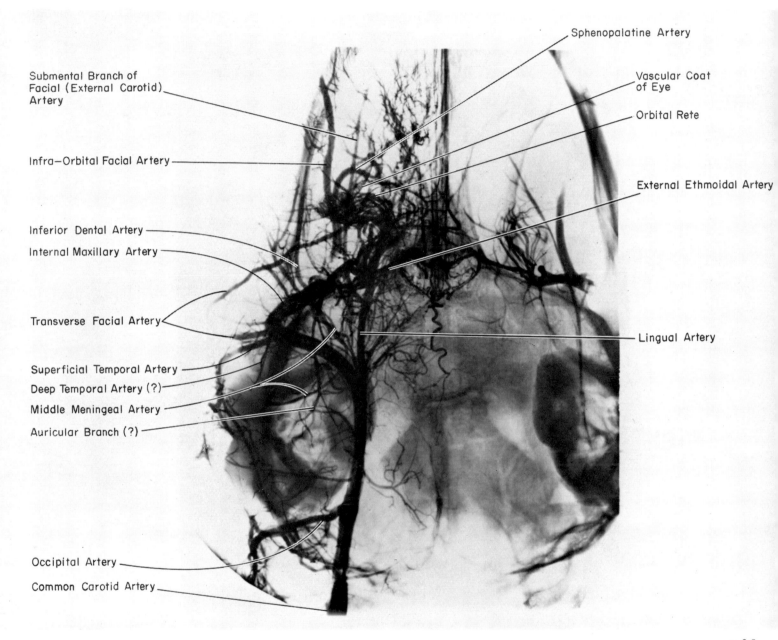

Submental Branch of Facial (External Carotid) Artery

Sphenopalatine Artery

Vascular Coat of Eye

Orbital Rete

Infra-Orbital Facial Artery

External Ethmoidal Artery

Inferior Dental Artery

Internal Maxillary Artery

Transverse Facial Artery

Lingual Artery

Superficial Temporal Artery

Deep Temporal Artery (?)

Middle Meningeal Artery

Auricular Branch (?)

Occipital Artery

Common Carotid Artery

× 0·8

The external carotid branches are so well filled that identification has become difficult in certain cases, for instance the posterior deep temporal artery in the ventro-dorsal view, the origin of the middle meningeal and the exact course of the facial (external maxillary artery). Neither the internal carotid nor the vertebral artery is outlined.

The general configuration is typical of seals. The posterior auricular artery is too small to be recognised. The transverse facial continues forwards as a frontal artery, the orbital rete is well developed and the middle meningeal enters the cranial cavity from the region of the orbit.

There is an artery, identified as the "auricular branch", the homologue of which in other mammals is not quite clear; but which evidently passes backwards on or in the under surface of the skull to supply the region of the inner ear. It would seem likely from the position and course of this artery that it runs for a part of its course within the pterygoid canal and it may well represent a portion of the inferior division of the stapedial artery in which flow has been reversed.

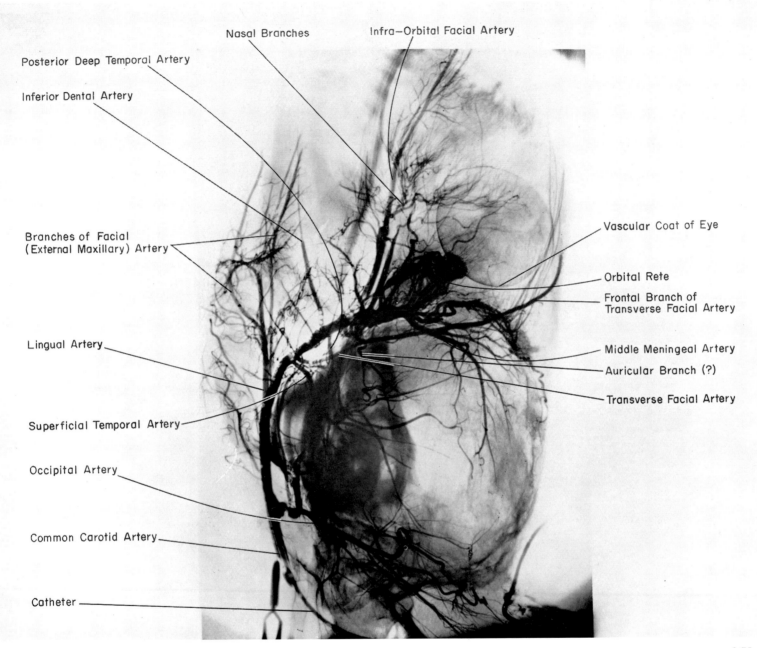

Nasal Branches

Infra—Orbital Facial Artery

Posterior Deep Temporal Artery

Inferior Dental Artery

Vascular Coat of Eye

Orbital Rete

Frontal Branch of
Transverse Facial Artery

Branches of Facial
(External Maxillary) Artery

Lingual Artery

Middle Meningeal Artery

Auricular Branch (?)

Transverse Facial Artery

Superficial Temporal Artery

Occipital Artery

Common Carotid Artery

Catheter

× 0·75

Orycteropus afer
Aardvark

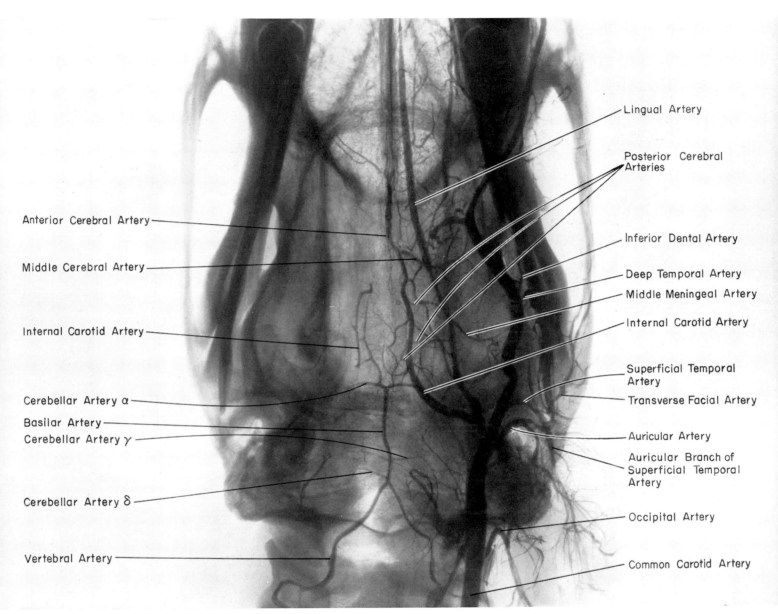

Lingual Artery

Posterior Cerebral Arteries

Anterior Cerebral Artery

Inferior Dental Artery

Middle Cerebral Artery

Deep Temporal Artery

Middle Meningeal Artery

Internal Carotid Artery

Internal Carotid Artery

Superficial Temporal Artery

Cerebellar Artery α

Transverse Facial Artery

Basilar Artery

Cerebellar Artery γ

Auricular Artery

Auricular Branch of Superficial Temporal Artery

Cerebellar Artery δ

Occipital Artery

Vertebral Artery

Common Carotid Artery

× 1·5

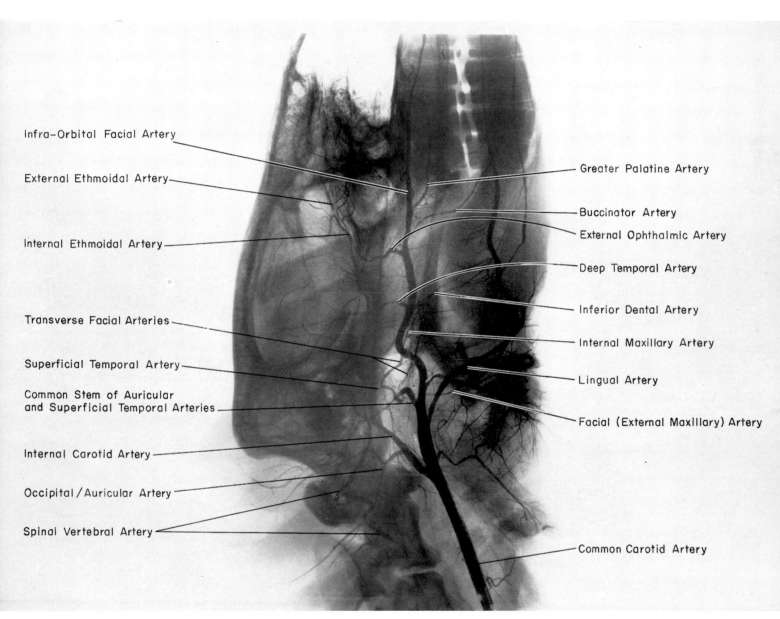

Infra-Orbital Facial Artery

External Ethmoidal Artery

Internal Ethmoidal Artery

Transverse Facial Arteries

Superficial Temporal Artery

Common Stem of Auricular
and Superficial Temporal Arteries

Internal Carotid Artery

Occipital/Auricular Artery

Spinal Vertebral Artery

Greater Palatine Artery

Buccinator Artery

External Ophthalmic Artery

Deep Temporal Artery

Inferior Dental Artery

Internal Maxillary Artery

Lingual Artery

Facial (External Maxillary) Artery

Common Carotid Artery

× 0·9

In the lateral view it is evident that the occipital artery arises from the internal carotid. Blood supply to the external ear derives partly from an auricular branch of the occipital artery and partly from a common stem for auricular and superficial temporal vessels.

There is a very considerable blood supply to the upper part of the neck, probably from superior thyroid and salivary branches of the external carotid artery.

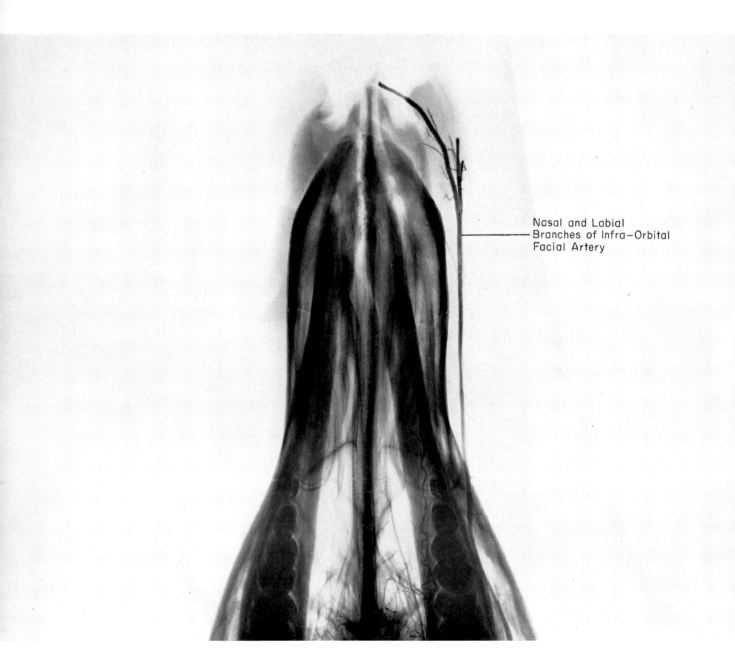

Nasal and Labial
Branches of Infra-Orbital
Facial Artery

× 1·5

Proboscidea

It is strange that our search of the literature has revealed no proper account of the cerebral arteries of the Indian Elephant and no account at all of the cranial arteries of the African (*Loxodonta africana*) beyond the common carotid, which is mentioned by Sikes (1971).

Allen Muller recorded that much for the Indian Elephant in 1682 when he described his dissection of an elephant accidentally burnt in Dublin on Friday, June 17th in the year 1681, saying "The Carotide Arterie of this animal was very large: for it readily received a large cane into it".

The next significant contribution to knowledge of the anatomy of the cranial arteries of the Indian Elephant (*Elephas maximus*) came from Watson in 1875 and is given here in precis form because we have been unable to find any other.

The common carotid arteries of both sides arise from the trunk of the innominate. They divide into internal and external carotids close to the angle of the jaw.

The external carotid passes outwards and upwards to the posterior aspect of the temporo-mandibular joint where it divides into the superficial temporal and the internal maxillary.

The external carotid supplies the following branches:

Lingual artery. This large artery supplies not only the tongue but provides two large branches to the soft palate.

Facial (external maxillary) artery. This comes off immediately in front of the lingual, runs downward and forward to turn around the angle of the jaw and then divide into two. One branch runs forward, anastamoses with the *mental* artery and supplies the lower lip. The other branch passes backward and supplies the buccinator muscle. The facial artery also gives off a branch which runs forward on the surface of the mylo-hyoid muscle which it supplies. Watson called this the *sublingual* branch.

Internal maxillary artery. This is the largest of the three anterior branches of the external carotid. Having reached the base of the skull it passes through the spheno-palatine canal, runs below the orbit and emerges from the infra-orbital canal to supply the trunk, running along the lateral margin to the tip. It gives many branches to the trunk, one in particular leaves the artery immediately above the incisor tooth and runs along the dorsal aspect.

The internal maxillary gives off several branches:

The *middle meningeal* arises before the internal maxillary enters the spheno-palatine canal. Watson says that it supplies not only the meninges but the mucous membrane of the multitudinous air-sinuses of the skull. His statement ought to be checked.

Posterior deep temporal artery.

Anterior deep temporal artery, arising after the internal maxillary artery has passed through the spheno-palatine canal.

A small *pterygoid* artery.

A large *buccal* artery describes a curve downward and forward and is distributed to the buccinator muscle.

External ophthalmic artery. This is a large vessel which is given off just before the artery enters the infra-orbital canal. Several of its branches (presumably palpebral and frontal) emerge on the face.

Superior dental artery. This leaves the infra-orbital canal by way of the superior dental canal and is distributed to the teeth of the upper jaw.

Superficial temporal artery. This passes straight up behind the temporo-mandibular joint under cover of the parotid gland as far as the zygoma where it divides into two terminal branches. The posterior, the smaller, passes up to the vertex whilst the anterior, considerably larger, runs upward and forward in the direction of the orbit. These branches are the main source of supply to the temporal gland.

The superficial temporal artery supplies:

A large *posterior auricular* which also supplies the parotid gland and the *stylo-mastoid* artery.

The *inferior dental* artery which, having passed through the dental canal, emerges as the *mental* artery.

The sub-zygomatic artery which immediately divides into the *masseteric* and the *transverse facial*.

Watson's account of the intracranial vessels is very short and open to question because what he describes is so unlike other mammals. Most of those who have dissected elephants have commented upon the putrefaction which sets in before the brain is reached. Therein may lie the clue to the inadequacy of Watson's description.

He says that the internal carotid divides into two branches, the *anterior cerebral* which runs forward and into the longitudinal fissure where it is united to the opposite anterior cerebral by the anterior communicating, and a posterior branch which anastamoses directly with the vertebral artery.

The vertebral artery, after entering a foramen transversarium of one of the cervical vertebrae posterior to the 5th runs up until it reaches a deep groove in the arch of the atlas which it perforates in order to enter the cranial cavity where it anastamoses with the posterior branch of the internal carotid. The vertebral artery in the neck provides many muscular branches, one of which is especially large and replaces the occipital branch of the carotid.

Within the head Watson states that the vertebral artery provides branches to supply the cerebellum and the posterior lobes of the cerebrum.

No conclusions can be drawn from Watson's failure to describe the middle cerebral artery but his positive comments about the vertebral should be taken seriously. It may well be that the basilar artery in the elephant is a paired structure.

Our own radiographs of the injection of *Elephas maximus*, poor though they are, support Watson's account of the external carotid branches; but unfortunately give no information about the cerebral vessels.

Hyracoidea

Two species are illustrated. In the case of the Rock hyrax there are pictures of two specimens. They serve as a reminder of the great variations between individuals.

B

Deep Ter

Inferior C

Pterygoic

Internal I
Artery

Lingual A

more like
of deer,
maxillary
The C
carotid a

Hyracoidea

Two species are illustrated. In the case of the Rock hyrax there are pictures of two specimens. They serve as a reminder of the great variations between individuals.

Procavia capensis
Rock Hyrax

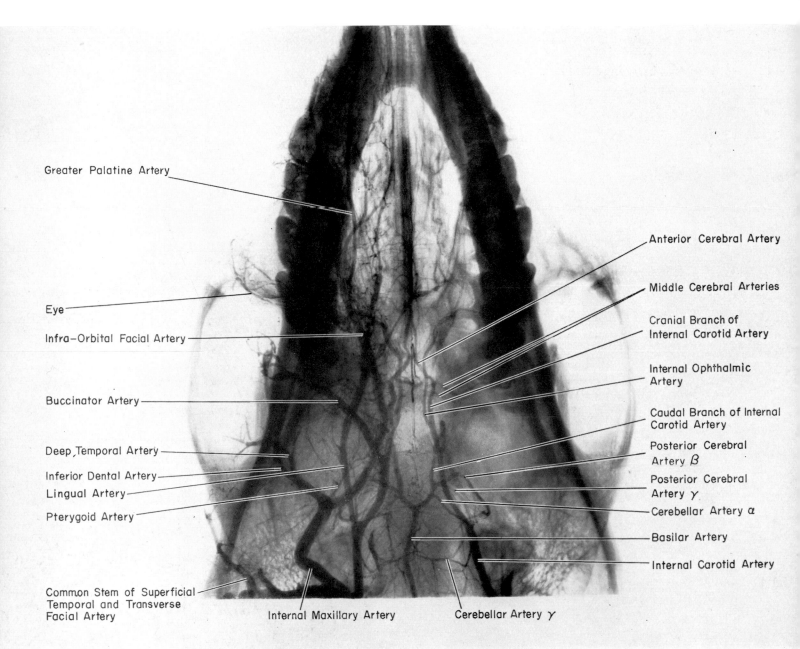

Greater Palatine Artery

Eye

Infra–Orbital Facial Artery

Buccinator Artery

Deep Temporal Artery

Inferior Dental Artery

Lingual Artery

Pterygoid Artery

Common Stem of Superficial
Temporal and Transverse
Facial Artery

Internal Maxillary Artery

Anterior Cerebral Artery

Middle Cerebral Arteries

Cranial Branch of
Internal Carotid Artery

Internal Ophthalmic
Artery

Caudal Branch of Internal
Carotid Artery

Posterior Cerebral
Artery β

Posterior Cerebral
Artery γ

Cerebellar Artery α

Basilar Artery

Internal Carotid Artery

Cerebellar Artery γ

$\times 2{\cdot}5$

Previous descriptions of the major cranial arteries by Lindahl and Lundberg (1946) and by George (1874), do not entirely agree with the present injection studies, though the disagreement is partly that of terminology.

For instance, although unfortunately the bifurcation of the common carotid has been distorted by the catheter in one specimen, it is almost certain that the occipital artery arises from the external carotid, not the common carotid. The next major branch of the external carotid has been given various names; but seems to represent the common origin of the auricular (posterior auricular) and superficial temporal arteries. One of the animals has a transverse facial springing

from the superficial temporal. In the other animal filling of this vessel is poor in the lateral view.

There is no sign of a facial (external maxillary) artery in either animal.

In one the posterior deep temporal arises from the inferior dental. In the other it is not definitely filled but may have the same origin.

A very large buccinator artery is found, perhaps because other arteries to the region of the cheek are so poorly developed.

The infra-orbital facial supplies a vessel which may be called the external ophthalmic though its point of origin is

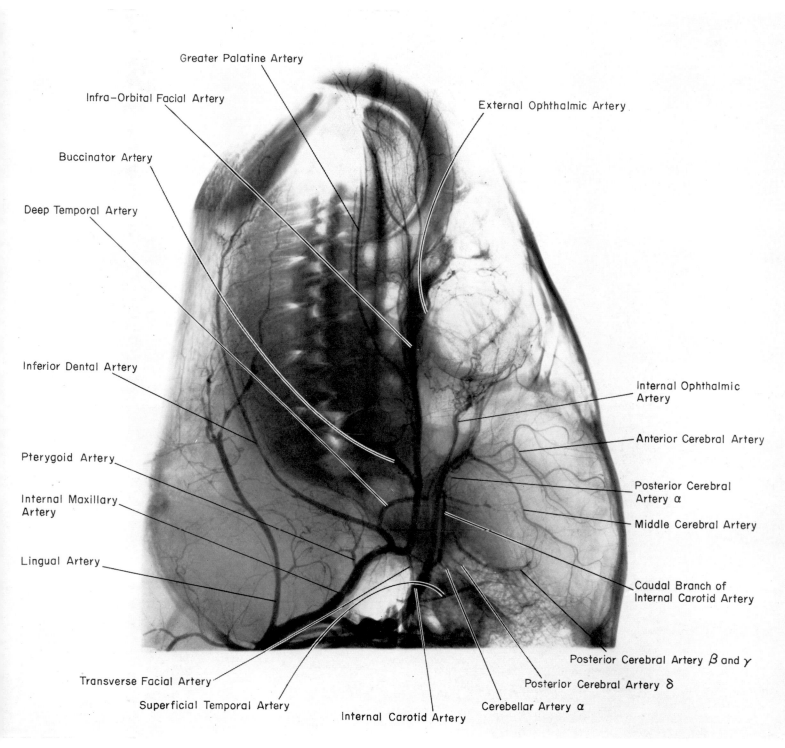

Greater Palatine Artery

Infra–Orbital Facial Artery

Buccinator Artery

Deep Temporal Artery

External Ophthalmic Artery

Inferior Dental Artery

Internal Ophthalmic Artery

Anterior Cerebral Artery

Pterygoid Artery

Posterior Cerebral Artery α

Internal Maxillary Artery

Middle Cerebral Artery

Lingual Artery

Caudal Branch of Internal Carotid Artery

Posterior Cerebral Artery β and γ

Transverse Facial Artery

Posterior Cerebral Artery δ

Superficial Temporal Artery

Internal Carotid Artery

Cerebellar Artery α

× 2·0

more like that of the angular artery when, as in many species of deer, that artery does not spring from the facial (external maxillary).

The Circle of Willis has direct supply from the internal carotid arteries. There is no rete. The basilar artery appears to continue downwards as the anterior spinal artery at least to the level of C2 without any major contribution from the vertebral or the occipital arteries. Previous authors are silent on this point.

One of the specimens shows a leash of vessels arising from

Procavia capensis

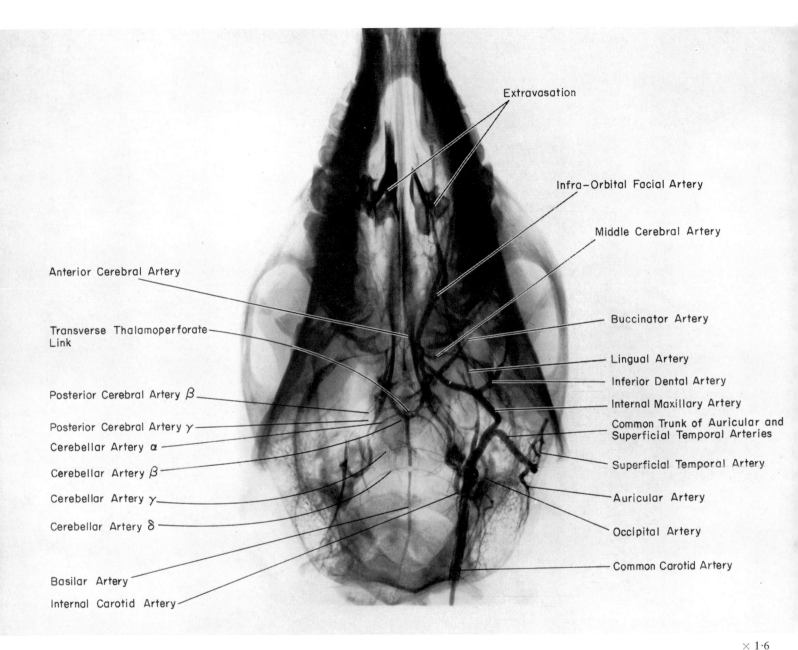

Extravasation

Infra-Orbital Facial Artery

Middle Cerebral Artery

Anterior Cerebral Artery

Transverse Thalamoperforate Link

Buccinator Artery

Lingual Artery

Inferior Dental Artery

Posterior Cerebral Artery β

Internal Maxillary Artery

Posterior Cerebral Artery γ

Common Trunk of Auricular and Superficial Temporal Arteries

Cerebellar Artery α

Cerebellar Artery β

Superficial Temporal Artery

Cerebellar Artery γ

Cerebellar Artery δ

Auricular Artery

Occipital Artery

Basilar Artery

Common Carotid Artery

Internal Carotid Artery

× 1·6

the caudal branches of the carotid close to their junction with the top of the basilar artery and forming side-to-side communications. Presumably these are the thalamo-perforate arteries.

In one animal; but not in the other, the middle cerebral arteries originate as two vessels on each side.

The posterior cerebral vessels are well shown. Both animals show α arteries (anterior choroidal) and a pair of arteries, presumably β and γ having a common origin. On one side of one animal a posterior cerebral δ has been filled.

There is a large internal ophthalmic artery.

Procavia capensis has many unique features; but we would agree with Beddard (1904) that there are some resemblances to the Perissodactyla.

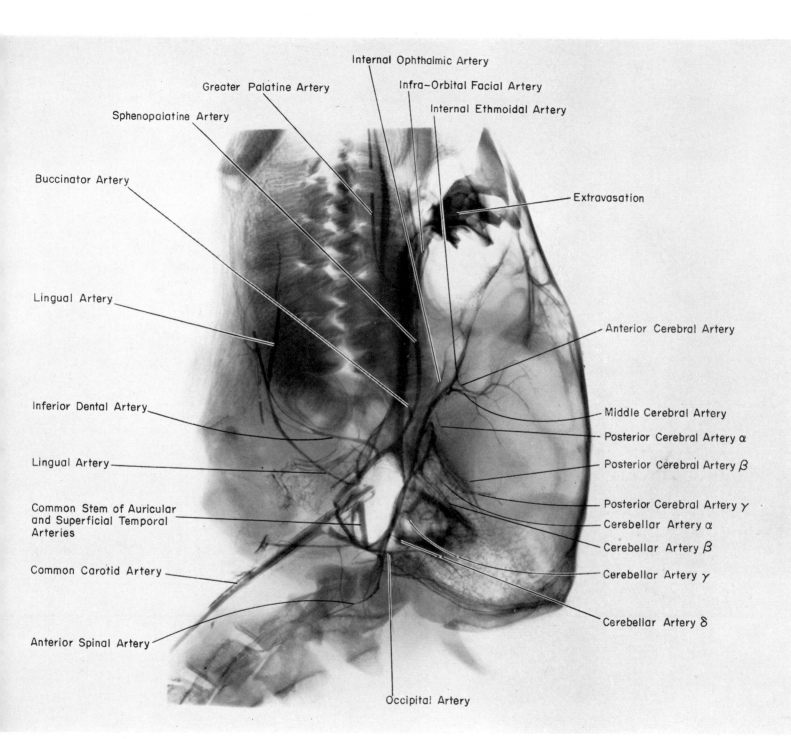

Internal Ophthalmic Artery

Greater Palatine Artery

Infra-Orbital Facial Artery

Sphenopalatine Artery

Internal Ethmoidal Artery

Buccinator Artery

Extravasation

Lingual Artery

Anterior Cerebral Artery

Inferior Dental Artery

Middle Cerebral Artery

Posterior Cerebral Artery α

Lingual Artery

Posterior Cerebral Artery β

Posterior Cerebral Artery γ

Common Stem of Auricular
and Superficial Temporal
Arteries

Cerebellar Artery α

Cerebellar Artery β

Common Carotid Artery

Cerebellar Artery γ

Cerebellar Artery δ

Anterior Spinal Artery

Occipital Artery

× 1·6

Dendrohyrax dorsalis
Beecroft's Hyrax

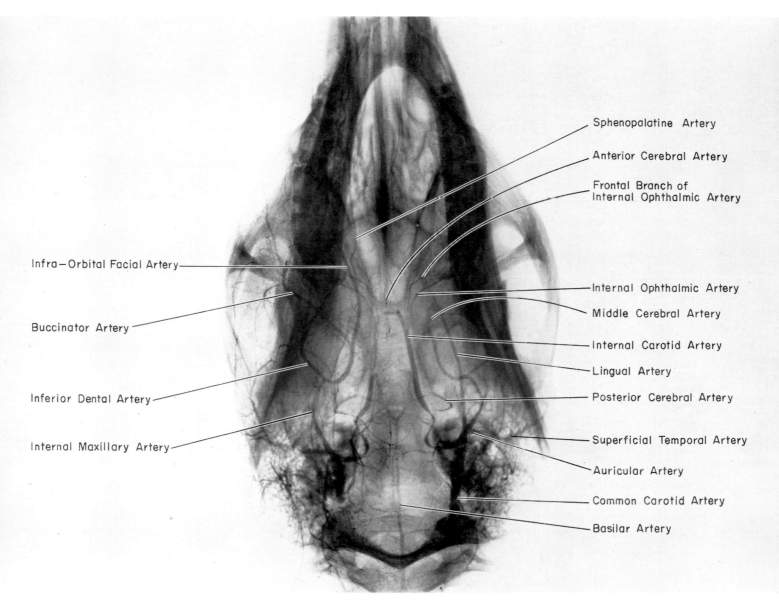

Sphenopalatine Artery

Anterior Cerebral Artery

Frontal Branch of
Internal Ophthalmic Artery

Infra—Orbital Facial Artery

Internal Ophthalmic Artery

Middle Cerebral Artery

Buccinator Artery

Internal Carotid Artery

Lingual Artery

Inferior Dental Artery

Posterior Cerebral Artery

Superficial Temporal Artery

Internal Maxillary Artery

Auricular Artery

Common Carotid Artery

Basilar Artery

× 1·25

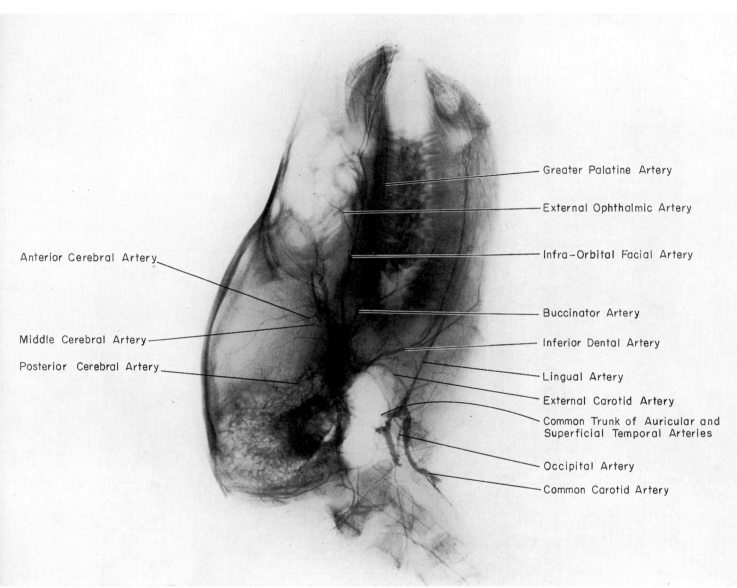

Anterior Cerebral Artery

Middle Cerebral Artery

Posterior Cerebral Artery

Greater Palatine Artery

External Ophthalmic Artery

Infra-Orbital Facial Artery

Buccinator Artery

Inferior Dental Artery

Lingual Artery

External Carotid Artery

Common Trunk of Auricular and
Superficial Temporal Arteries

Occipital Artery

Common Carotid Artery

$\times$ 1·25

The arrangement of the vessels is very similar to *Procavia capensis*, only the early division of the internal ophthalmic artery being strikingly different.

The anastomosis between the two posterior cerebral arteries on the dorsal surface of the midbrain, seen in the ventro-dorsal view, is interesting.

Sirenia

During the nineteenth century there was a dispute about the vascular arrangements of the manatee, Huxley (1860) and Owen (1868) denying that it possessed an arterial retial system. Murie (1874), however, described in some detail how the major systemic arteries break up quickly into bundles and leashes of smaller parallel vessels. Fawcett in 1942 confirmed Murie's work.

We have been unable to examine a specimen ourselves and the existing descriptions which we have been able to find give no information about the cerebral vessels. Murie's account of the extracranial arteries, however, may be of considerable help. Some of it is quoted here. The similarity to the cetacean system is clear.

Murie found the stem of a fair-sized common carotid which was branchless until it lay opposite the deep hollow in front of the shoulder where a transverse humeral artery ran into a broad, radiating rete covering the subscapularis, supraspinatus, etc. More anteriorly, on a level with the cricoid, the common carotid divided as into internal and external carotid arteries. The internal, in Murie's words, "dips among rete mirabile at the posterior base of the skull just behind the cranial series of plexuses. Among others one occupies the posterior portion of the great fissure between the occipital and tympano-perotic bones and whilst mingling with the cervical and spinal rete, complex branches are lodged within the skull at what corresponds to a groove or recess of the lateral sinus, where also venous channels obtain.

The external carotid at the stylo-hyal and under cover of the digastric and parotid gland bifurcates; and plexuses are derived from both of these. The branch agreeing with the facial runs towards the angle of the mandible and at the concavity of the body of the bone, turns upwards and is distributed with a plexiform arrangement on the face. From its proximal end and in fact enwrapping it, are retia which may be regarded as submaxillary, submental, etc. subdivisions".

In fact, every branch of what would otherwise be a conventional mammalian external carotid tree ends in the same retial pattern.

Perissodactyla

The horse, *Equus caballus*, as the type animal was described in detail by Tandler (1899) and the following account is taken principally from him.

(Similarities between horse, zebra and tapir are obvious.)

After the origin of the thyroid artery the common carotid runs cranially and divides into three branches, the rather narrow internal carotid, the occipital artery and the large external carotid artery.

The external carotid, after a short course, gives rise to a very short common trunk for the lingual and facial (external maxillary) arteries. It then continues up to the level of the mandibular condyle where, giving off a large posterior auricular artery and a small anterior auricular as well as a number of glandular branches, it becomes the internal maxillary artery. The internal maxillary, running forwards, supplies by another common trunk the superficial temporal and transverse facial vessels. Further anteriorly still it loses the inferior dental and deep temporal arteries and enters the pterygoid canal. At the anterior end of the pterygoid canal the internal maxillary gives rise to a large orbital or external ophthalmic artery which penetrates the orbital wall, supplies muscular branches and a ciliary artery and ends by dividing into the lachrymal, frontal and ethmoidal branches. An anastomosis is formed within the orbit between the external and internal ophthalmic arteries. The internal maxillary also supplies the well-developed spheno-palatine and the buccinator arteries. It then continues forwards into the infra-orbital canal as the infra-orbital facial artery.

The occipital artery, whose precise relations with the other two main terminal branches of the common carotid vary from animal to animal, runs dorsally and cranially from its origin. It first gives off a number of branches to the neck muscles, then divides into an ascending mastoid artery and a descending anastomotic ramus. Both of these have muscular twigs: but their principle destinations are, for one the mastoid diploe and for the other a wide connection with the cerebral vertebral artery via a hole in the atlas homologous with the foramen transversarium.

The internal carotid is a relatively small vessel which arrives at the skull base by coursing around the medial side of the mastoid bulla. The internal carotid then penetrates the cartilage which fills in foramen lacerum and its surrounding bone-defect at the point of the petrous bone and enters the cavernous sinus. Within the cavernous sinus, while still subdural, the internal carotid gives off an anastomotic branch which crosses the clivus to join the similar branch of the other carotid, an anastomotic connection which varies in size from one animal to another. It seems to resemble in position, though not in size, the anastomosis which may exist between the origin of the tentorial arteries in man (El Gammal *et al.*, 1967).

After piercing the dura the internal carotid divides into cranial and caudal branches. From the former comes the internal ophthalmic and then a division into middle and anterior cerebral vessels. From the caudal branch arise the posterior cerebral arteries (usually β, γ and δ) and the cerebellar artery before it unites with its fellow at the upper end of the basilar.

The basilar, itself, tapers as it passes caudally; but does have a functional connection with the cerebral vertebral artery. A pair of cerebellar arteries γ is usually found.

Accounts of the cranial arteries of the horse are also given in general text-books such as Sisson (1938), Jenke (1919), Nickel and Schwarz (1903).

Equus caballus
The Horse

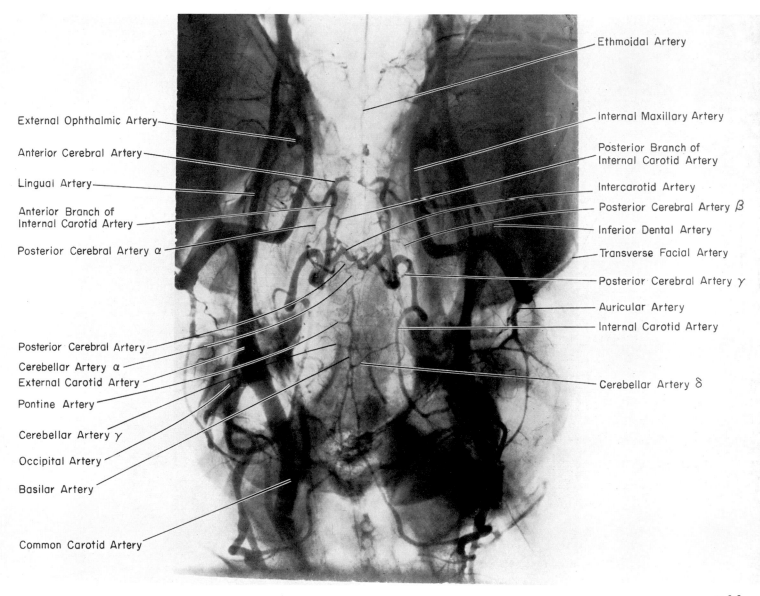

Ethmoidal Artery

External Ophthalmic Artery

Anterior Cerebral Artery

Lingual Artery

Anterior Branch of
Internal Carotid Artery

Posterior Cerebral Artery α

Internal Maxillary Artery

Posterior Branch of
Internal Carotid Artery

Intercarotid Artery

Posterior Cerebral Artery β

Inferior Dental Artery

Transverse Facial Artery

Posterior Cerebral Artery γ

Auricular Artery

Internal Carotid Artery

Posterior Cerebral Artery

Cerebellar Artery α

External Carotid Artery

Pontine Artery

Cerebellar Artery γ

Occipital Artery

Basilar Artery

Cerebellar Artery δ

Common Carotid Artery

$\times$ 0·5

In this example a variation of the origin of cerebellar artery γ is shown on one side, where its major source is from the δ position.

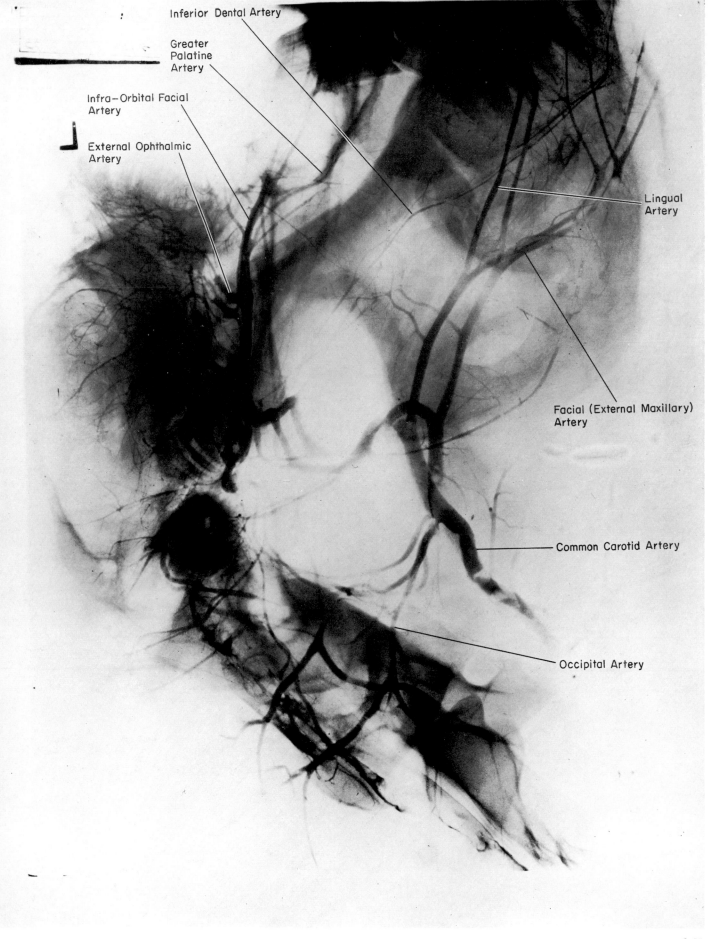

Inferior Dental Artery

Greater Palatine Artery

Infra—Orbital Facial Artery

External Ophthalmic Artery

Lingual Artery

Facial (External Maxillary) Artery

Common Carotid Artery

Occipital Artery

× 0·55

Equus caballus

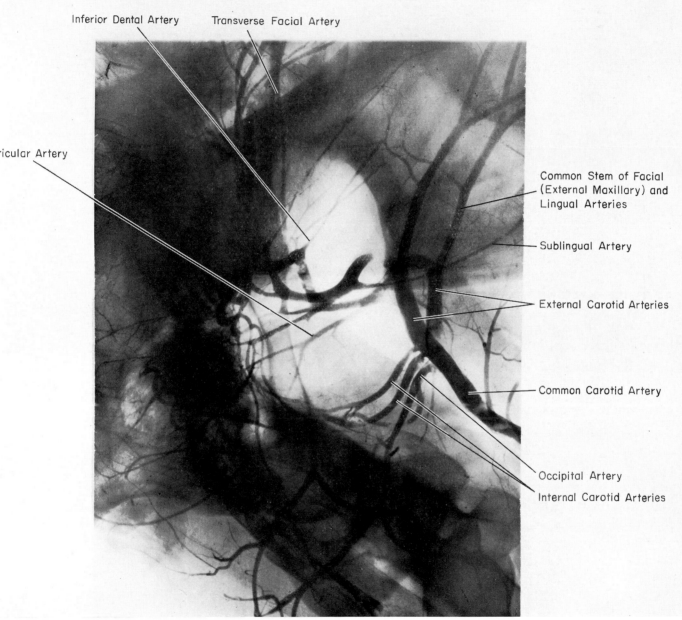

Inferior Dental Artery

Transverse Facial Artery

Auricular Artery

Common Stem of Facial (External Maxillary) and Lingual Arteries

Sublingual Artery

External Carotid Arteries

Common Carotid Artery

Occipital Artery

Internal Carotid Arteries

× 0·6

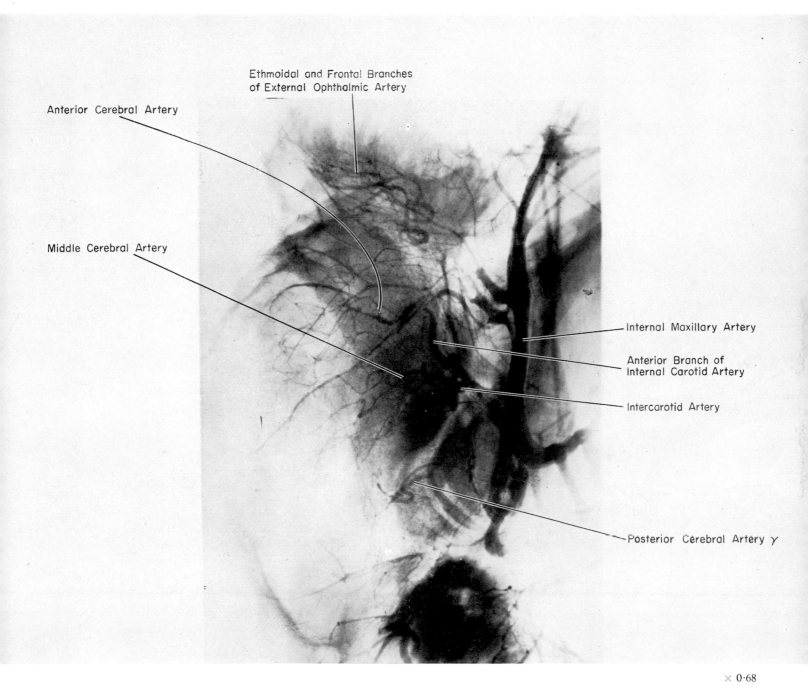

Ethmoidal and Frontal Branches
of External Ophthalmic Artery

Anterior Cerebral Artery

Middle Cerebral Artery

Internal Maxillary Artery

Anterior Branch of
Internal Carotid Artery

Intercarotid Artery

Posterior Cerebral Artery γ

× 0·68

Equus zebra burchelli
Common Zebra

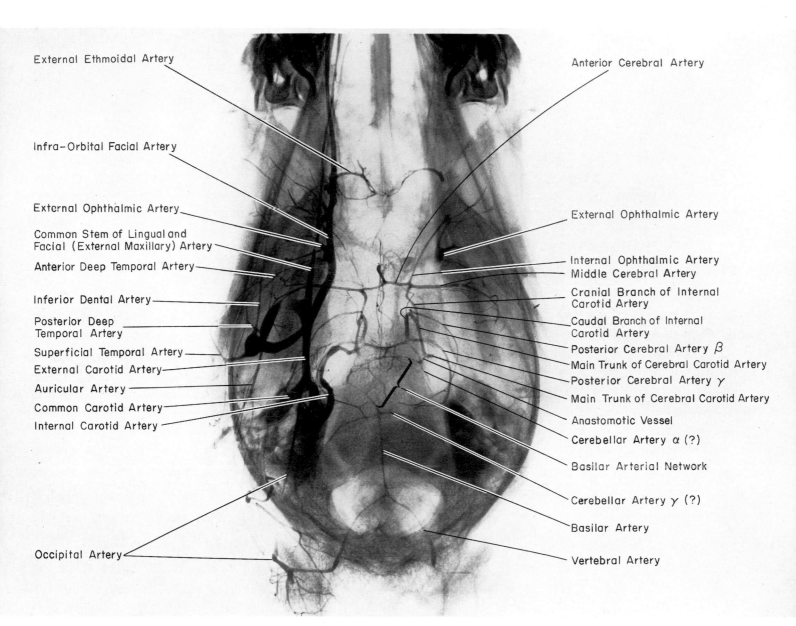

External Ethmoidal Artery

Infra-Orbital Facial Artery

External Ophthalmic Artery

Common Stem of Lingual and
Facial (External Maxillary) Artery

Anterior Deep Temporal Artery

Inferior Dental Artery

Posterior Deep
Temporal Artery

Superficial Temporal Artery

External Carotid Artery

Auricular Artery

Common Carotid Artery

Internal Carotid Artery

Occipital Artery

Anterior Cerebral Artery

External Ophthalmic Artery

Internal Ophthalmic Artery
Middle Cerebral Artery

Cranial Branch of Internal
Carotid Artery

Caudal Branch of Internal
Carotid Artery

Posterior Cerebral Artery β

Main Trunk of Cerebral Carotid Artery

Posterior Cerebral Artery γ

Main Trunk of Cerebral Carotid Artery

Anastomotic Vessel

Cerebellar Artery α (?)

Basilar Arterial Network

Cerebellar Artery γ (?)

Basilar Artery

Vertebral Artery

$\times$ 0·8

The anatomy of the extra- and intracranial arterial tree closely follows the description given by Tandler of the horse with one notable exception. The internal carotid, close to the point where it perforates the fibrocartilaginous skull base, supplies a branch, not as in the horse to join the opposite carotid, but to pierce the dura, forming an anastomotic channel to supply the network of vessels on the ventral surface of the brain-stem. The main line of the basilar artery is deviated from the centre and reinforced by small, somewhat indirect channels.

In this specimen the lingual and facial (external maxillary) arteries are not well shown; but the anastamosis between internal and external ophthalmic arteries is very clearly seen.

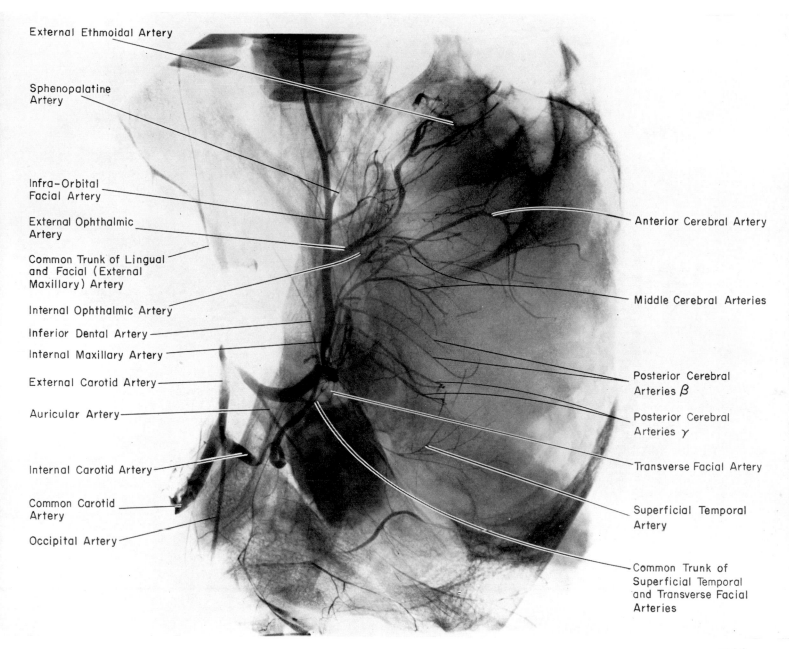

External Ethmoidal Artery

Sphenopalatine Artery

Infra-Orbital Facial Artery

External Ophthalmic Artery

Common Trunk of Lingual and Facial (External Maxillary) Artery

Internal Ophthalmic Artery

Inferior Dental Artery

Internal Maxillary Artery

External Carotid Artery

Auricular Artery

Internal Carotid Artery

Common Carotid Artery

Occipital Artery

Anterior Cerebral Artery

Middle Cerebral Arteries

Posterior Cerebral Arteries β

Posterior Cerebral Arteries γ

Transverse Facial Artery

Superficial Temporal Artery

Common Trunk of Superficial Temporal and Transverse Facial Arteries

$\times 1 \cdot 2$

Tapirus indicus
Malayan Tapir

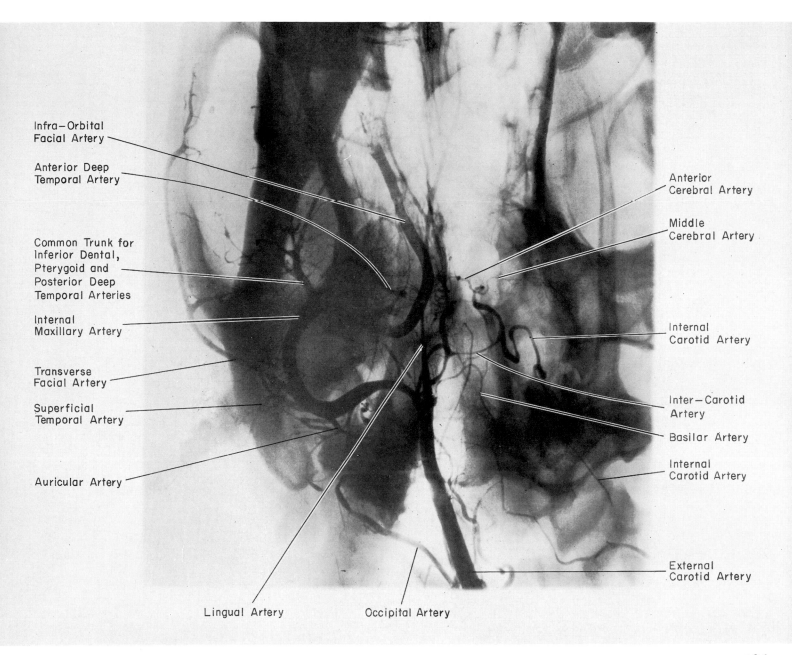

Infra–Orbital Facial Artery

Anterior Deep Temporal Artery

Common Trunk for Inferior Dental, Pterygoid and Posterior Deep Temporal Arteries

Internal Maxillary Artery

Transverse Facial Artery

Superficial Temporal Artery

Auricular Artery

Anterior Cerebral Artery

Middle Cerebral Artery

Internal Carotid Artery

Inter–Carotid Artery

Basilar Artery

Internal Carotid Artery

External Carotid Artery

Lingual Artery   Occipital Artery

× 0·6

Because of the size of the head it has not proved easy to see and therefore identify many of the arteries. Many have not been named. The inferior dental artery arises by a common stem with two large vessels which turn around the coronoid process of the mandible. These are presumed to be the pterygoid and masseteric arteries.

The external ophthalmic artery has been tentatively named. In an unpublished ventro-dorsal view, it ran in an antero-lateral direction.

In this ventro-dorsal view, a connection is seen between the internal carotid arteries at a point which corresponds well with the extradural connection described in horses.

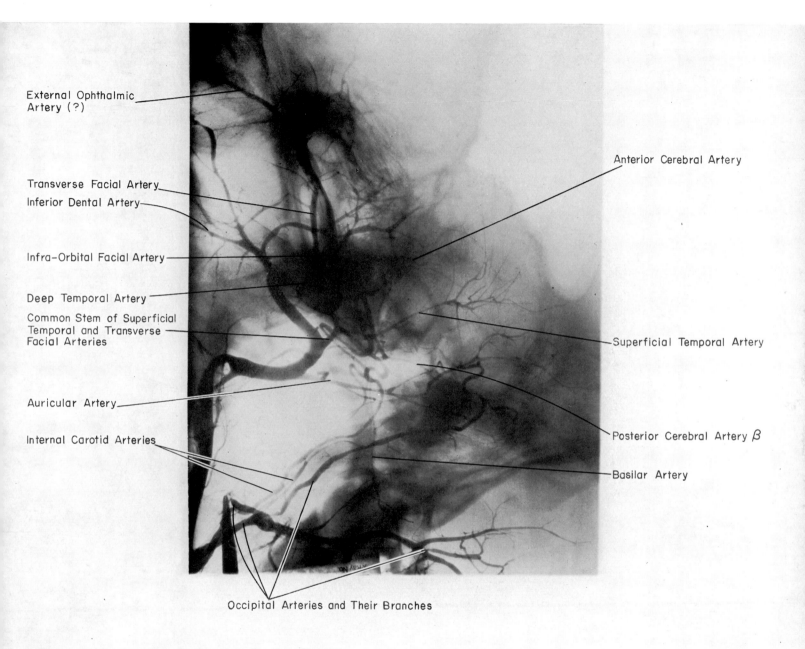

External Ophthalmic Artery (?)

Anterior Cerebral Artery

Transverse Facial Artery

Inferior Dental Artery

Infra-Orbital Facial Artery

Deep Temporal Artery

Common Stem of Superficial Temporal and Transverse Facial Arteries

Superficial Temporal Artery

Auricular Artery

Posterior Cerebral Artery β

Internal Carotid Arteries

Basilar Artery

Occipital Arteries and Their Branches

× 0·5

Artiodactyla

Without exception all Artiodactyla possess a specialised cerebral arterial system peculiar to themselves and different from other Ungulates.

The essential feature of the system is an extradural rete (Galen, A.D. 130–200; Tandler, 1899; Daniels *et al.*, 1953; Ask-Upmark, 1935) lying more or less completely within the cranial cavity. It consists of a large number of small arteries forming the only significant connection between the extra-cranial arterial supply and the intradural internal carotid. The retia are usually situated on either side of the basi-sphenoid and close to the pituitary fossa in the floor of the middle fossa. They receive their blood from the internal maxillary via two main vessels, an arteria anastomotica originating from or in close relationship with the external ophthalmic artery and a ramus anastomoticus sharing a common origin with the middle meningeal. The arteria anastomotica enters through the floor of the middle fossa.

By the time a foetus is at full term or shortly after birth the internal carotid which developed in an orthodox fashion has usually shrunk again to a narrow channel in its intra-osseous portion and has entirely disappeared in the neck. Not infre-quently, however, the ascending pharyngeal is large and has connections with the intracranial rete which pass through the floor of the skull.

The pathway from spinal vertebral arteries to basilar artery is also usually interrupted, the spinal vertebrals forming connections with the occipital arteries. The cranial vertebrals, which are in any case extremely narrow taper from their origin in the basilar.

Thus all or almost all of the cerebral blood flow is metred via a system where hydrodynamic properties must be different from those of a simple direct arterial supply.

In most Artiodactyla there is also an orbital rete through which runs the blood to the ciliary artery; but the cranial and orbital retia are not usually directly continuous with one another.

The retial system of Artiodactyla should be compared with that of the *Felidae* which shows a parallel evolutionary trend, and with that of *Lorisidae*.

One other feature held by most of the Artiodactyla in common is the retention of a long row of posterior cerebral and of cerebellar arteries, so that in many of the species almost all of the alternative origins of these vessels, as described by Hofmann (1900) are used.

Some of the individual characteristics of families, species and individuals appear in the following pages.

Sus scrofa
Wild Boar (adult)

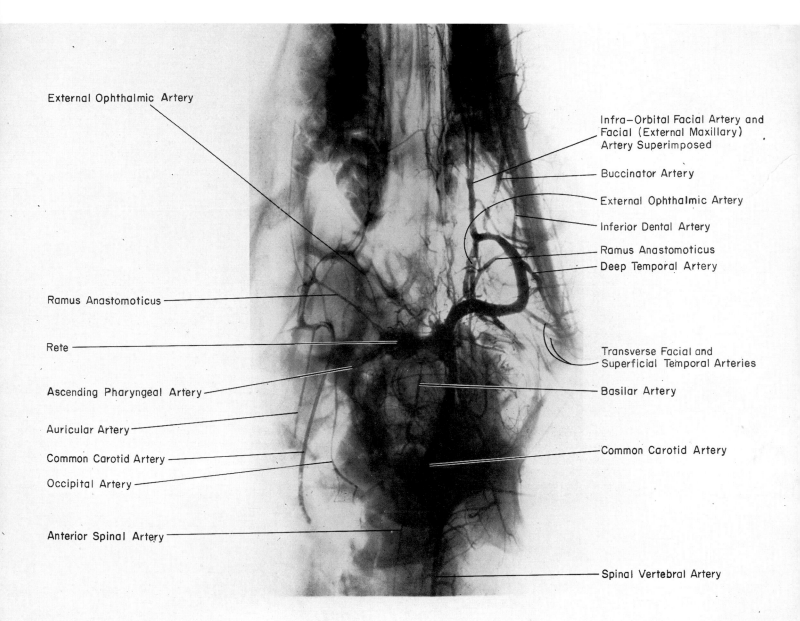

External Ophthalmic Artery

Infra-Orbital Facial Artery and Facial (External Maxillary) Artery Superimposed

Buccinator Artery

External Ophthalmic Artery

Inferior Dental Artery

Ramus Anastomoticus

Deep Temporal Artery

Ramus Anastomoticus

Rete

Transverse Facial and Superficial Temporal Arteries

Ascending Pharyngeal Artery

Basilar Artery

Auricular Artery

Common Carotid Artery

Occipital Artery

Common Carotid Artery

Anterior Spinal Artery

Spinal Vertebral Artery

× 0·62

Naming these arteries presented some difficulties. The large ascending pharyngeal artery on the better filled side is obscured in the basal view. The facial (external maxillary) artery is partly superimposed in this view on the external ophthalmic and on the infra-orbital facial. The arteria anastomotica arising from the external ophthalmic is hidden in the ventro-dorsal view.

The very large artery given off just before the inferior dental is presumed from its origin to be the posterior deep temporal, but it has unusually large branches.

It will be noted that we have followed Daniel *et al.* (1953) rather than Flechsig and Zintzsch (1969) and early authors in naming the major artery supplying the brain, the ascending pharyngeal, not the internal carotid. See also Diwo and Roth (1913).

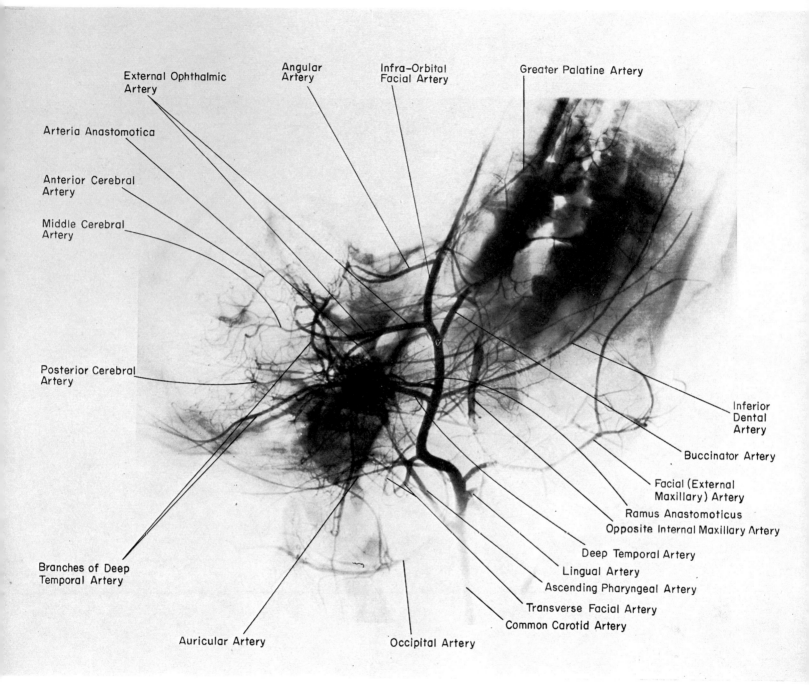

External Ophthalmic Artery

Angular Artery

Infra-Orbital Facial Artery

Greater Palatine Artery

Arteria Anastomotica

Anterior Cerebral Artery

Middle Cerebral Artery

Posterior Cerebral Artery

Inferior Dental Artery

Buccinator Artery

Facial (External Maxillary) Artery

Ramus Anastomoticus

Opposite Internal Maxillary Artery

Deep Temporal Artery

Lingual Artery

Ascending Pharyngeal Artery

Branches of Deep Temporal Artery

Transverse Facial Artery

Common Carotid Artery

Auricular Artery

Occipital Artery

× 0·76

Sus scrofa
Wild Boar (young)

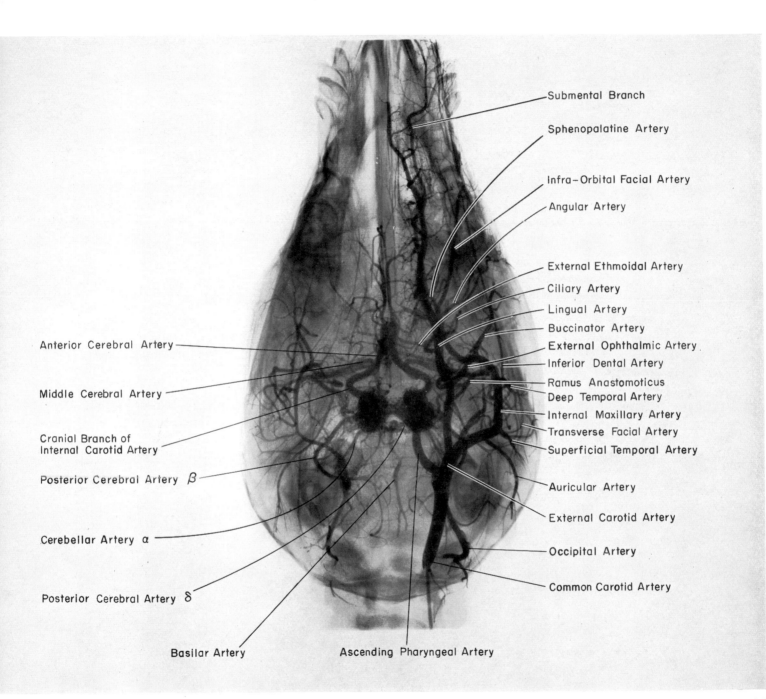

Submental Branch

Sphenopalatine Artery

Infra–Orbital Facial Artery

Angular Artery

External Ethmoidal Artery

Ciliary Artery

Lingual Artery

Buccinator Artery

External Ophthalmic Artery

Inferior Dental Artery

Ramus Anastomoticus

Deep Temporal Artery

Internal Maxillary Artery

Transverse Facial Artery

Superficial Temporal Artery

Auricular Artery

External Carotid Artery

Occipital Artery

Common Carotid Artery

Anterior Cerebral Artery

Middle Cerebral Artery

Cranial Branch of
Internal Carotid Artery

Posterior Cerebral Artery β

Cerebellar Artery α

Posterior Cerebral Artery δ

Basilar Artery

Ascending Pharyngeal Artery

$\times$ 1·3

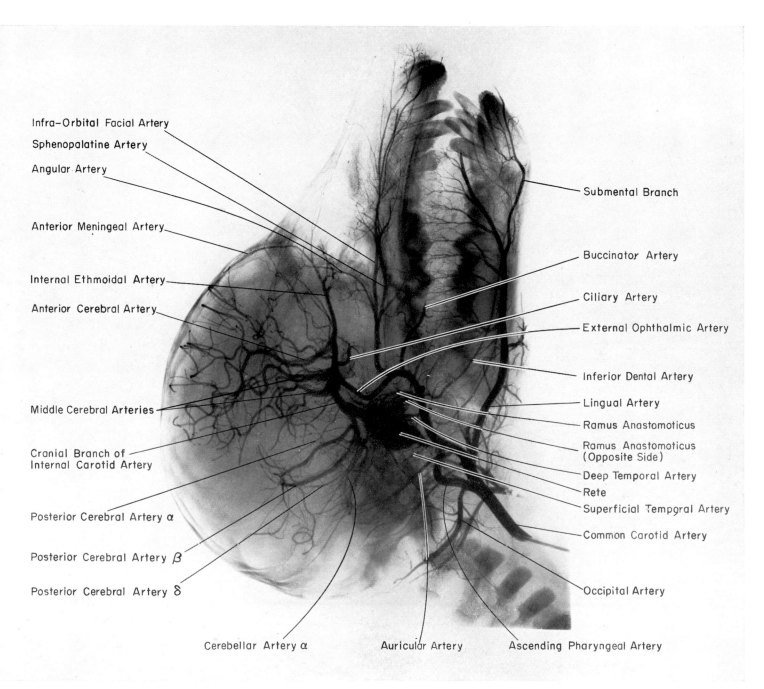

Infra–Orbital Facial Artery

Sphenopalatine Artery

Angular Artery

Anterior Meningeal Artery

Internal Ethmoidal Artery

Anterior Cerebral Artery

Middle Cerebral Arteries

Cranial Branch of
Internal Carotid Artery

Posterior Cerebral Artery α

Posterior Cerebral Artery β

Posterior Cerebral Artery δ

Cerebellar Artery α

Auricular Artery

Ascending Pharyngeal Artery

Submental Branch

Buccinator Artery

Ciliary Artery

External Ophthalmic Artery

Inferior Dental Artery

Lingual Artery

Ramus Anastomoticus

Ramus Anastomoticus
(Opposite Side)

Deep Temporal Artery

Rete

Superficial Temporal Artery

Common Carotid Artery

Occipital Artery

× 1·3

In this young animal it is very much easier to see the arrangement of the intracranial arteries.

Hippopotamus amphibius
Hippopotamus

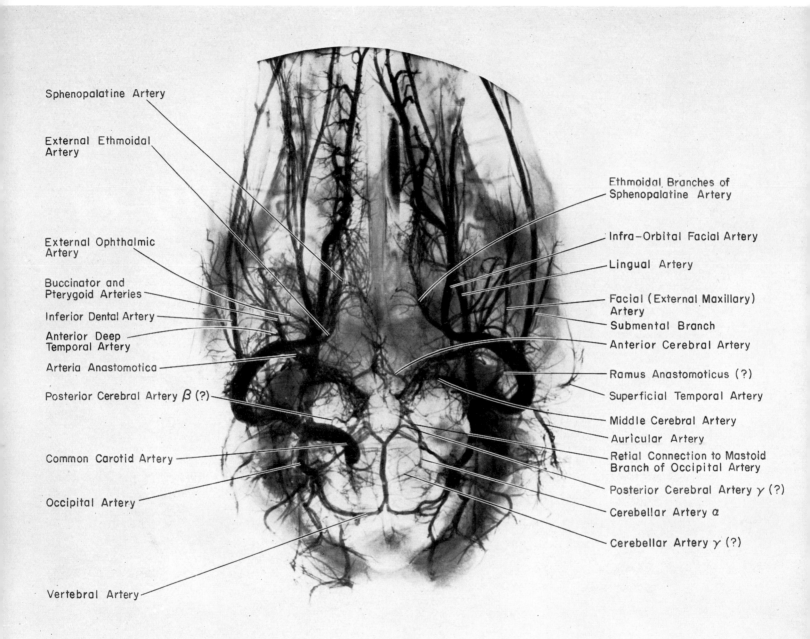

Sphenopalatine Artery

External Ethmoidal Artery

External Ophthalmic Artery

Buccinator and Pterygoid Arteries

Inferior Dental Artery

Anterior Deep Temporal Artery

Arteria Anastomotica

Posterior Cerebral Artery β (?)

Common Carotid Artery

Occipital Artery

Vertebral Artery

Ethmoidal Branches of Sphenopalatine Artery

Infra-Orbital Facial Artery

Lingual Artery

Facial (External Maxillary) Artery

Submental Branch

Anterior Cerebral Artery

Ramus Anastomoticus (?)

Superficial Temporal Artery

Middle Cerebral Artery

Auricular Artery

Retial Connection to Mastoid Branch of Occipital Artery

Posterior Cerebral Artery γ (?)

Cerebellar Artery α

Cerebellar Artery γ (?)

× 0·75

This young animal shows most of the typical features of all Artiodactyla. The principal arterial supply to the Circle of Willis for instance, comes from a very large arteria anastomotica. There is some doubt whether the branch opposite the inferior dental artery is a ramus anastomoticus with a middle meningeal continuation (as it has been labelled in the picture) or whether it might possibly be the posterior deep temporal artery.

The other connections of the Circle of Willis are interesting. There is a narrow, rather tortuous vessel on each side connecting the posterior part of the rete with the mastoid branch of the occipital artery.

The cranial ends of the vertebral arteries also have several large communications with the occipital arteries, a system which constitutes another simple rete.

There are several asymmetrical features. The spheno-palatine and external ethmoidal arteries seem to arise from a common stem on one side. The posterior cerebral arteries are also asymmetrical.

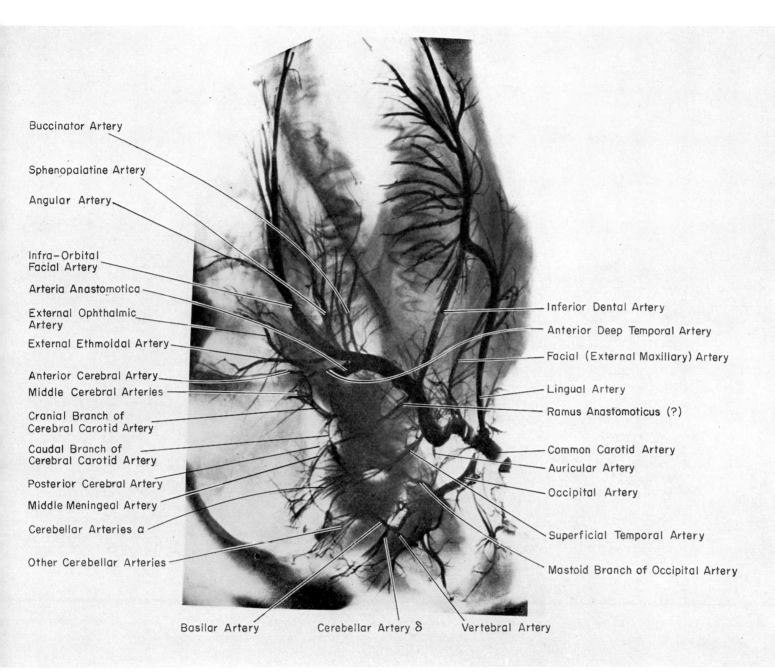

Buccinator Artery

Sphenopalatine Artery

Angular Artery

Infra-Orbital Facial Artery

Arteria Anastomotica

External Ophthalmic Artery

External Ethmoidal Artery

Anterior Cerebral Artery

Middle Cerebral Arteries

Cranial Branch of Cerebral Carotid Artery

Caudal Branch of Cerebral Carotid Artery

Posterior Cerebral Artery

Middle Meningeal Artery

Cerebellar Arteries α

Other Cerebellar Arteries

Inferior Dental Artery

Anterior Deep Temporal Artery

Facial (External Maxillary) Artery

Lingual Artery

Ramus Anastomoticus (?)

Common Carotid Artery

Auricular Artery

Occipital Artery

Superficial Temporal Artery

Mastoid Branch of Occipital Artery

Basilar Artery   Cerebellar Artery δ   Vertebral Artery

× 0·8

Camelus bactrianus
Bactrian Camel

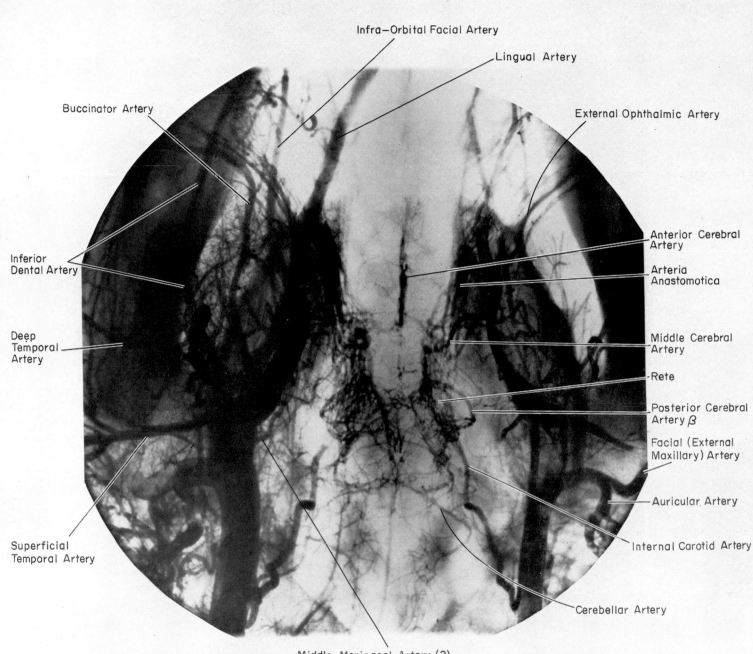

Infra—Orbital Facial Artery

Lingual Artery

Buccinator Artery

External Ophthalmic Artery

Inferior
Dental Artery

Anterior Cerebral
Artery

Arteria
Anastomotica

Deep
Temporal
Artery

Middle Cerebral
Artery

Rete

Posterior Cerebral
Artery β

Facial (External
Maxillary) Artery

Auricular Artery

Superficial
Temporal Artery

Internal Carotid Artery

Cerebellar Artery

Middle Meningeal Artery (?)

× 0·76

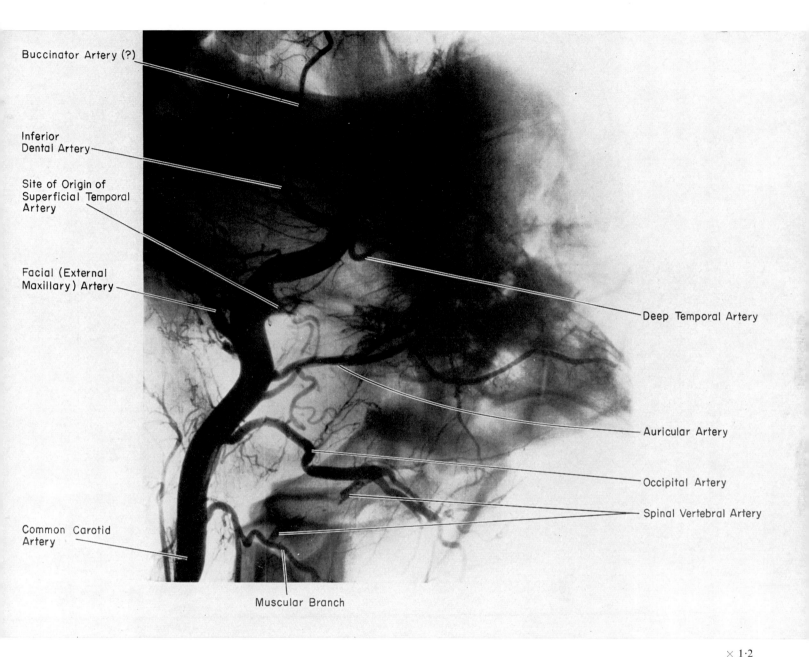

Buccinator Artery (?)

Inferior Dental Artery

Site of Origin of Superficial Temporal Artery

Facial (External Maxillary) Artery

Common Carotid Artery

Muscular Branch

Deep Temporal Artery

Auricular Artery

Occipital Artery

Spinal Vertebral Artery

× 1·2

The camel's head is so large that a number of different regions have been selected for illustrations which are taken from several different animals.

Tandler (1899) in describing a new-born specimen of *Camelus dromedarius* speaks of the internal carotid artery in the neck but notes that it was so small that he expected it would soon have closed altogether. He also said that it arose from the common carotid after the lingual and occipital arteries had been given off.

The identity of this artery, seen also by us in two of these animals, needs proof because of its unusually distal origin. Nevertheless its course as Tandler described across the wall of the bulla seems more in accord with that of the usual internal carotid than with the ascending pharyngeal. One should be inclined to follow Tandler.

The buccinator artery is not well identified in any of the pictures.

There is a reduplicated arteria anastomotica. The internal maxillary undergoes a kind of trifurcation. According to Tandler the medial branch would be the arteria anastomotica.

Camelus bactrianus

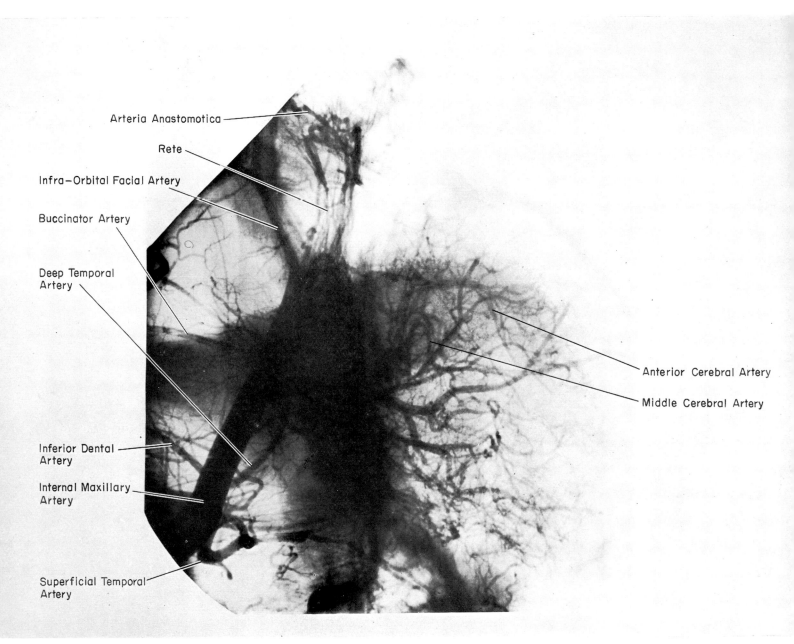

Arteria Anastomotica

Rete

Infra-Orbital Facial Artery

Buccinator Artery

Deep Temporal Artery

Inferior Dental Artery

Internal Maxillary Artery

Superficial Temporal Artery

Anterior Cerebral Artery

Middle Cerebral Artery

× 0·79

The lateral branch of the internal maxillary at this point is said to give rise to the lachrymal and frontal arteries. The middle branch is the infraorbital facial artery.

The auricular (posterior auricular) and facial (external maxillary) may arise from a common stem.

Tayeb (1951) and Kanan (1970) give their own account of the anatomy.

Kanan has shown that the posterior communicating arteries are also directly connected to the retia; there is another, more direct link between internal carotid and a lateral branch of the posterior cerebral. The direct link between cervical vertebral and basilar is preserved.

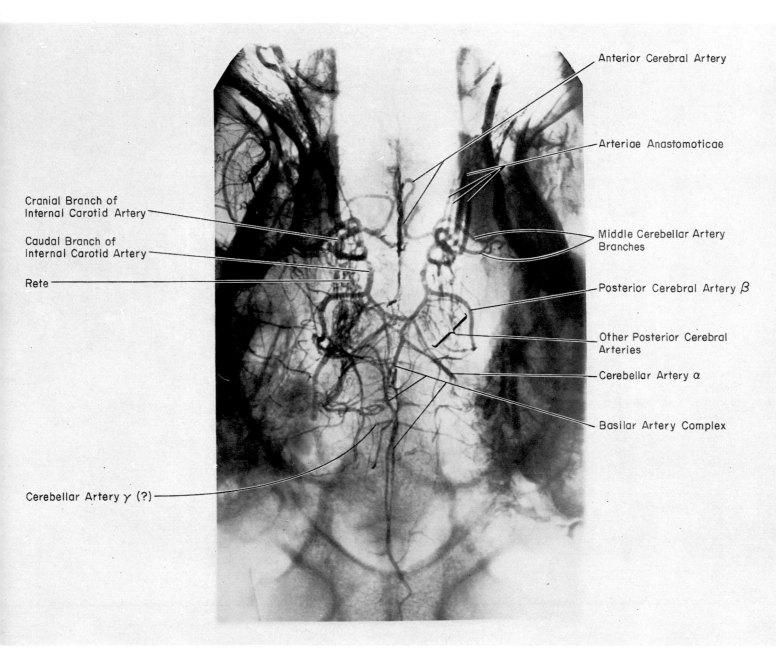

Anterior Cerebral Artery

Arteriae Anastomoticae

Cranial Branch of
Internal Carotid Artery

Caudal Branch of
Internal Carotid Artery

Rete

Middle Cerebellar Artery
Branches

Posterior Cerebral Artery β

Other Posterior Cerebral
Arteries

Cerebellar Artery α

Basilar Artery Complex

Cerebellar Artery γ (?)

$\times$ 0·7

Camelus bactrianus

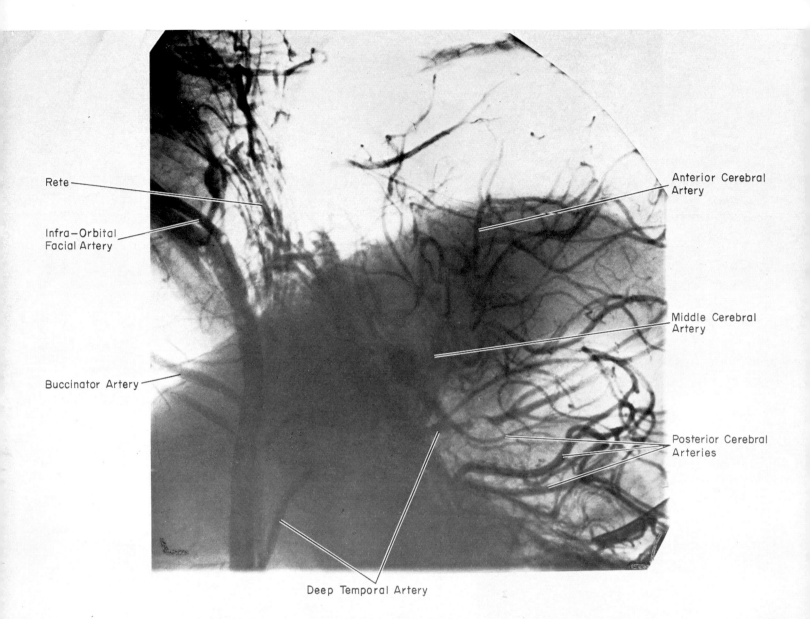

Rete

Infra–Orbital
Facial Artery

Buccinator Artery

Anterior Cerebral
Artery

Middle Cerebral
Artery

Posterior Cerebral
Arteries

Deep Temporal Artery

× 0·6

Dama dama
Black Fallow Deer

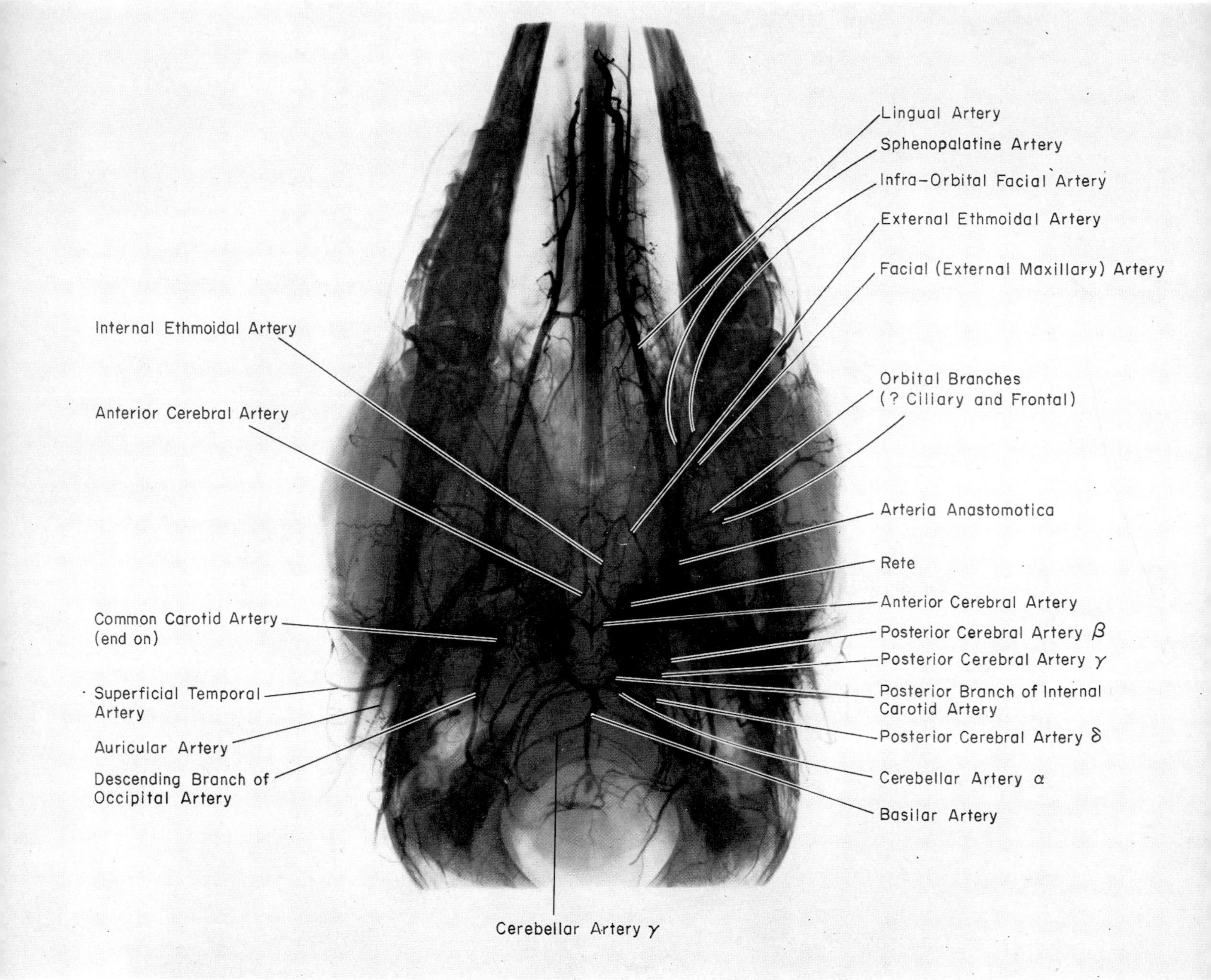

Lingual Artery

Sphenopalatine Artery

Infra–Orbital Facial Artery

External Ethmoidal Artery

Facial (External Maxillary) Artery

Orbital Branches
(? Ciliary and Frontal)

Arteria Anastomotica

Rete

Anterior Cerebral Artery

Posterior Cerebral Artery β

Posterior Cerebral Artery γ

Posterior Branch of Internal
Carotid Artery

Posterior Cerebral Artery δ

Cerebellar Artery α

Basilar Artery

Internal Ethmoidal Artery

Anterior Cerebral Artery

Common Carotid Artery
(end on)

Superficial Temporal
Artery

Auricular Artery

Descending Branch of
Occipital Artery

Cerebellar Artery γ

$\times$ 1·0

This injection specimen is included because it shows so
well the anastamosis between internal and external ethmoidal
arteries.

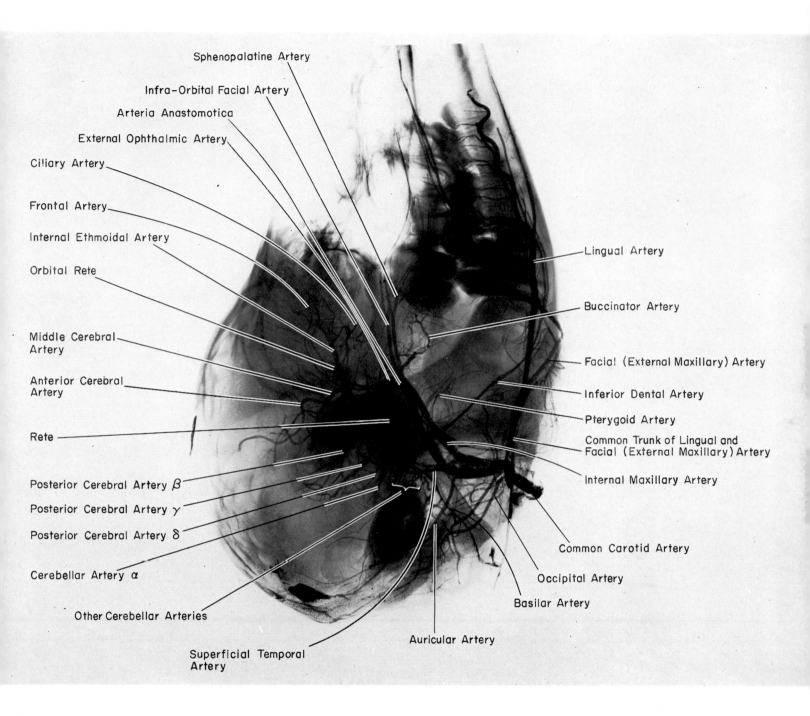

Sphenopalatine Artery

Infra-Orbital Facial Artery

Arteria Anastomotica

External Ophthalmic Artery

Ciliary Artery

Frontal Artery

Internal Ethmoidal Artery

Orbital Rete

Middle Cerebral Artery

Anterior Cerebral Artery

Rete

Posterior Cerebral Artery β

Posterior Cerebral Artery γ

Posterior Cerebral Artery δ

Cerebellar Artery α

Other Cerebellar Arteries

Superficial Temporal Artery

Auricular Artery

Basilar Artery

Occipital Artery

Common Carotid Artery

Internal Maxillary Artery

Common Trunk of Lingual and Facial (External Maxillary) Artery

Pterygoid Artery

Inferior Dental Artery

Facial (External Maxillary) Artery

Buccinator Artery

Lingual Artery

× 1·0

Cervus nippon
Formosan Deer

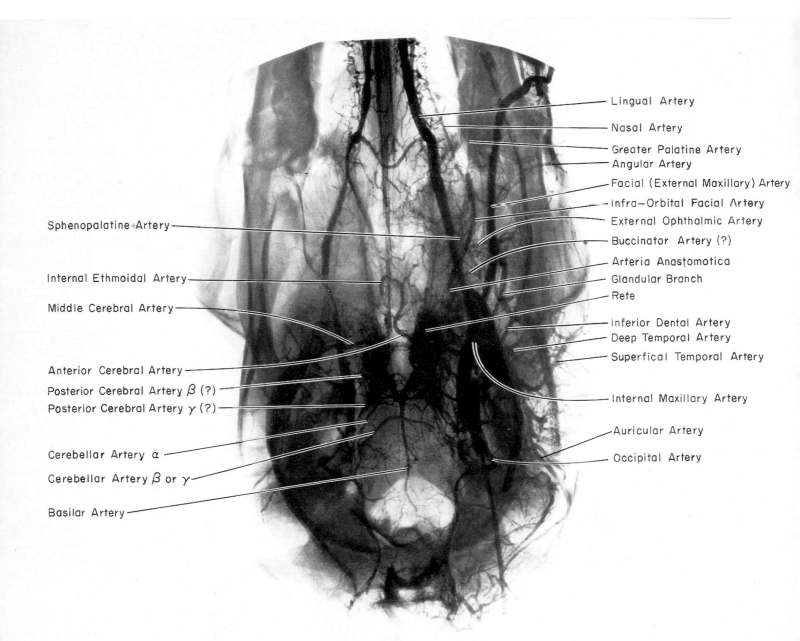

Lingual Artery

Nasal Artery

Greater Palatine Artery

Angular Artery

Facial (External Maxillary) Artery

Infra—Orbital Facial Artery

External Ophthalmic Artery

Buccinator Artery (?)

Arteria Anastomotica

Glandular Branch

Rete

Inferior Dental Artery

Deep Temporal Artery

Superfical Temporal Artery

Internal Maxillary Artery

Auricular Artery

Occipital Artery

Sphenopalatine Artery

Internal Ethmoidal Artery

Middle Cerebral Artery

Anterior Cerebral Artery

Posterior Cerebral Artery β (?)

Posterior Cerebral Artery γ (?)

Cerebellar Artery α

Cerebellar Artery β or γ

Basilar Artery

× 0·92

A segment of the external carotid artery is rather poorly outlined.

The facial (external maxillary) artery is well developed. Perhaps in consequence of this neither the infra-orbital facial nor the buccinator artery is very large.

No attempt has been made to name muscular branches such as pterygoid arteries; but they are filled.

The exact identification of posterior cerebral and cerebellar arteries by Hofmann's classification is tentative.

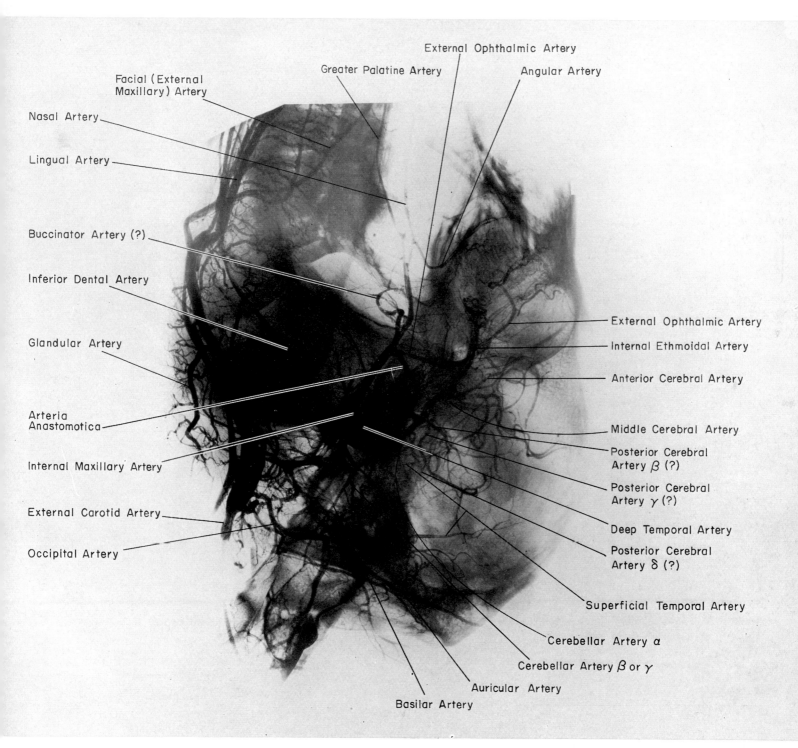

External Ophthalmic Artery

Greater Palatine Artery

Angular Artery

Facial (External Maxillary) Artery

Nasal Artery

Lingual Artery

Buccinator Artery (?)

Inferior Dental Artery

Glandular Artery

Arteria Anastomotica

Internal Maxillary Artery

External Carotid Artery

Occipital Artery

External Ophthalmic Artery

Internal Ethmoidal Artery

Anterior Cerebral Artery

Middle Cerebral Artery

Posterior Cerebral Artery β (?)

Posterior Cerebral Artery γ (?)

Deep Temporal Artery

Posterior Cerebral Artery δ (?)

Superficial Temporal Artery

Cerebellar Artery α

Cerebellar Artery β or γ

Auricular Artery

Basilar Artery

$\times$ 0·82

Cervus elaphus
Red Deer (adult)

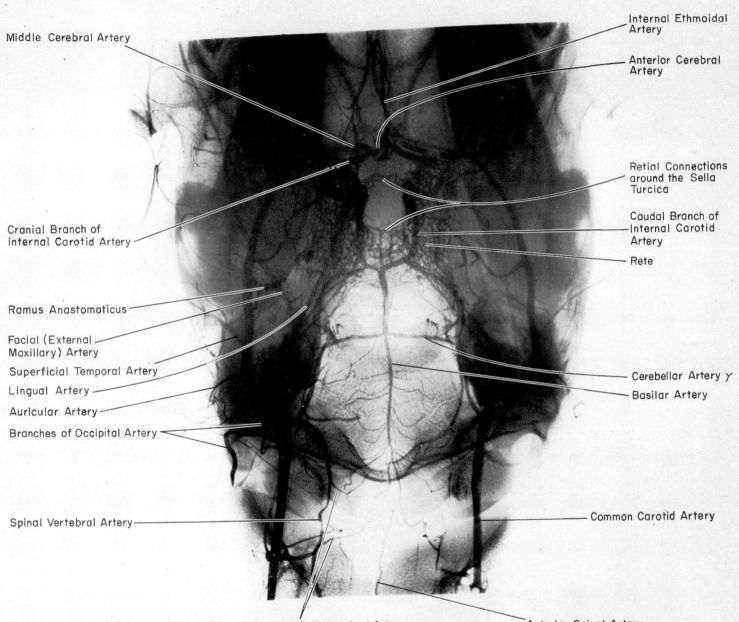

Middle Cerebral Artery

Internal Ethmoidal Artery

Anterior Cerebral Artery

Retial Connections around the Sella Turcica

Cranial Branch of Internal Carotid Artery

Caudal Branch of Internal Carotid Artery

Rete

Ramus Anastomoticus

Facial (External Maxillary) Artery

Superficial Temporal Artery

Lingual Artery

Cerebellar Artery γ

Basilar Artery

Auricular Artery

Branches of Occipital Artery

Spinal Vertebral Artery

Common Carotid Artery

Connections between Anterior Spinal Arterial Complex and Vertebral Artery

Anterior Spinal Artery

× 1·4

The ventro-dorsal view does not show well the majority of the external carotid branches; but reveals the pattern of the rete and the main intracranial arterial tree. Note the long row of pontine, cerebellar and medullary arteries. All except cerebellar arteries α and γ, the presumed homologues of the superior and anterior inferior cerebellar arteries, are approximately the same size.

Narrow connections exist between the basilar artery, anterior spinal arterial complex and spinal vertebral arteries. See Godynicki (1968).

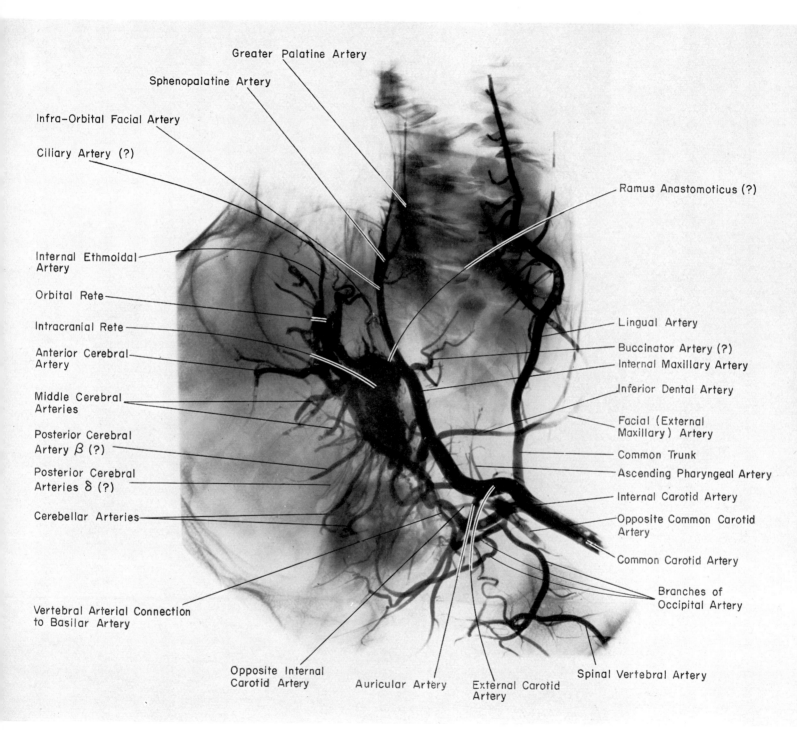

Greater Palatine Artery

Sphenopalatine Artery

Infra-Orbital Facial Artery

Ciliary Artery (?)

Ramus Anastomoticus (?)

Internal Ethmoidal Artery

Orbital Rete

Intracranial Rete

Lingual Artery

Anterior Cerebral Artery

Buccinator Artery (?)

Internal Maxillary Artery

Inferior Dental Artery

Middle Cerebral Arteries

Facial (External Maxillary) Artery

Posterior Cerebral Artery β (?)

Common Trunk

Ascending Pharyngeal Artery

Posterior Cerebral Arteries δ (?)

Internal Carotid Artery

Opposite Common Carotid Artery

Cerebellar Arteries

Common Carotid Artery

Branches of Occipital Artery

Vertebral Arterial Connection to Basilar Artery

Opposite Internal Carotid Artery

Auricular Artery

External Carotid Artery

Spinal Vertebral Artery

× 1·0

Cervus elaphus
Red Deer (young)

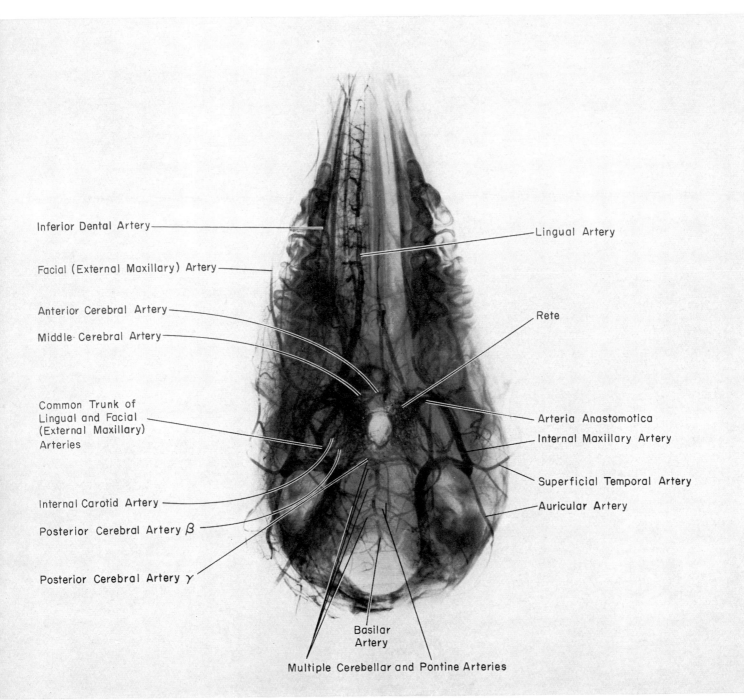

Inferior Dental Artery

Facial (External Maxillary) Artery

Anterior Cerebral Artery

Middle Cerebral Artery

Common Trunk of
Lingual and Facial
(External Maxillary)
Arteries

Internal Carotid Artery

Posterior Cerebral Artery β

Posterior Cerebral Artery γ

Lingual Artery

Rete

Arteria Anastomotica

Internal Maxillary Artery

Superficial Temporal Artery

Auricular Artery

Basilar
Artery

Multiple Cerebellar and Pontine Arteries

× 0·9

The injection of this very young animal shows beyond doubt that even after birth the internal carotid artery may be a major source of blood supply to the brain. Barium has run up one internal carotid and down the other.

The ascending pharyngeal arteries are small and have no connection with the retia.

The spinal vertebral arteries with their occipital arterial reinforcement continue upwards to join the basilar artery.

Identification of the arteria anastomotica is doubtful in the lateral view because of superimposition.

In the basal view a long row of cerebellar and pontine arteries is revealed making individual identification impossible.

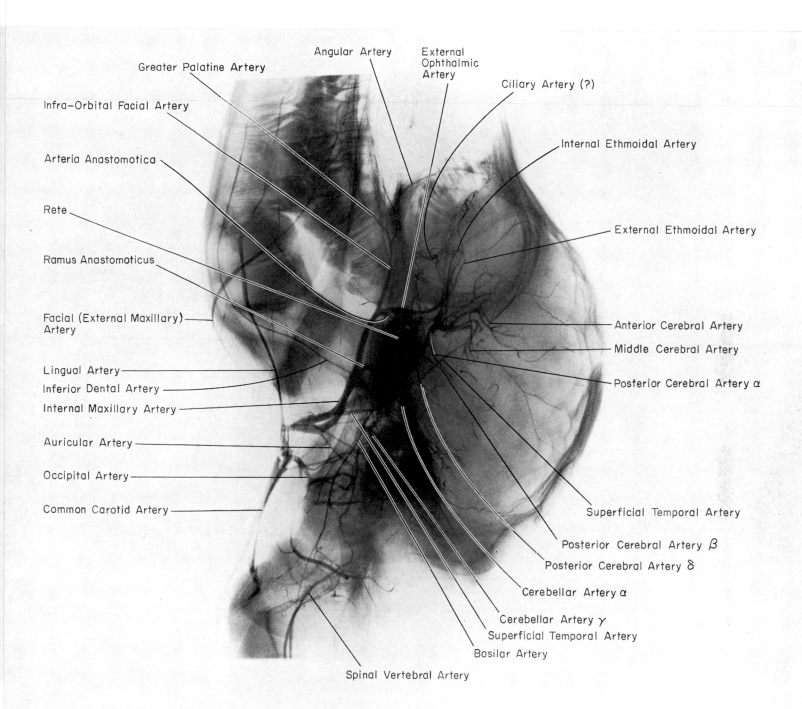

Greater Palatine Artery

Angular Artery

External Ophthalmic Artery

Ciliary Artery (?)

Infra-Orbital Facial Artery

Internal Ethmoidal Artery

Arteria Anastomotica

Rete

External Ethmoidal Artery

Ramus Anastomoticus

Facial (External Maxillary) Artery

Anterior Cerebral Artery

Middle Cerebral Artery

Lingual Artery

Posterior Cerebral Artery α

Inferior Dental Artery

Internal Maxillary Artery

Auricular Artery

Occipital Artery

Common Carotid Artery

Superficial Temporal Artery

Posterior Cerebral Artery β

Posterior Cerebral Artery δ

Cerebellar Artery α

Cerebellar Artery γ

Superficial Temporal Artery

Basilar Artery

Spinal Vertebral Artery

× 1·5

Bison bonasus

European Bison

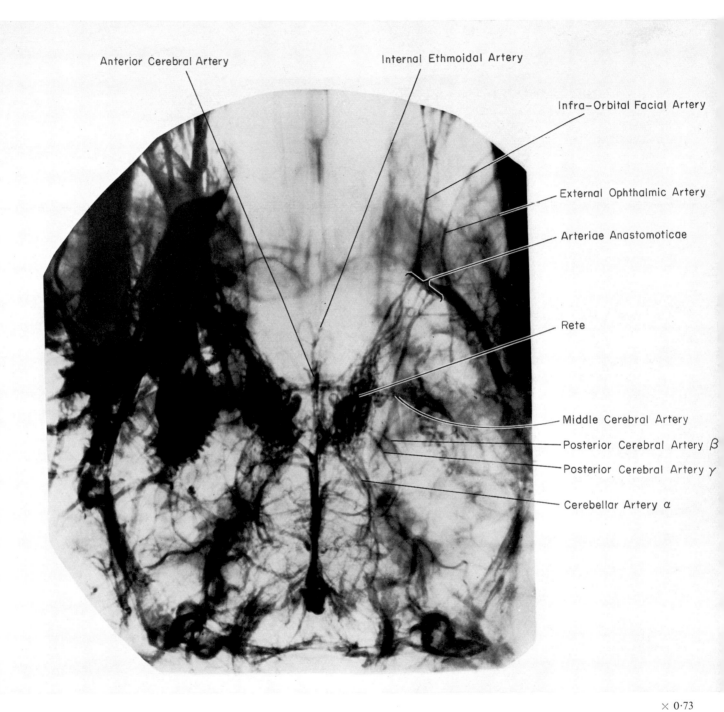

Anterior Cerebral Artery

Internal Ethmoidal Artery

Infra–Orbital Facial Artery

External Ophthalmic Artery

Arteriae Anastomoticae

Rete

Middle Cerebral Artery

Posterior Cerebral Artery β

Posterior Cerebral Artery γ

Cerebellar Artery α

× 0·73

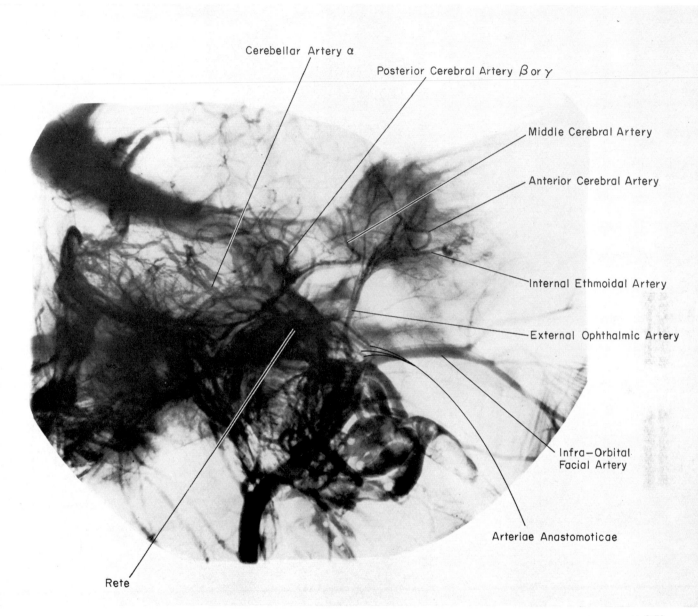

Cerebellar Artery α

Posterior Cerebral Artery β or γ

Middle Cerebral Artery

Anterior Cerebral Artery

Internal Ethmoidal Artery

External Ophthalmic Artery

Infra—Orbital Facial Artery

Arteriae Anastomoticae

Rete

× 0·73

This is mixed arterial and venous injection. In the ventro-dorsal view, for instance, the basilar artery is obscured by the superior sagittal sinus.

Note the multiplicity of arteries representing the arteria anastomotica.

Aepyceros melampus
Impala

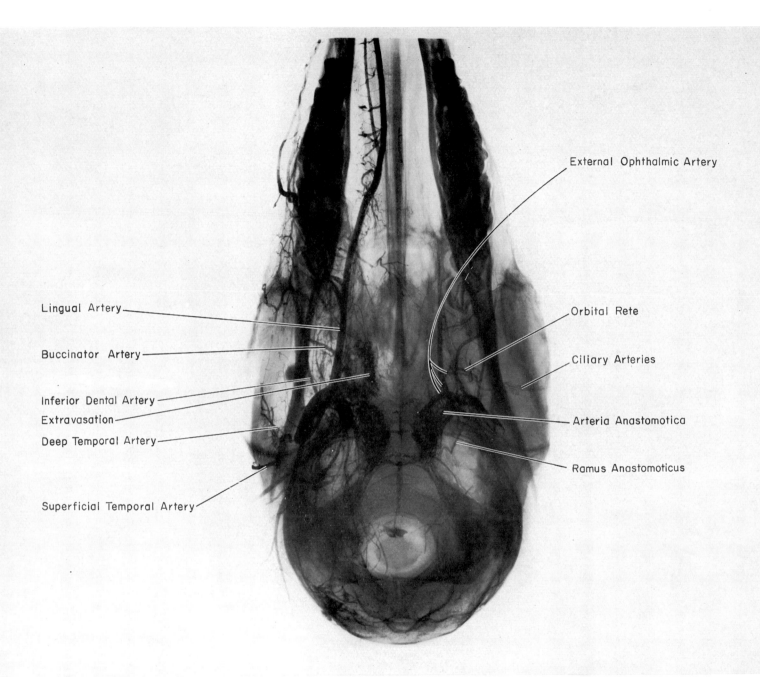

External Ophthalmic Artery

Lingual Artery

Buccinator Artery

Inferior Dental Artery

Extravasation

Deep Temporal Artery

Superficial Temporal Artery

Orbital Rete

Ciliary Arteries

Arteria Anastomotica

Ramus Anastomoticus

× 1·0

The density of the skull base and the fact that extravasation of contrast medium took place in the posterior nares makes it difficult to follow some of the arteries. It seems clear, however, that the deep temporal extends unusually far forwards to supply the superficial soft tissues of the upper and posterior parts of the orbit.

The arrangement of posterior cerebral arteries is very much as Hoffman described it for *Cervus elephas*. There is an α artery which serves rather more than the choroid plexus, a very large β artery and a moderate size δ posterior cerebral.

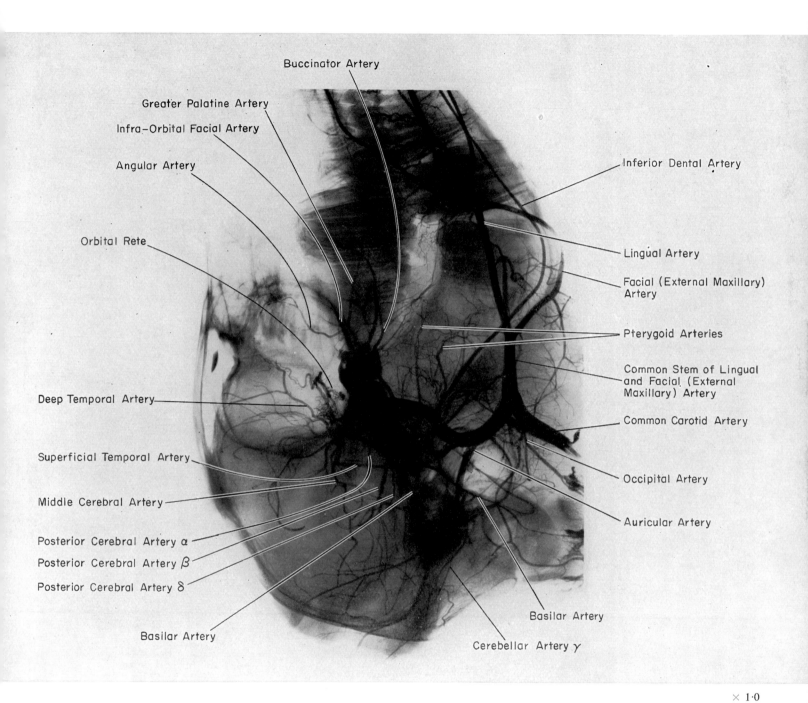

Buccinator Artery

Greater Palatine Artery

Infra–Orbital Facial Artery

Angular Artery

Orbital Rete

Deep Temporal Artery

Superficial Temporal Artery

Middle Cerebral Artery

Posterior Cerebral Artery α

Posterior Cerebral Artery β

Posterior Cerebral Artery δ

Basilar Artery

Inferior Dental Artery

Lingual Artery

Facial (External Maxillary) Artery

Pterygoid Arteries

Common Stem of Lingual and Facial (External Maxillary) Artery

Common Carotid Artery

Occipital Artery

Auricular Artery

Basilar Artery

Cerebellar Artery γ

× 1·0

Gazella thomsoni
Thompson's Gazelle

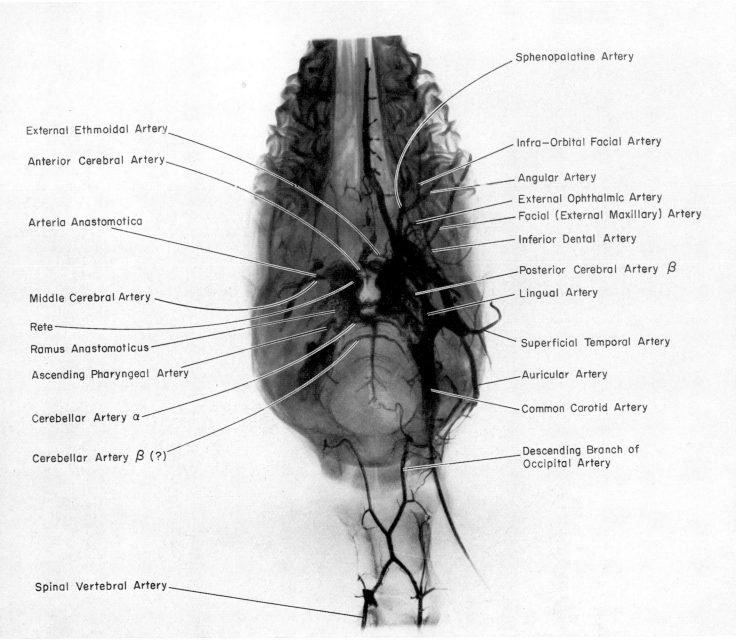

External Ethmoidal Artery

Anterior Cerebral Artery

Arteria Anastomotica

Middle Cerebral Artery

Rete

Ramus Anastomoticus

Ascending Pharyngeal Artery

Cerebellar Artery α

Cerebellar Artery β (?)

Spinal Vertebral Artery

Sphenopalatine Artery

Infra–Orbital Facial Artery

Angular Artery

External Ophthalmic Artery

Facial (External Maxillary) Artery

Inferior Dental Artery

Posterior Cerebral Artery β

Lingual Artery

Superficial Temporal Artery

Auricular Artery

Common Carotid Artery

Descending Branch of Occipital Artery

× 0·9

The occipital arteries have been excluded by decapitation. The general arrangement of vessels is characteristic of deer.

Tributaries of the orbital rete have only been named provisionally but probably include a large external ophthalmic artery and a connection between the orbital and intracranial retia, which should be the arteria anastomotica.

The ventro-dorsal view also shows quite well that there are patent vessels supplying the retia directly from the neck. These appear to be ascending pharyngeal arteries.

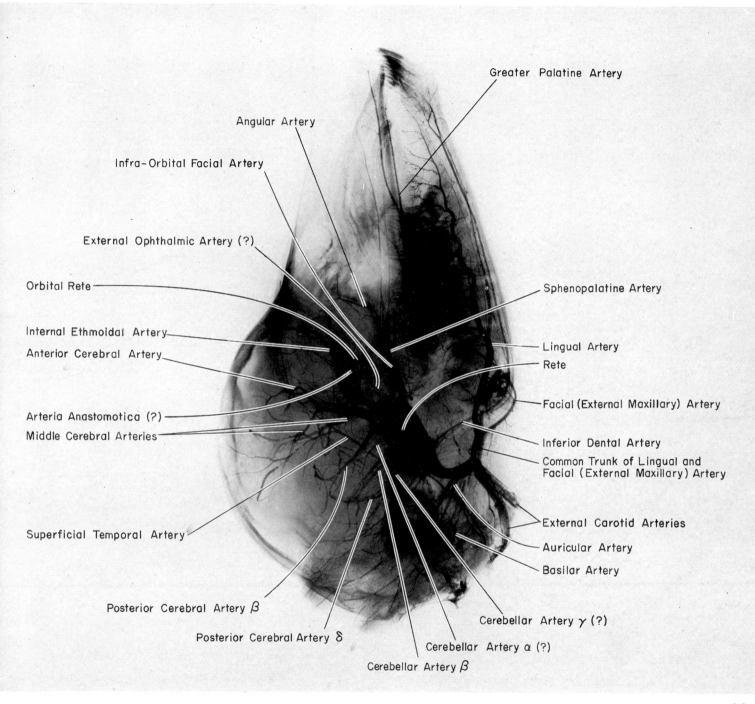

Greater Palatine Artery

Angular Artery

Infra-Orbital Facial Artery

External Ophthalmic Artery (?)

Orbital Rete

Sphenopalatine Artery

Internal Ethmoidal Artery

Anterior Cerebral Artery

Lingual Artery

Rete

Facial (External Maxillary) Artery

Arteria Anastomotica (?)

Middle Cerebral Arteries

Inferior Dental Artery

Common Trunk of Lingual and
Facial (External Maxillary) Artery

External Carotid Arteries

Superficial Temporal Artery

Auricular Artery

Basilar Artery

Posterior Cerebral Artery β

Cerebellar Artery γ (?)

Posterior Cerebral Artery δ

Cerebellar Artery α (?)

Cerebellar Artery β

$\times$ 1·0

Capra hircus
Goat

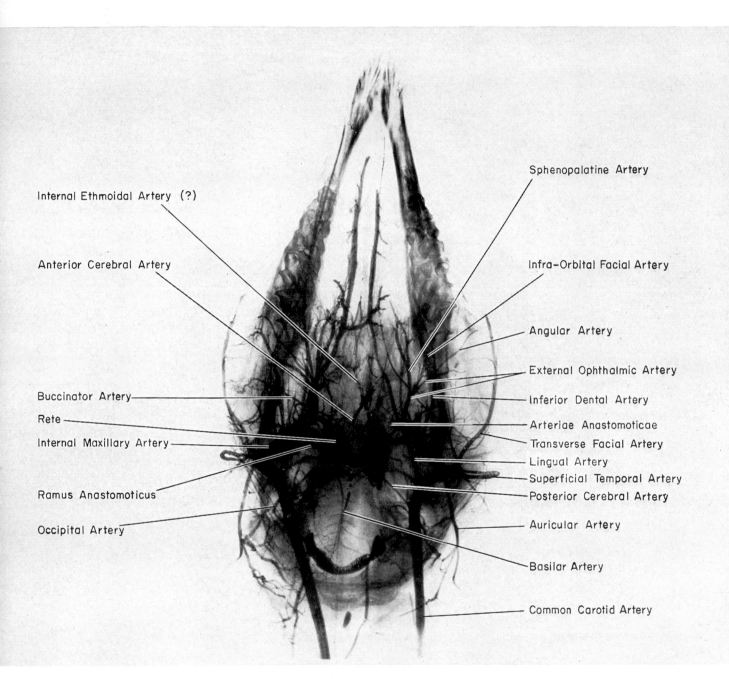

Internal Ethmoidal Artery (?)

Sphenopalatine Artery

Anterior Cerebral Artery

Infra-Orbital Facial Artery

Angular Artery

External Ophthalmic Artery

Buccinator Artery

Inferior Dental Artery

Rete

Arteriae Anastomoticae

Internal Maxillary Artery

Transverse Facial Artery

Lingual Artery

Superficial Temporal Artery

Posterior Cerebral Artery

Ramus Anastomoticus

Auricular Artery

Occipital Artery

Basilar Artery

Common Carotid Artery

× 0·7

This animal had had a myelogram prior to death and some of the contrast medium is lying in the upper cervical canal.

In the ventro-dorsal view the small facial (external maxillary) artery is invisible. Note how the lateral part of the face is principally supplied by the transverse facial and the angular branch of the external ophthalmic artery.

The long row of branches of the basilar artery consists of cerebellar arteries β, γ and δ as well as pontine arteries and possibly a separate internal auditory artery.

Ovis aries
Sheep

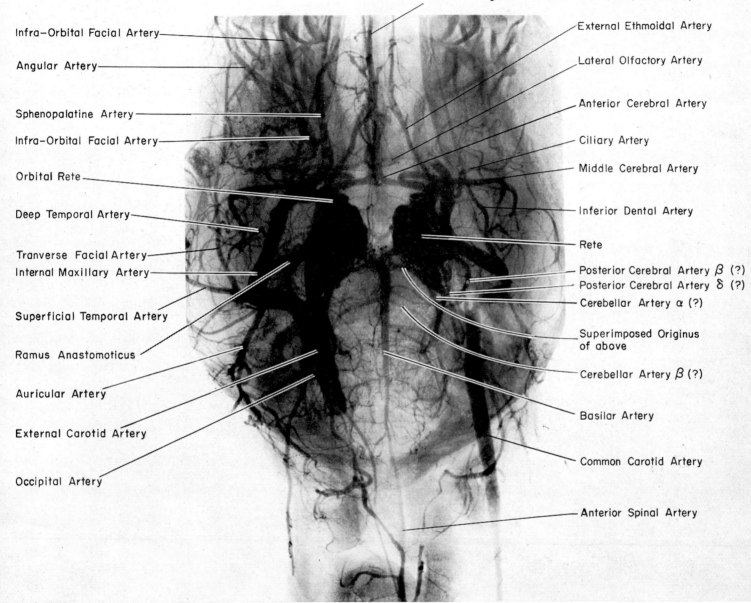

Internal Ethmoidal or Marginal Branch of Anterior Cerebral Artery

Infra–Orbital Facial Artery

Angular Artery

Sphenopalatine Artery

Infra–Orbital Facial Artery

Orbital Rete

Deep Temporal Artery

Tranverse Facial Artery

Internal Maxillary Artery

Superficial Temporal Artery

Ramus Anastomoticus

Auricular Artery

External Carotid Artery

Occipital Artery

External Ethmoidal Artery

Lateral Olfactory Artery

Anterior Cerebral Artery

Ciliary Artery

Middle Cerebral Artery

Inferior Dental Artery

Rete

Posterior Cerebral Artery β (?)

Posterior Cerebral Artery δ (?)

Cerebellar Artery α (?)

Superimposed Originus of above

Cerebellar Artery β (?)

Basilar Artery

Common Carotid Artery

Anterior Spinal Artery

$\times$ 1·0

Superimposition causes some difficulties of interpretation, for instance in the recognition of the various posterior cerebral arteries.

The arteria anastomotica is completely invisible; hidden by the rete. The ramus anastomoticus is enormous. The ascending pharyngeal artery is probably still patent and still connected to the rete.

The way in which the basilar artery tapers from front to back is well shown, more of its branches are filled than can be named with any confidence.

Ovis aries
Domestic Sheep (young)

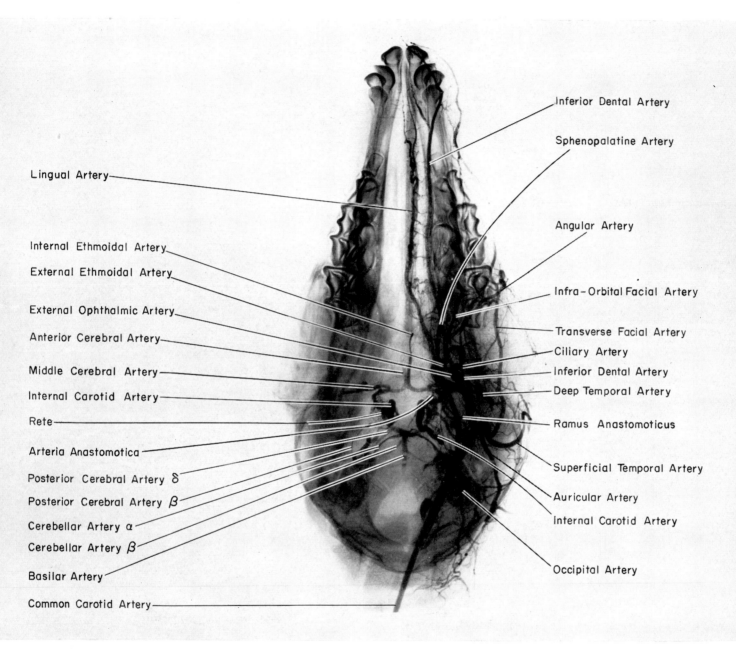

Inferior Dental Artery

Sphenopalatine Artery

Lingual Artery

Angular Artery

Internal Ethmoidal Artery

External Ethmoidal Artery

Infra-Orbital Facial Artery

External Ophthalmic Artery

Transverse Facial Artery

Anterior Cerebral Artery

Ciliary Artery

Middle Cerebral Artery

Inferior Dental Artery

Internal Carotid Artery

Deep Temporal Artery

Rete

Ramus Anastomoticus

Arteria Anastomotica

Posterior Cerebral Artery δ

Posterior Cerebral Artery β

Superficial Temporal Artery

Cerebellar Artery α

Auricular Artery

Cerebellar Artery β

Internal Carotid Artery

Basilar Artery

Common Carotid Artery

Occipital Artery

× 1·1

This very young lamb still possesses a functional internal carotid, but it exhibits several extremely narrow segments in the upper part of the neck.

The ascending pharyngeal artery is very small, but is visible in the original radiograph.

The lingual and facial (external maxillary) arteries were said by Tandler to have a common stem; but the facial here is represented only by its submental branch. The angular artery springs instead from the infra-orbital facial.

The posterior cerebral arteries seem to be β and δ, resembling the deer; but α has not been identified.

Cerebellar arteries α, β and perhaps γ have been identified and another pair of smaller vessels presumably medullary running laterally from the basilar cranial to the cerebellar artery γ. Below this point the basilar artery is unfilled.

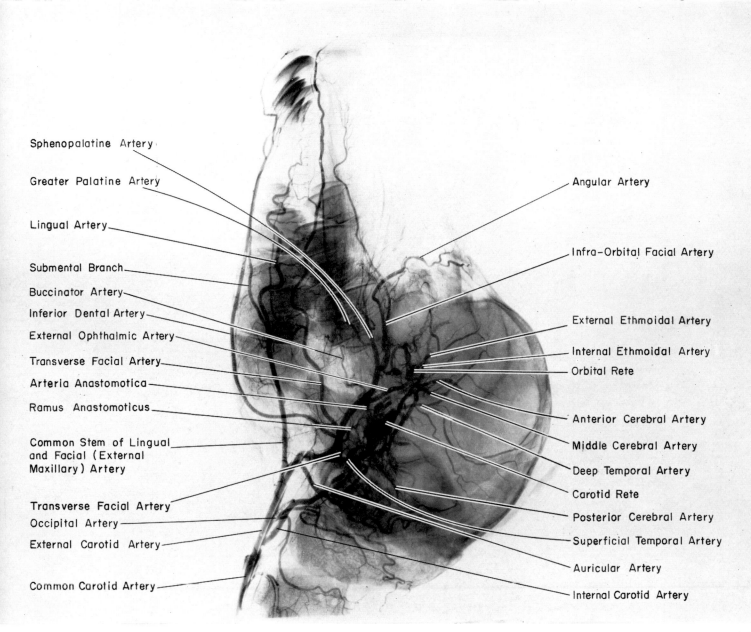

Sphenopalatine Artery

Greater Palatine Artery

Lingual Artery

Submental Branch

Buccinator Artery

Inferior Dental Artery

External Ophthalmic Artery

Transverse Facial Artery

Arteria Anastomotica

Ramus Anastomoticus

Common Stem of Lingual and Facial (External Maxillary) Artery

Transverse Facial Artery

Occipital Artery

External Carotid Artery

Common Carotid Artery

Angular Artery

Infra-Orbital Facial Artery

External Ethmoidal Artery

Internal Ethmoidal Artery

Orbital Rete

Anterior Cerebral Artery

Middle Cerebral Artery

Deep Temporal Artery

Carotid Rete

Posterior Cerebral Artery

Superficial Temporal Artery

Auricular Artery

Internal Carotid Artery

× 1·1

Ovis aries
Norfolk Horned Sheep (Ram)

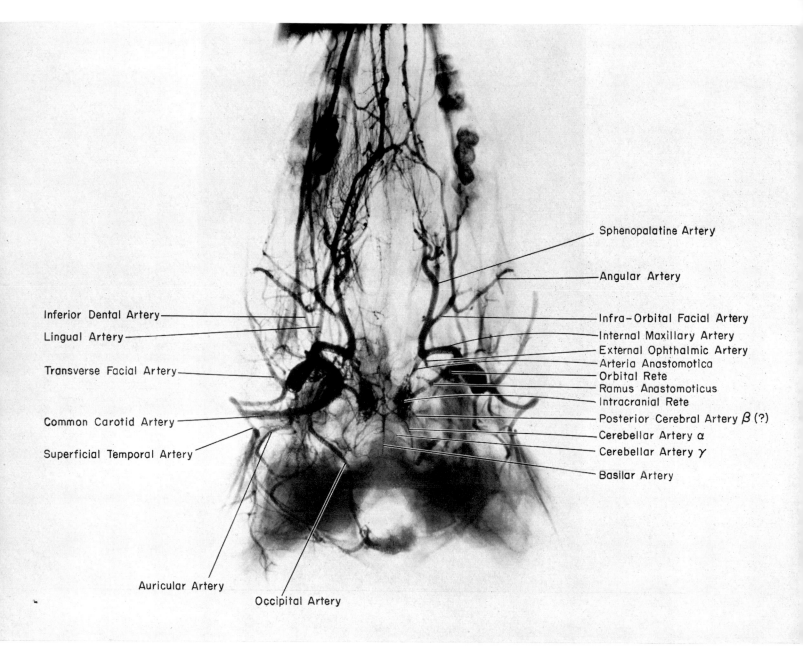

Inferior Dental Artery

Lingual Artery

Transverse Facial Artery

Common Carotid Artery

Superficial Temporal Artery

Auricular Artery

Occipital Artery

Sphenopalatine Artery

Angular Artery

Infra-Orbital Facial Artery

Internal Maxillary Artery

External Ophthalmic Artery

Arteria Anastomotica

Orbital Rete

Ramus Anastomoticus

Intracranial Rete

Posterior Cerebral Artery β (?)

Cerebellar Artery α

Cerebellar Artery γ

Basilar Artery

$\times$ 0·7

The very large blood supply from the superficial temporal to the horns dominates the lateral view. In the ventro-dorsal view the presence of the horns has dictated an overtilt to the head position.

No vestige of the extracranial internal carotid remains. The intracranial rete is supplied by the large ramus anastomoticus and arteria anastomotica.

The external ophthalmic running to the orbital rete is clearly demonstrated.

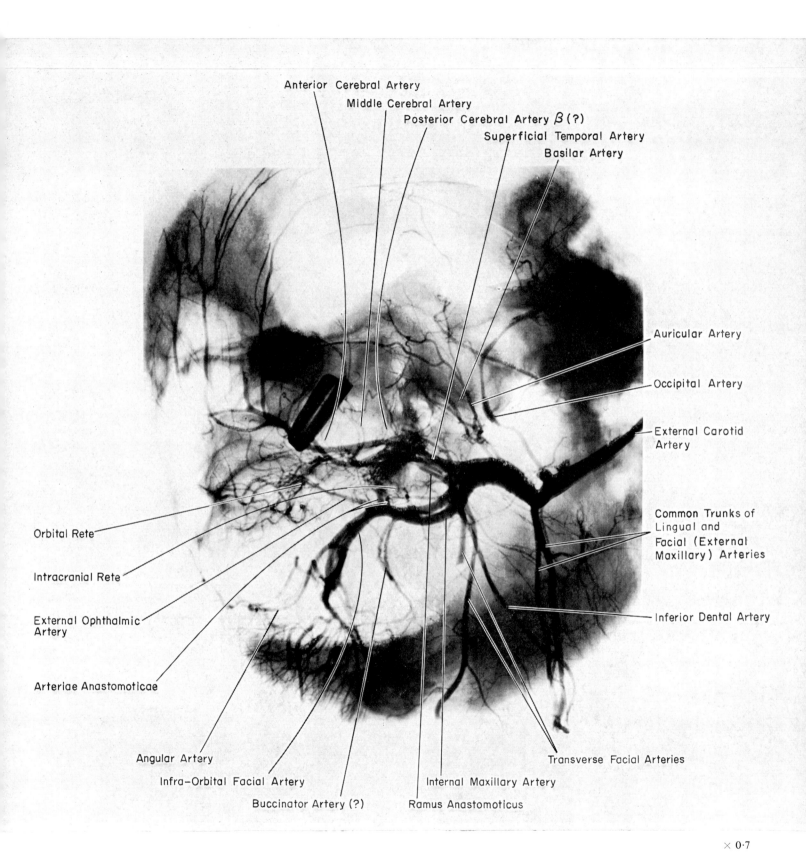

Anterior Cerebral Artery

Middle Cerebral Artery

Posterior Cerebral Artery β (?)

Superficial Temporal Artery

Basilar Artery

Auricular Artery

Occipital Artery

External Carotid Artery

Common Trunks of Lingual and Facial (External Maxillary) Arteries

Inferior Dental Artery

Orbital Rete

Intracranial Rete

External Ophthalmic Artery

Arteriae Anastomoticae

Angular Artery

Infra–Orbital Facial Artery

Buccinator Artery (?)

Ramus Anastomoticus

Internal Maxillary Artery

Transverse Facial Arteries

× 0·7

Ovis musimon
Mouflon

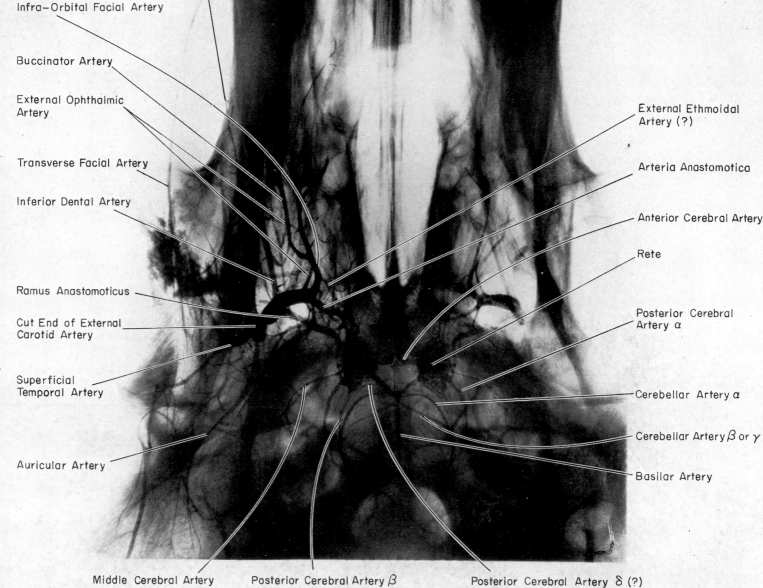

Angular Artery

Infra–Orbital Facial Artery

Buccinator Artery

External Ophthalmic Artery

Transverse Facial Artery

Inferior Dental Artery

Ramus Anastomoticus

Cut End of External Carotid Artery

Superficial Temporal Artery

Auricular Artery

External Ethmoidal Artery (?)

Arteria Anastomotica

Anterior Cerebral Artery

Rete

Posterior Cerebral Artery α

Cerebellar Artery α

Cerebellar Artery β or γ

Basilar Artery

Middle Cerebral Artery   Posterior Cerebral Artery β   Posterior Cerebral Artery δ (?)

× 1·2

The external carotid had been severed on the cranial side of the origins of the lingual, facial (external maxillary) and occipital arteries.

This injection gives a good view of the two large contributors to the rete, the arterial anastomotica and the ramus anastomoticus.

There is some extravasation of contrast medium in the postero-lateral part of the orbit.

The animal had well-developed horns, the blood supply of one can be seen coming from the superficial temporal artery. There is also a very large transverse facial artery.

Because of the projection the upper part of the basilar artery is foreshortened in the ventro-dorsal view and there may be a greater distance than appears between the upper end of the basilar artery and the cerebellar branches labelled as β or γ (in which case the designation γ would be appropriate).

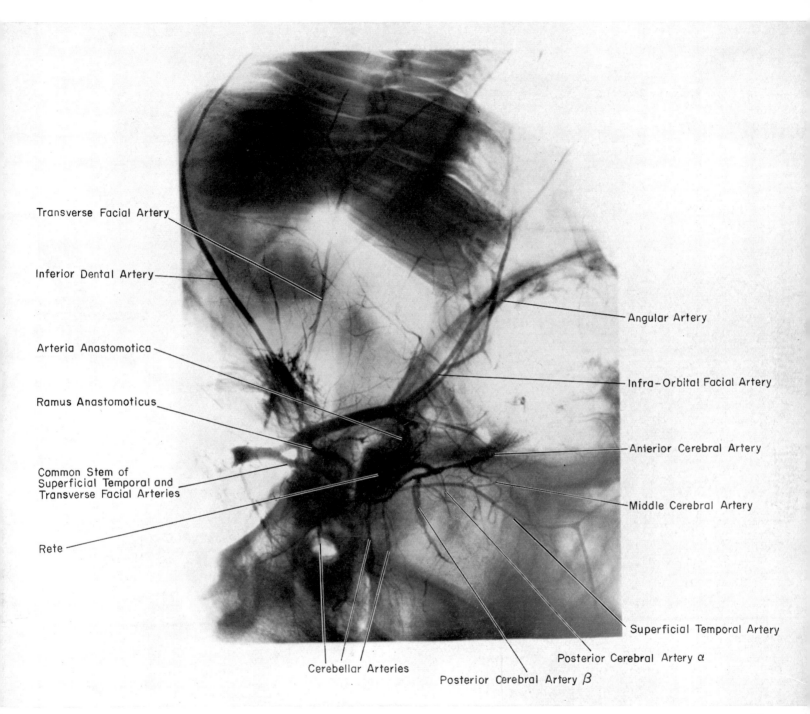

Transverse Facial Artery

Inferior Dental Artery

Angular Artery

Arteria Anastomotica

Infra–Orbital Facial Artery

Ramus Anastomoticus

Anterior Cerebral Artery

Common Stem of
Superficial Temporal and
Transverse Facial Arteries

Middle Cerebral Artery

Rete

Superficial Temporal Artery

Posterior Cerebral Artery α

Cerebellar Arteries

Posterior Cerebral Artery β

× 1·2

Bibliography

Aaron, C., Doyon, D., Fischgold, H., Metzger, J. and Richard, J.
1970 Arteriographie de la Carotide Externe, pp 46–54.
Masson et Cie, Paris.

Adams, W. E.
1957 The extracranial carotid rete and carotid fork in *Nycticebus coucang*.
Ann. Zool. 2: pp 21–38.

Adams, W. E.
1957 On the possible homologies of the occipital artery in mammals, with some remarks on the phylogeny and certain anomalies of the subclavian and carotid arteries.
Acta anat., 29: pp 90–113.

Adams, W. E.
1957 The carotid sinus complex in the hedgehog (*Erinaceus europaeus*).
J. Anat. Lond., 91: pp 207–227.

Adams, J. H., Daniel, P. M. and Prichard, M. M. I.
1969 Blood supply to pituitary gland of ferret with special reference to infarction after stalk section.
J. Anat., 104: pp 209–225.

Ask-Upmark, E.
1935 Rete Mirabile Caroticum.
Acta Psychiatria, 6: pp 126–181.

Ask-Upmark, E.
1935 The Carotid Sinus and the Cerebral Circulation.
Acta Psychiat. Neurol. Lund, Supp. 6: pp 1–374.

Ask-Upmark, E.
1953 On the entrance of the carotid artery into the cranial cavity in *Stenops gracilis* and *Otolicnus crassicaudatus*.
Acta anat., 19: pp 101–103.

Baldwin, B. A. and Bell, F. R.
1963 The anatomy of the cerebral circulation of the sheep and ox. The dynamic distribution of the blood supplied by the carotid and vertebral arteries to cranial regions.
J. Anat. Lond., 97: pp 203–215.

Bardenfleth, K. S.
1913 On the systematic position of *Aeluropus melanoleucus*.
Mindeskr. Jaetus Steenstrup; art. 17: pp 1–15.

Barkow, H. C. L.
1866 Die Blutgefässe, vorzuglich die Schlagadern der Säugethiere in ihren wesentlichsten Verschiedenheiten dargestelt.
In: Comparative Morphologie des Menschen und der menschenähnlichen Thiere, Vol. 4. Breslau.

Baumel, J. J. and Gerchman, L.
1968 The avian intercarotid anastomosis and its homologue in other vertebrates.
Amer. J. Anat., 122: pp 1–18.

Beart, R., Fishman, M. C. and Szidon, J. P.
1968 Anatomical observations in the harbour seal *Phoca vitulina*.
Bull. Mt. Desert Isl. biol. lab. 8: pp 6–7.

Beauregard, H.
1892 Le Canal Carotidien des Roussettes.
C.r. Soc. Biol., pp 914–916.

Becker, H.
1960 Arterien und Venen am Kopf des Schweines.
Vet. Med. Diss., Hanover.

Beddard, F. E.
1893 on—The Brain of the African Elephant.
Proc. Zool. Soc. London, pp 311–315.

Beddard, F. E.
1904 Note on the Brains of the Potto (*Perodicticus potto*) and the Slow Loris (*Nycticebus tardigradus*), with some observations upon the arteries of the Brain in certain Primates.
Proc. Zool. Soc. London.

Beddard, F. E.
1909 On some points in the structure of the lesser anteater (*Tamandua tetradactyla*) with notes on the cerebral arteries of Myrmecophaga and on the postcaval of Orycteropus.
Proc. Zool. Soc. London, pp 683–703.

Bender, W.
1969 Die Gefässversogung des Balkensund der Ammonoformation im Gehirn des Rhesusaffen.
Gegenbaurs. morph. Jb., 113: pp 214–228.

Berlinerblau, F.
1875 "Über den directen Übergang von Arterien in Venen."
Archiv. fur Anatomie, Physiologie und Wissenschaftliche Medizin, pp 177–188.

Bianchini, B.
1903 Osservazioni anatomiche sulle arterie encefaliche corticali del cavallo e del cane in rapporto a quelle degli altri mammiferi domestici.
Boll. Soc., Zool. Ital. (2) iii: pp 21–55.

Breschet, M. G.
1836 Histoire Anatomique et Physiologique d'un Organe de Nature Vasculaire Découvert Dans les Cétàce's Paris: Nechet.

Brown, J. O.
1968 Some observations on the cerebral arterial circles of mink (*Mustela vison*).
Anat. Rec., 161: pp 311–324.

Buchanan, G. D. and Arata, A. A.
1967 Cranial vasculature in certain neotropical bats.
Anat. Rec., 157: p 221.

Buchanan, G. D. and Arata, A. A.
1969 Cranial vasculature of a neotropical fruit-eating bat *Artibeus lituratus*.
Anat. Anz., 124: pp 314–325.

Bugge, J.
1967 The Arterial supply of the middle ear of the rabbit with special reference to the contribution of the stapedial artery to the development of the superior tympanic artery and the petrosal branch.
Acta anat., 67: pp 208–220.

Bugge, J.
1968 The Arterial supply of the rabbit nose and oral cavity.
Acta Rec., 161: pp 311–324.

Bugge, J.
1969 The cephalic arterial system in the rabbit with special reference to muscles of mastication and the temporo-mandibular joint.
Acta anat., 72: pp 109–122.

Bugge, J.
1971 The cephalic arterial system in New and Old World hystricomorphs, and in bathyergoids, with special reference to the systematic classification of rodents.
Acta anat. 80: pp 516–536.

Burne, R. H.
1952 Cetacean Dissection.
Published 1952—The Trustees of the British Museum, London.

Cabrera, A.
1925 Genera Mammalium. Insectivora Galeopithecia.
Madrid.

Calsson, A.
1926 Ueber *Ailurus fulgens*.
Acta Zool., 6: pp 269–305.

Castelli, W. A. and Huelke, D. F.
1965 "The arterial system of the head and neck of the rhesus monkey with emphasis on the external carotid system."
Amer. J. Anat., 116: pp 149–170.

Castelli, W. A. and Huelke, D. F.
1965 The arterial supply of the dura mater of the Rhesus monkey.
Anat. Rec., 152: pp 155–160.

Chapmis, G.
1966 Contribution a l'étude de l'artère carotide interne des carnivores.
Mammalia, 30: pp 82–96.

Chauveau, A. and Arloing, S.
1891 "The Comparative Anatomy of The Domesticated Animals."
Trans. G. Fleming. London, Churchill.

Coceani, F. and Gloor, P.
1966 The distribution of the internal carotid circulation in the brain of the macaque monkey (*Macaca mulatta*).
J. Comp. Neurol., 128: pp 419–430.

Coupin, F., Hindzé, B. and Lafont, M.
1928 Contribution a l'étude de deux jeunes Gorilles.
(1) Introduction; (2) Le cerveau; (3) Artères de l'encephale par B. Hindzé. pp 147–158.

Daniel, P. M., Dawes, J. D. K. and Prichard, M. M. L.
1953 Studies of the carotid rete and its associated arteries.
Philos. Trans., Royal Society London, 237B: pp 173–208.

Davies, D. V.
1947 The cardio-vascular system of the Slow Loris (*Nyctice-bus tardigradus malaianus*).
Proc. Zool. Soc. London, 117: pp 377–410.

Davis, D. D.
1964 The Giant Panda. A morphological study of evolutionary mechanism.
Fieldiana: Zool. Mem., 3: pp 1–399.

Davis, D. D. and Story, H. E.
1943 The carotid circulation in the Domestic Cat.
Field Mus. Nat. Hist., Chicago, Zool. Ser. 28: pp 1–47.

Decérisy, J. L.
1950 Les artères de bulbe et de la protubérance chez certain singes du Nouveau Monde (Genres Ateles, Lagothrix, Eriodes).
Bull. Mus. Hist. nat., Paris, 22: pp 431–437.

Decérisy, J. L.
1951 Les artères du bulbe et de la protubérance chez certain singes du Nouveau Monde (Genres Ateles, Lagothrix, Eriodes).
Bull. Mus. Hist. nat., Paris (2) 23: pp 62–65.

Decérisy, J. L.
1952 Remarques a propos du Cercle de Willis des Primates.
Mammalia, Paris, 16: pp 213–215.

Dekock, L. L.
1956 The Carotid body of the pilot whale (*Globicephala melaena*).
Nature, London, 177: pp 1084–1085.

Dekock, L. L.
1959 The arterial vessels of the neck in the pilot whale (*Globicephala melaena Traill*) and the porpoise (*Phocaena phocaena* L.) in relation to the carotid body.
Acta anat., 36: pp 274–292.

de la Torre, E., Netsky, M. G. and Meschan, I.
1959 Intracranial and Extracranial Circulation in the Dog: Anatomic and Angiographic Studies.
Amer. J. Anat., 105: pp 343–382.

de la Torre, E. and Netsky, M. G.
1960 Study of Persistent Primitive Maxillary Artery in Human Fetus: Some Homologies of Cranial Arteries in Man and Dog.
Amer. J. Anat., 106: pp 185–195.

de Vries, B.
1905 Sur la signification morphologique des artères cérebrales.
Arch. de Biol., 2–: pp 357–457.

Diwo, A. and Roth, J.
1913 Die Kopfarterien des Schweines.
Osten, Wschr. Rierheilk, 38: pp 437–440.

Dyrud, J.
1944 The external carotid artery of the Rhesus Monkey (*Macaca mulatta*).
Anat. Rec. Philadelphia, 90: pp 17–22.

Elze, C.
1910 Ueber das Verhalten der Arteria basilaris bei verscheidenen Species des Genus Ateles.
Anat. Anz. Jena, 37: pp 33–38.

Fawcett, D. W.
1942 A Comparative Study of the Blood-Vascular Bundles in the Florida Manatee (*Trichechus latirostris*) and in certain Cetaceans and Edentates.
J. Morph., 71: pp 105–124.

Fazzari, I.
1929 Die Arterien des Kleinhirns.
Anat. Anz. Jena, 67: pp 497–501.

Finelli, R., Caputo, G. and Rascio, L.
1966 Aspetti anatomici e correlazioni fiscologiche sulla circulazione encefalica di mirabile carotidea nel *Bubalus buffalas*.
Boll. Soc. ital. Biol. sper., 42: pp 2016–2018.

Flechsig, G. F. and Zintzsch, I.
1969 Die Arterien der Schädelbasis des Schweines.
Anat. Ans., 125: pp 206–219.

Francaviglia, M. C.
1893 Notisie anatomiche sul *Bradypus tridactylus* L., var. netus, lesson.
Boll. Soc. Rom. Zool. ii: pp 126–137.

Franklin, K. J. and Haynes, F.
1927 The Histology of The Giraffes Carotid Functionally Considered.
J. Anat., 62: p 115.

Freisenhausen, H. D.
1965 Gefässanordung und Kapillardichte im Gehirn des Kaninchens.
Acta anat., 62: pp 539–562.

Fujimoto, T.
1959 Stereological anatomy of several ducts and vessels by injection methods of acrylic resin. V. Arterial distribution of the temporal muscle in some mammals.
Okajimas Folia Anat. Jap., 33: pp 389–424.

Galen.
AD 130–200 De usu partium corpus humane. [Medicorum Graecorum Opera Quae Exstant, KUHN, C. G. (1821–1833), Vol. III: lib. IX, cap. IV, p 684.
Publisher—Cnoblock, Leipzeig].

Galliano, R. E., Morgane, P. J., McFarland, W. L., Nagel, E. L. and Catherman, R. L.
1966 The anatomy of the cervico-thoracic arterial system in the bottlenose dolphin (*Tursiops truncatus*) with a surgical approach suitable for guided angiography.
Anat. Record, 155: (3) pp 325–338.

George, M.
1875 Monographie anatomique des mammiferes due Genre Daman.
An. Scienc. Nat., 1:

Gillilan, L. A.
1969 The Arterial and Venous Blood Supplies to the Cerebellum of Primates.
J. Neuropathology and Experimental Neurology, Vol. XXVIII, No. 2: pp 295–307.

Godynicki, S.
1968 Arteries of the head in the red deer.
Pr. Korn. Nank. roln. lesn. Poznan, 26: pp 77–113.

Goss, C. M.
1961 On anatomy of veins and arteries by Galen of Pergamos.
Anat. Rec., 141: pp 355–366.

Greene, E. C.
1935 Anatomy of the rat.
Trans. Amer. Philos. Soc., New Series, 27: pp 1–370.

Gregory, W. K.
1936 On the phylogenetic relationships of the giant panda (*Ailuropda*) to other arctoid carnivora.
Amer. Mus. Nov. No. 878: pp 1–29.

Grosser, O.
1901 Zur Anatomie und Entwicklungsgeschichte des Gefässsystems der Chiropteren.
Zschr. f. Anat. u. Entwicklungsgesch., 17: pp 203–424.

Guthrie, D. A.
1963 The carotid circulation in the Rodentia.
Bull. Mus. Comp. Zool. Harvard Univ., 128: pp 455–482.

Guthrie, D. A.
1969 Carotid circulation in *Aplodontia rufa*.
J. Mammal., 50: pp 1–7.

Hafforl, A.
1933 Das Arteriensystem—Vol. 6: pp 563 in—Handbuch der vergleichenden Anatomie der Wirbeltiere: ed. Urban and Schwarzenberg. Berlin.

Hata, Y.
1967 Stereological studies on several ducts and vessels by injection method of acrylic resin.
18: On the buccal artery in some mammals.
Okajimas Folia anat. jap., 43: pp 331–361.

Hata, Y., Takashima, T. and Kitamura, H.
1965 Stereological studies on several ducts and vessels by injection method of acrylic resin.
14: On the A. alveolaris superior posterior of the rabbit.
Okajimas Folia anat. jap., 41: pp 213–220.

Henson, C. H.
1923 The Brachial Vessels and their Derivations in the Pig.
Contribution to Embr. 15.

Hill, W. C. O.
1953–1966 Primates, Vol. 1–6.
Edinburgh University Press.

Hill, W. C. O.
1967 Taxonomy of the baboon in—Vatbòrg, "The Baboon in Medical Research".
H. K. Lewis, London.

Hill, W. C. O.
1969 Vascular supply of face in long-snouted primates (Mandrillus, Papio), pp 155–159—in: Recent Advances in Primatology: ed. H. O. Hofer.
(Proc. 2nd Internat. Congress on Primatology, Atlanta, Georgia, 1968, Vol. 2).

Hochstetter, F.
1896 Beiträge zur Anatomie und Entwicklungsgeschichte der Blutgefäss-systems der Monotremen.
Denk. Gas. Jena, V: p 191.

Hofer, H. and Tigges, J.
1964 Makromorphologie des Zentralnervensystems. 1. Morphogenese, Häute, Blutversorgung, Ventrikelsystem und Rückenmach.
Handbuch. Zool. Berlin 8, Band 34, Lief 1, Teil 7 Beitr: 1–42.

Hofmann, M.
1900 Zeitschrift für Morphologie und Anthropologie, 2: p 247.

Hunter, John.
1787 Observations on the structure and oeconomy of Whales.
Phil. Trans. Roy. Soc., London, 77: p 371.

Hunter, John.
1787 Quoted by Cushing—1930 in Neurophysiological Mechanisms from a clinical standpoint.
Lister Memorial Lecture.
Lancet, 219: pp 119–175.

Hürlimann, Rud.
1912 Die arteriellen Kopfgefässe der Katse.
Internat. Mondtschr. Anat., 29: pp 371–442.

Huxley, J.
1866 Lectures at The Royal College of Surgeons.
The Lancet, Vol. 1: pp 880 and 381.

Hworostuchin, W.
1911 Zur Frage uber den Bau des Plexus chorioideus.
Arch. mikr. Anat., Bonn, 77: Abt. 1, pp 232–244.

Hyrtl, J.
1853 Das arterielle Gefäss-system der Monotremen Denkschriften der math.-naturw.
Klasse der K. Akademie der Wissenschaftern, Bd. V: p 191.

Hyrtl, J.
1854 Das Arterielle Gefäss-system der Edentaten.
Denkschrift. Kais. Akad. Wiss, Wien, 6: p 21.

Hyrtl, J.
1864 Neue Wundernetse und Geflechte bei Vögeln und Säugethieren.
Denkschr. Akad. Wiss. 22: pp 113–152.

Ivanova, E. I.
1967 New data on the nature of the rete mirabile and derivative apparatuses in some semi-aquatic mammals.
Dokl. (Proc.) Acad. Sci. U.S.S.R. (biol.), 173: pp 1–3.

Jellinger, K.
1966 Zur Frage der Arterienklappen in Nagergehirn.
Anat. Anz., 119: pp 246–258.

Jenke, W.
1919 Die Gehirnarterien des Pferdes, Hundes, Rindes und Schweines, vergleichen mit denen des Menschen.
Vet. Med. Diss., Dresden.

Jeppson, P. G. and Olin, T.
1960 Cerebral angiography in the rabbit. An investigation of vascular anatomy and variation in circulatory pattern with conditions of injection.
Lund Univ. Arsskr. N.F. 2 56 14: pp 1–56.

Jewell, P. A.
1952 The anastomoses between internal and external carotid circulation in the dog.
J. Anat. London, 86: pp 83–94.

Kanagasuntherami, R. and Krichnamarti, A.
1965 Observations on the carotid rete in the lesser bushbaby *Galago senegalensis*.
J. Anat., 99: pp 861–875.

Kanan, C. V.
1970 The Cerebral Arteries of the *Camelus dromedarius*.
Acta Anat. Basel, 77: pp 605–616.

Kassell, N. F. and Langfitt, T. W.
1965 Variation in the Circle of Willis in *Macaca mulatta*.
Anat. Rec., 152: pp 257–263.

Lamberton, C.
1947 Quelques traits de l'evolution de la circulation endo- et exocranienne chez les Primates.
Bull. Acad. Malgache N.S., 26: pp 141–142.

Lawrence, W. E. and Rewell, R. E.
1948 Cerebral blood supply in the Giraffidae.
Proc. Zool. Soc. London, 118: pp 202–212.

Lehmann, H.
1905 On the embryonic history of the aortic arches in mammals.
Anat. Anz., 26: p 406.

Lierse, W.
1957 Die Gefässversorgung der Stammganglien im Gehirn der Katze.
Anat. Anz., 109: pp 358–368.

Lindahl, E. and Lundberg, M.
1946 Hyrax, *Procovia capensis*. Arteries in the head and their development.
Acta Zool., 27: (Hefte 2–3) pp 101–153.

Linebach, P.
1933 "The vascular system" in The Anatomy of the Rhesus Monkey, ed. C. G. Hartman & W. C. Straus; pp 248–265.
The William and Wilkins Co., Baltimore.

Mackay, J. J.
1886 The arteries of the head and neck and the rete mirabile of the porpoise (*Phocaena communis*).
Proc. Phil. Soc., Glasgow, 17: pp 366–376.

Martin, P.
1923 Lehrbuch der Anatomie der Haustiere. Bd. 4, Anatomie d. Schweines, d. Hundes u.d. Katse, Stuttgart.

Martinez, P.
1965 Le system artérial de la base du cerveau et l'origine des artère hypophysaries chez le chat.
Acta anat. 61: pp 511–546.

Martinez-Martinez, P.
1967 Le réseau admirable extracranien et la circulation cérébrale.
C.r. Ass. Anat. 51: pp 671–680.

May, N. D. S.
1968 Experimental studies of collateral circulation in head and neck of sheep (*Ovis aries*).
J. Anat., 103: pp 171–181.

McCoy, H. A.
1963 Arterial variability of carotid pattern in the Rhesus monkey (*Macaca mulatta*).
Amer. J. Phys. Anthrop., 21: p 424.

McCoy, H. A.
1967 The external carotid artery of the baboon and the rhesus monkey; branching pattern and distribution.
Vol. 2: pp 151–179—in: The Baboon In Medical Research: ed. Vagtborg. (Proc. 2nd Inter. Symp.)
Univ. Texas Press, Austin and London.

Meek, Walter J.
1906 A study of the choroid plexus (Abstract).
Des Moines Proc. Iowa Acad. Sci., 13: pp 245–249.

Mergner, H.
1961 Die Blutversorgung der lamina terminalis bei einigen Affen.
Z. Wiss. Zool., 165: pp 140–185.

Michel, G. and Rothkegel, R.
1960 Die Augswergung der A. carotis communis beim Syn. Goldhamster (*Mesocricetus auratus* W.).
Anat. Anz., 108: pp 260–271.

Miller, E. M., Christensen, G. C. and Evans, H. E.
1964 Anatomy of the Dog, Chapter 8—the Brain; Herman Meyer.
W. B. Saunders and Co., Philadelphia and London.

Mivart, St. George.
1881 The Cat.
Murray, London.

Morgane, P. J., McFarland, W. L., Nagel, E. L., Viamonte, M. and Galliano, R. E.
1966 Arterial supply to the brain of the dolphin, *Tursiops truncatus*.
Physiologist, 9: p 249.

Morgane, P. J., Nagel, E. L., Galliano, R. E. and Viamonte, M.
1967 Angiography and blood supply to the brain of the dolphin, *Tursiops truncatus*.
Anat. Record, 157: p 290.

Moris, F.
1969 Etude anatomique de la region cephalique *Phocaena marsouin phocaena* L. du cetace adortocete.
Mammalia, 33: pp 666–726.

Muller, A.
1682 "An Anatomical Account of the Elephant accidentally burnt in Dublin on Friday, June 17th in the year 1681."
London. Printed for Sam Smith, Bookseller at The Prince's Arms in St. Paul's Church Yard, 1682.

Murie, J.
1873 On the organisation of the Caaing Whale, *Globicephalus melar*.
Trans. Zool. Soc. London, 8. 4. 235.

Murie, J.
1874 Researches upon the Anatomy of the Pinnipeda, Part III. Descriptive Anatomy of the Sea-Lion (*Otariajubata*).
Trans. Zool. Soc. London, 8. 9. 501.

Murie, J.
1874 On the form and structure of the Manatee.
Trans. Zool. Soc., 8: pp 127–202.

Nagel, E. L., Morgane, P. J., McFarland, W. L. and Galliano, R. E.
1968 Rete mirabile of dolphin: its pressure-damping effect on cerebral circulation.
Science, N.Y., 161: pp 898–900.

Nair, V., Palm, D. and Roth, L. J.
1960 Relative vascularity of certain anatomical areas of the brain and other organs of the rat.
Nature. Lond., 188: pp 497–498.

Nickel, R. and Schwarz, R.
1903 Vergleichende Betrachtungen der Kopfarterien der Haussäugetiere (Katze, Hund, Schwein, Rind, Schof, Ziege, Pferd).
Zbl. Vet. Med., 10: pp 89–120.

Nilges, R. G.
1944 The arteries of the mammalian cornu ammonis.
J. Comp. Neurol. Philadelphia, 80: pp 177–190.

Norris, H. W.
1906 The Carotid Arteries and their Relation to the Circle of Willis in The Cat.
Des Moines Proc. Iowa Acad. Sci., 13: pp 251–255.

Ommanney, F. D.
1932 The vascular network (rete mirabile) of the fin whale (*Balaenoptera physalus*).
Discovery Rept., 5: pp 327–362.

Owen, R.
1841 Notes on the Anatomy of the Nubian Giraffe.
Trans. Zool. Soc., London, 2: p 217.

Owen, R.
1868 Comparative anatomy and physiology of vertebrates.
Mammals (London), Vol. 3. p 915.

Ozaki, A.
1968 Study of spheno-palatine artery by injection of acrylic resin.
Okajimas Folia anat. jap., 44: pp 301–336.

Pardi, F.
1910 Illustrazione ed interpetrazione di un ramo collaterale non ancora descritto della arteria carotide eesterna.
Arteria della glandula sottomascellare.
Piser Atti. Soc. Tose se Nat. Proc. Verb. 19: pp 12–19.

Platzer, W.
1960 "Das Arterien und Venensystems" Primatologica III/2:
pp 273–387. ed. H. Hofer, A. H. Schultz, D. Starck.
Karger. Basel/New York.

Pocock, R. I.
1916 On the course of the internal carotid artery and the
foramina connected therewith in the skull of Felidae and
Viverridae.
Ann. Mag. Nat. Hist., London, 17: pp 261–269.

Pogorzelski, J. K.
1962 Studies of vascular system of choroid plexuses in brain,
lateral ventricles and of pia mater of some laboratory animals.
Folia Morph. Warszawa, 21: pp 21–42 and 145–163.

Popesko, P. and Stryhal, M.
1959 Das Gefäss-system des Schweinekopfes vom systemati-
schen und topographischen Standpunkt (Tschech).
Folia Vet. 3: pp 25–35.

Rapp.
1827 Ueber das Wundernets.
Meckels Arch. f. Anat. und Physiol.

Reighard, J. and Jennings, H. S.
1901 Anatomy of the Cat.
Henry Holt, New York.

Reighard, J. and Jennings, H. S.
1935 3rd ed.

Rojecki, F.
1889 "Sur la circulation arterielle chez *Macacus cynomolgus*
et le *Macacus sinicus* comparee a celle des singes anthropo-
morphes et l'homme".
J. Anat., Paris, 25: pp 245–386.

Rosen, W. C.
1967 The Morphology of valves in the cerebral vessels of the
rat.
Anat. Rec., 157: pp 481–487.

Rossatti, B.
1956 Observations of the blood-supply of the rabbits ear and
on the experimental new formation of arteriovenous anastomoses.
J. Anat., London, 90: pp 318–328.

Salzer, H.
1895 Ueber die Entwicklung der Kopfvenen der Meer-
schweinchens.
Morph. Jahrb. XXIII: pp 232–255.

Samano Bishop, M.
1965 Persistencia de la arteria estapedica en quicopteras
muraelagos.
An. Inst. Biol. Univ. Mex., 36: (1966) pp 303–317.

Schanklin, W. M. and Azzam, N. A.
1963 A study of the valves in the arteries of the rodent brain.
Anat. Rec., 147: pp 407–414.

Schaurer, E.
1940 Arteries and veins in the Mammalian brain.
Anat. Rec., Philadelphia, 78: pp 173–196.

Schlesinger, B.
1941 The angio-architecture of the thalamus in the Rabbit.
J. Ant., London, 75: pp 176–196.

Schummer, A. and Zimmermann, G.
1937 Weitere Ubtersuchungen über die Sinus durae matris,
Dip!oe und Kopfven des Hundes mittels der Korrosion
methode.
Z. anat. Entw-Gesch., 107: pp 1–6.

Shellshear, J. L.
1929 A study of the arteries of the brain of the spiny ant-
eater to illustrate the principles of arterial distribution.
Philos. Trans., London, 218B: pp 1–36.

Shimizu, E.
1968 Stereological studies on several ducts and vessels by
injection method of acrylic resin.
20: On the Ethmoidal artery in some Mammals.
Okajimas Folia anat. jap., 45: pp 99–141.

Sikes, S. K.
1971 Natural History of The African Elephant.
Weidenfeld and Nicolson, London.

Sisson, S. (Revised J. D. Grossman).
1938 The anatomy of the domestic animals.
Philadelphia and London.

Slijper, E. J.
1936 Die Cetacean Vergleichendanatomisch und Systema-
tisch.
Capita Zoologica, The Hague, Vol. 7, pp 1–304 and 305–590.

Slijper, E. J.
1958 On the vascular system of cetacea.
Proc. Intern. Congr. Zool. 15th, Sect. III 38: pp 1–3.

Slijper, E. J.
1959 On the vascular system of Cetacea.
Proc. Int. Congr. Zool., 15: pp 309–311.

Smith, C.
1924 The origin and development of the carotid body.
Amer. J. Anat., 34: pp 87–131.

Sonntag, C. F.
1925 A Monograph of *Orycteropus afer*.
Proc. Zool. Soc., London, 25: pp 331–437.

Spaltehols, W.
1913 Handatlas der Anatomie des Menschen.
S. Hirsel, Leipsig.

Steuerwald, E. A.
1969 Review of the phylogenetic position of the Tree Shrew
(*Tupaia glis* Diard), with new observations on the arteria
carotis interna.
Diss. Abstr. Int. 30B: p 2510.

Story, H. E.
1951 The carotid arteries in the Procyonidae.
Fieldiana: Zoology, 32: pp 475–577.

Sunder-Plassman, P.
1930 Untersuchungen über den Bulbus carotidis bei Mensch und Tier im Hinblick aud die "Sinusreflexe" nach H. E. Hering: ein Vergleich mit anderen Gefässtrecken; die Histopathologie des Bulbus carotidis; das Glomus caroticum.
Z. Anat. EntwGesch., Berlin, 93: pp 567–622.

Tandler, J.
1899 Zur vergleichenden Anatomie der Kopfarterien bei den Mammalia.
Denkschriften d. Kaiserl. Akad. d. Wiss. Wien, 67: pp 677–784.

Tandler, J.
1901 Zur vergleichenden Anatomie der Kopfarterien bei den Mammalia.
Anat. Hefte. 18.

Tandler, J.
1902 Zur Entwicklungsgeschichte der Kopfarterien bei den Mammalia.
Gegenbaur. Morph. Jahrb. 6: 30, pp 275–373.

Tandler, J.
1906 Zur Entwicklungsgeschichte der arteriellen Wundernetse.
Anat. Hefte. 31: pp 237–265.

Taslitz, N.
1965 The Arterial supply of the monkey brain.
Diss. Abstr. 26: pp 1279–1280.

Tayeb, M. A. F.
1951 A study on the blood supply of the camel's head.
Brit. vet. J., 107 3 pp 147–155.

Taylor, C. R.
1966 The vascularity and possible thermoregulatory function of the horns in Goats.
Physiol. Zool., 39: pp 127–139.

Teh-Cheng, J.
1968 Anatomical studies of the vascular system of the brain of *Macaca cyclopis* Swinhoe.
J. Formosan med. Ass., 67: pp 240–257.

Theile, F. W.
1852 Über das Arteriensystem von *Simia inuus* Untersucht.
Arch. Anat. Physiol. Wiss. Med. pp 419–489.

Vesalius, Andreas.
1543 De Humani Corporis Fabrica libri septem.
Basel.

Viamonte, M., Morgane, P. J., Galliano, R. E., Nagel, E. L. and McFarland, W. L.
1968 Angiography in the living dolphin and observation on the blood supply to the brain.
Am. J. Physiol., 214: pp 1225–1249.

Von Citters, R. L., Kemper, W. S. and Franklin, D. L.
1968 Blood flow and pressure in the giraffe carotid artery.
Comp. Biochem. Physiol. 24: pp 1035–1042.

Waldo, C. M., Wislocki, G. B. and Fawcett, D. W.
1949 Observation on the blood supply of growing antlers.
Amer. J. Anat. Philadelphia, 84: pp 27–61.

Walmsley, R.
1938 Some observations of the vascular system of a female fetal finback.
Carnegie Contrib. to Embryol., 27: p 107.

Watson, M.
1875 Contributions to the Anatomy of the Indian Elephant. Part IV. Muscles and blood vessels of the face and head.
J. Anat., 9: pp 118–133.

Weinstein, J. D. and Hedges, T. R.
1962 Studies of intracranial and orbital vasculature of the Rhesus monkey (*Macaca mulatta*).
Anat. Rec., 144: pp 37–42.

Werner, L.
1969 Angioarchitektonic des Rhombencephalon und cerebellum, 1. Leptomeningeale Gefässe von *Tupaia glis*.
Z. mikrosk. Anat. Forsch., 80: pp 379–398.

Wiedersheim, R.
1883 Lehrbuch der vergleicheichen Anatomie der Wirbelthiere, auf Grundlage der Entwicklungsgeschichte.
Jena (8 vo).

Wiland, C.
1966 The Basilar artery of the brain in foxes.
Folia morph., 25: pp 645–649.

Wiland, C.
1968 The basal arteries of the brain in the domestic rabbit.
Folia morph., 27: pp 329–336.

Willis, Thomas.
1684 Dr. Willis' Practice of Physick, being the whole medical works of that renowned and famous Physician. Translated into English by S. Pordage, London.

Wilson, H. S.
1879 The rete mirabile of the narwhal.
J. Anat. Physiol., 14: pp 377–400.

Wislocki, G. B.
1937 The vascular supply of the Hypophysis Cerebri of the Cat.
Anat. Rec. 69: pp 361–387.

Wislocki, G. B.
1940 Peculiarities of the cerebral blood vessels of the Opossum: diencephalon, area postrema and retina.
Anat. Rec., Philadelphia, 78: pp 119–137.

Wislocki, G. B. and Straus, W. C. Jr.
1932 On the Blood-Vascular Bundles in the limbs of certain Edentates and lemurs.
Bull. Mus. Comp. Zool., 74: pp 1–15.

Woolard, H. H.
1926 A monograph of *Orycteropus afer* II.
Proc. Zool. Soc., London. Part 3.

Yü-Ch'üan Tsang.
1949 The superficial arterial pattern of the ruminant brain.
Peking Nat. Hist. Bull. 18: pp 107–117.

Ziehen, T.
1897 Das centralnervensystem der Monotremen und Marsupialier.
Semon Zool. Forsch in Australia und dem Malayischen Archipel.
Zietzschmann, O.
1943 Die Arterien—in Ellenberger und Baum: Handbuch d. vergl.
Anatomie d. Haustiere. Berlin.

Index of Species

Index of Common Names

Index of Common Names
continued)

Index of Families